American College of Physicians

MKSAP® 15

Medical Knowledge Self-Assessment Program®

Cardiovascular Medicine

Cardiovascular Medicine

Contributors

Catherine M. Otto, MD, FACP, Book Editor[1]
J. Ward Kennedy-Hamilton Endowed Professor of
  Cardiology
Professor of Medicine
Director, Cardiology Fellowship Programs
University of Washington School of Medicine
Seattle, Washington

Howard H. Weitz, MD, FACP, Associate Editor[2]
Professor of Medicine
Director, Division of Cardiology
Vice-Chairman, Department of Medicine
Jefferson Medical College, Thomas Jefferson University
Philadelphia, Pennsylvania

R. Michael Benitez, MD[1]
Associate Professor of Medicine
Fellowship Program Director
Division of Cardiology
University of Maryland School of Medicine
Baltimore, Maryland

Heidi M. Connolly, MD[1]
Professor of Medicine
Mayo Clinic College of Medicine
Rochester, Minnesota

Rosario V. Freeman, MD, MS[2]
Associate Professor
Division of Cardiology
University of Washington
Seattle, Washington

Kristen K. Patton, MD[2]
Assistant Professor
Division of Cardiology
University of Washington
Seattle, Washington

David M. Shavelle, MD[2]
Associate Clinical Professor
David Geffen School of Medicine at UCLA
Division of Cardiology
Director, Interventional Cardiology
Director, Interventional Cardiology Fellowship
Los Angeles County/Harbor-UCLA Medical Center
Torrance, California

Marcus F. Stoddard, MD[1]
Professor of Medicine
Clinical Chief
Division of Cardiovascular Medicine
Department of Medicine
The University of Louisville
Louisville, Kentucky

Andrew Wang, MD[2]
Associate Professor of Medicine
Director, Fellowship Training Program
Division of Cardiovascular Medicine
Duke University Medical Center
Durham, North Carolina

Audrey H. Wu, MD, MPH[1]
Clinical Assistant Professor
Division of Cardiovascular Medicine
University of Michigan Health System
Ann Arbor, Michigan

Editor-in-Chief

Patrick C. Alguire, MD, FACP[1]
Director, Education and Career Development
American College of Physicians
Philadelphia, Pennsylvania

Cardiovascular Medicine Reviewers

Philip Altus, MD, MACP[2]
Gloria Fioravanti, DO, FACP[1]
John D. Goldman, MD, FACP[2]
Jose A. Joglar, MD[1]
Warren J. Manning, MD, FACP[1]
Michael W. Peterson, MD, FACP[1]
Ileana L. Piña, MD[2]
Mark D. Siegel, MD[1]

Cardiovascular Medicine ACP Editorial Staff

Becky Krumm, Senior Staff Editor
Sean McKinney, Director, Self-Assessment Programs
Margaret Wells, Managing Editor
Charles Rossi, Senior Associate of Clinical Content
  Development
John Murray, Editorial Coordinator

ACP Principal Staff

Steven E. Weinberger, MD, FACP[2]
Deputy Executive Vice President
Senior Vice President, Medical Education and Publishing

D. Theresa Kanya, MBA[1]
Vice President, Medical Education and Publishing

Sean McKinney[1]
Director, Self-Assessment Programs

Margaret Wells[1]
Managing Editor

Charles Rossi[1]
Senior Associate of Clinical Content Development

Becky Krumm[1]
Senior Staff Editor

Ellen McDonald, PhD[1]
Senior Staff Editor

Amanda Neiley[1]
Staff Editor

Katie Idell[1]
Production Administrator/Editor

Valerie Dangovetsky[1]
Program Administrator

John Murray[1]
Editorial Coordinator

Shannon O'Sullivan[1]
Editorial Coordinator

Developed by the American College of Physicians

1. Has no relationships with any entity producing, marketing, re-selling, or distributing health care goods or services consumed by, or used on, patients.

2. Has disclosed relationships with entities producing, marketing, re-selling, or distributing health care goods or services consumed by, or used on, patients. See below.

Conflicts of Interest

The following contributors and ACP staff members have disclosed relationships with commercial companies:

Philip Altus, MD, MACP
Consultantship
King Pharmaceuticals, Sanofi-Aventis
Speakers Bureau
Bristol-Myers Squibb, King Pharmaceuticals, Sanofi-Aventis

Rosario V. Freeman, MD, MS
Employment (Spouse)
Philips Medical Systems

John D. Goldman, MD, FACP
Employment
Pinnacle Health

Kristen K. Patton, MD
Research Grants/Contracts
Boston Scientific (includes Guidant products), Medtronic, Inc.

Ileana L. Piña, MD
Speakers Bureau
AstraZeneca, GlaxoSmithKline, Novartis, Sanofi-Aventis

David M. Shavelle, MD
Research Grants/Contracts
Takeda, GlaxoSmithKline, eV3, Inc., Boston Scientific, Abbott Vascular, Atritech, Inc., St. Jude, Inc., Possis, Inc., Cordis, Inc., Boehringer Ingelheim, AstraZeneca, Cardiomems

Andrew Wang, MD
Research Grants/Contracts
Evalve, Inc., Radiant Medical, Medtronic, Inc.

Steven E. Weinberger, MD, FACP
Stock Options/Holdings
Abbott, GlaxoSmithKline

Howard H. Weitz, MD, FACP
Other
GlaxoSmithKline (member of adverse events review committee of a clinical research trial)

Acknowledgments

The American College of Physicians (ACP) gratefully acknowledges the special contributions to the development and production of the 15th edition of the Medical Knowledge Self-Assessment Program® (MKSAP 15) of Scott Thomas Hurd (Senior Systems Analyst/Developer), Ricki Jo Kauffman (Manager, Systems Development), Michael Ripca (Technical Administrator/Graphics Designer), and Lisa Torrieri (Graphic Designer). The Digital version (CD-ROM and Online components) was developed within the ACP's Interactive Product Development Department by Steven Spadt (Director), Christopher Forrest (Senior Software Developer), Ryan Hinkel (Senior Software Developer), John McKnight (Software Developer), Sean O'Donnell (Senior Software Developer), and Brian Sweigard (Senior Software Developer). Computer scoring and reporting are being performed by ACT, Inc., Iowa City, Iowa. The College also wishes to acknowledge that many other persons, too numerous to mention, have contributed to the production of this program. Without their dedicated efforts, this program would not have been possible.

Continuing Medical Education

The American College of Physicians is accredited by the Accreditation Council for Continuing Medical Education (ACCME) to provide continuing medical education for physicians.

The American College of Physicians designates this educational activity for a maximum of 166 *AMA PRA Category 1 Credits*™. Physicians should only claim credit commensurate with the extent of their participation in the activity.

AMA PRA Category 1 Credit™ is available from July 31, 2009, to July 31, 2012.

Learning Objectives

The learning objectives of MKSAP 15 are to:
- Close gaps between actual care in your practice and preferred standards of care, based on best evidence
- Diagnose disease states that are less common and sometimes overlooked and confusing
- Improve management of comorbidities that can complicate patient care
- Determine when to refer patients for surgery or care by subspecialists
- Pass the ABIM certification examination
- Pass the ABIM maintenance of certification examination

Target Audience

- General internists and primary care physicians
- Subspecialists who need to remain up-to-date in internal medicine
- Residents preparing for the certifying examination in internal medicine
- Physicians preparing for maintenance of certification in internal medicine (recertification)

How to Submit for CME Credits

To earn CME credits, complete a MKSAP 15 answer sheet. Use the enclosed, self-addressed envelope to mail your completed answer sheet(s) to the MKSAP Processing Center for scoring. Remember to provide your MKSAP 15 order and ACP ID numbers in the appropriate spaces on the answer sheet. The order and ACP ID numbers are printed on your mailing label. If you have not received these numbers with your MKSAP 15 purchase, you will need to acquire them to earn CME credits. E-mail ACP's customer service center at custserv@acponline.org. In the subject line, write "MKSAP 15 order/ACP ID numbers." In the body of the e-mail, make sure you include your e-mail address as well as your full name, address, city, state, ZIP code, country, and telephone number. Also identify where you have made your MKSAP 15 purchase. You will receive your MKSAP 15 order and ACP ID numbers by e-mail within 72 business hours.

Disclosure Policy

It is the policy of the American College of Physicians (ACP) to ensure balance, independence, objectivity, and scientific rigor in all its educational activities. To this end, and consistent with the policies of the ACP and the Accreditation Council for Continuing Medical Education (ACCME), contributors to all ACP continuing medical education activities are required to disclose all relevant financial relationships with any entity producing, marketing, re-selling, or distributing health care goods or services consumed by, or used on, patients. Contributors are required to use generic names in the discussion of therapeutic options and are required to identify any unapproved, off-label, or investigative use of commercial products or devices. Where a trade name is used, all available trade names for the same product type are also included. If trade-name products manufactured by companies with whom contributors have relationships are discussed, contributors are asked to provide evidence-based citations in support of the discussion. The information is reviewed by the committee responsible for producing this text. If necessary, adjustments to topics or contributors' roles in content development are made to balance the discussion. Further, all readers of this text are asked to evaluate the content for evidence of commercial bias so that future decisions about content and contributors can be made in light of this information.

Resolution of Conflicts

To resolve all conflicts of interest and influences of vested interests, the ACP precluded members of the content-creation committee from deciding on any content issues that involved generic or trade-name products associated with proprietary entities with which these committee members had relationships. In addition, content was based on best evidence and updated clinical care guidelines, when such evidence and guidelines were available. Contributors' disclosure information can be found with the list of contributors' names and those of ACP principal staff listed in the beginning of this book.

Educational Disclaimer

The editors and publisher of MKSAP 15 recognize that the development of new material offers many opportunities for error. Despite our best efforts, some errors may persist in print. Drug dosage schedules are, we believe, accurate and in accordance with current standards. Readers are advised, however, to ensure that the recommended dosages in MKSAP 15 concur with the information provided in the product information material. This is especially important in cases of new, infrequently used, or highly toxic drugs. Application of the information in MKSAP 15 remains the professional responsibility of the practitioner.

The primary purpose of MKSAP 15 is educational. Information presented, as well as publications, technologies, products, and/or services discussed, is intended to inform subscribers about the knowledge, techniques, and experiences of the contributors. A diversity of professional opinion exists, and the views of the contributors are their own and not those of the ACP. Inclusion of any material in the program does not constitute endorsement or recommendation by the ACP. The ACP does not warrant the safety, reliability, accuracy, completeness, or usefulness of and disclaims any and all liability for damages and claims that may result from the use of information, publications, technologies, products, and/or services discussed in this program.

Publisher's Information

Unauthorized Use of This Book Is Against the Law

MKSAP 15 ISBN: 978-1-934465-25-7
Cardiovascular Medicine ISBN: 978-1-934465-28-8

Printed in the United States of America.

For order information in the U.S. or Canada call 800-523-1546, extension 2600. All other countries call 215-351-2600. Fax inquiries to 215-351-2799 or e-mail to custserv@acponline.org.

Errata and Norm Tables

Errata for MKSAP 15 will be posted at http://mksap.acponline.org/errata as new information becomes known to the editors.

MKSAP 15 Performance Interpretation Guidelines with Norm Tables, available December 31, 2010, will reflect the knowledge of physicians who have completed the self-assessment tests before the program was published. These physicians took the tests without being able to refer to the syllabus, answers, and critiques. For your convenience, the tables are available in a printable PDF file at http://mksap.acponline.org/normtables.

Table of Contents

Epidemiology of Cardiovascular Disease

Overview 1
Women and Cardiovascular Disease 1
Ethnicity and Cardiovascular Disease 2
Diabetes Mellitus and Cardiovascular Disease 2
Metabolic Syndrome and Cardiovascular Disease 2
Cancer and Cardiovascular Disease 2
Systemic Inflammatory Conditions and Cardiovascular Disease 3
Lifestyle Factors and Cardiovascular Disease 4

Extensions of the Physical Examination

Introduction 4
Structural Heart Disease 4
Coronary Artery Disease 6
Cardiac Arrhythmias 7

Coronary Artery Disease

Risk Factors for Coronary Artery Disease 10
    Conventional Risk Factors 10
    Conditional Risk Factors 11
    Cardiovascular Risk Reduction 12
    Cardiovascular Disease and Depression 12
Chronic Stable Coronary Artery Disease 12
    Diagnosis of Coronary Artery Disease 12
    Medical Treatment of Chronic Stable Coronary Artery Disease 14
    Coronary Revascularization 16
    Medically Refractory Angina 17
    Follow-Up Care 17
Acute Coronary Syndromes 18
    Clinical Presentation and Classification 18
    Initial Medical Treatment of Acute Coronary Syndromes 19
    Non–ST-Elevation Myocardial Infarction and Unstable Angina 19
    ST-Elevation Myocardial Infarction 21
Coronary Artery Disease in Women 26
    Presentation and Evaluation 26
    Medical Treatment 26
    Invasive Treatment 27
Coronary Artery Disease in Patients with Diabetes Mellitus 27
    Prevention of Cardiovascular Complications 27
    Diagnosis of Coronary Artery Disease in Patients with Diabetes 27
    Pharmacologic Treatment and Secondary Prevention . 27
    Invasive Approaches in Patients with Diabetes 28

Heart Failure

Diagnosis and Evaluation of Heart Failure 29
    Clinical Evaluation 29
    Diagnostic Testing 29
Therapeutic Options for Heart Failure 31
    Initiation and Titration of Medical Therapy 31
    Treatment of Heart Failure with Preserved Systolic Function 35
    Device Therapy 35
Management of Chronic Heart Failure 36
    Disease Management Team Approach 36
    Serial Assessment 36
    Assessing Prognosis 37
Acute Exacerbation of Chronic Heart Failure 37
    Cardiogenic Shock 37
Advanced Refractory Heart Failure 39
Investigational Therapies for Heart Failure 40
Specific Cardiomyopathies 40
    Takotsubo Cardiomyopathy 40
    Acute Myocarditis 41
    Tachycardia-Mediated Cardiomyopathy 41
    Arrhythmogenic Right Ventricular Dysplasia 41
    Giant Cell Myocarditis 41

Myocardial Disease

Restrictive Cardiomyopathy 41
    Clinical Presentation and Evaluation 42
    Differentiating Restrictive Cardiomyopathy from Constrictive Pericarditis 43
    Treatment 43
Hypertrophic Cardiomyopathy 44
    Clinical Presentation and Evaluation 44
    Clinical Course 45
    Management 46
Cardiac Tumors 47
    Pathophysiology 47
    Clinical Presentation and Evaluation 48
    Management 48

Arrhythmias

Approach to the Patient with Bradycardia 49
    Clinical Presentation and Evaluation 49
    Sick Sinus Syndrome 49
    Atrioventricular Block 49
Approach to the Patient with Tachycardia 50
    Evaluation and Initial Management 50
    Antiarrhythmic Drugs 52
Atrial Fibrillation 53
    Clinical Presentation and Evaluation 53
    Acute Management 53
    Long-Term Management 54
Atrial Flutter 55
    Clinical Presentation and Evaluation 55
    Acute Management 56
    Chronic Management 56
Supraventricular Tachycardias 56
    Epidemiology and Electrophysiology 56
    Clinical Presentation and Evaluation 56
    Acute Management 56
    Long-Term Management 57
    Wolff-Parkinson-White Syndrome 57
Premature Ventricular Complexes 58
Nonsustained Ventricular Tachycardia 59
Sustained Ventricular Tachycardia 59
    Ventricular Tachycardia with Structural Heart Disease 59
    Idiopathic Ventricular Tachycardia 59
Sudden Cardiac Death 59
    Epidemiology and Risk Factors 59
    Genetics 60
    Acute Management 61
    Long-Term Management and Secondary Prevention 61

Pericardial Disease

Acute and Recurrent Pericarditis 62
    Clinical Presentation 62
    Evaluation 63
    Management 64
Pericardial Effusion Without Cardiac Compression 66
    Clinical Presentation and Evaluation 66
    Management 66
Cardiac Tamponade 66
    Clinical Presentation and Evaluation 66
    Management 67
Constrictive Pericarditis 68
    Clinical Presentation and Evaluation 68
    Management 69

Valvular Heart Disease

Diagnosis and Evaluation of Valvular Heart Disease 69
    History and Physical Examination 69
    Diagnostic Evaluation 70
General Principles of Management of Valvular Heart Disease 70
Aortic Stenosis 72
    Pathophysiology 72
    Clinical Presentation 74
    Management 74
Mitral Stenosis 74
    Pathophysiology 74
    Clinical Presentation 74
    Management 75
Acute Valvular Regurgitation 76
    Acute Aortic Regurgitation 76
    Acute Mitral Regurgitation 76
Chronic Valvular Regurgitation 76
    Chronic Aortic Regurgitation 77
    Chronic Mitral Regurgitation 77
    Mitral Valve Prolapse 78
Tricuspid Valve Disease 78
Endocarditis 79
    Diagnosis 79
    Management 79
    Prophylaxis 79
Prosthetic Valves 80

Adult Congenital Heart Disease

Epidemiology 81
Newly Diagnosed Congenital Heart Disease in Adults 81
    Atrial Septal Defect 81
    Patent Foramen Ovale 83
    Ventricular Septal Defect 84
    Coarctation of the Aorta 85
    Patent Ductus Arteriosus 86
    Pulmonary Stenosis 86
Previously Operated Congenital Heart Disease 87
    Postoperative or Postintervention Atrial Septal Defect 87
    Postoperative Ventricular Septal Defect 87
    Postoperative Aortic Coarctation 87
    Tetralogy of Fallot 87
Adults with Cyanotic Congenital Heart Disease 88
    General Management 88
    Eisenmenger Syndrome 88

Diseases of the Aorta

Introduction 89

Aortic Atheroma...89

Abdominal Aortic Aneurysm 90

    Clinical Presentation and Natural History 90

    Screening...90

    Management 90

Thoracic Aortic Aneurysm 90

Marfan Syndrome 91

    Pathophysiology and Clinical Presentation 91

    Management 91

Takayasu Arteritis..92

Acute Aortic Syndromes 92

    Pathophysiology and Clinical Presentation 92

    Diagnosis...92

    Treatment..92

Peripheral Arterial Disease

Evaluation of Peripheral Arterial Disease 93

    Clinical Presentation and Differential Diagnosis 93

    Physical Examination and Diagnostic Studies 94

Management of Peripheral Arterial Disease 94

    Cardiovascular Risk Factor Modification 94

    Medical Treatment of Symptomatic Patients 96

    Endovascular and Surgical Management 96

Acute Limb Ischemia 97

    Pathogenesis 97

    Management 97

Pregnancy and Cardiovascular Disease

Cardiovascular Changes with Pregnancy 98

Prepregnancy Evaluation....................................98

Management of Cardiovascular Disease During Pregnancy..99

    Peripartum Cardiomyopathy....................................99

    Medication Use during Pregnancy 100

    Anticoagulation during Pregnancy 100

Cardiovascular Medicine

Epidemiology of Cardiovascular Disease

Overview

More than 80 million adult Americans (1 in 3) have cardiovascular disease, with approximately 47% of these persons older than 60 years. If high blood pressure is excluded, approximately 10% of the adult U.S. population has cardiovascular disease (coronary artery disease, heart failure, stroke).

The incidence of a first cardiovascular event increases directly with age, occurring in 10 per 1000 men between ages 45 and 54 years and increasing to 59 per 1000 men for ages 75 to 84 years (**Figure 1**). The incidence of a first cardiovascular event for women also increases substantially with age, with a delay of approximately one decade in rates compared with men.

Cardiovascular disease is the most common cause of death in the United States; although cancer-related deaths slightly exceed deaths related to cardiovascular disease for persons ages 45 to 74 years, deaths due to cardiovascular disease are more than twice as frequent as cancer-related deaths for persons older than 74 years.

KEY POINT

- Cardiovascular disease is the leading cause of death in the United States, and among persons 75 years and older, more than twice as many die from cardiovascular disease than from cancer-related causes.

Women and Cardiovascular Disease

Women develop cardiovascular disease at later ages than men, but the prevalence of cardiovascular disease is similar for both sexes. The average lifetime risk for a woman to develop cardiovascular disease is approximately 1 in 2. Cardiovascular disease is the leading cause of death among women; 1 of 3 women die of cardiovascular disease, compared with 1 of 5 women dying from cancer-related causes. More women than men in the United States die of cardiovascular disease each year. Over the past 25 years, the number of cardiovascular deaths among men has declined significantly, but the number among women has remained essentially unchanged.

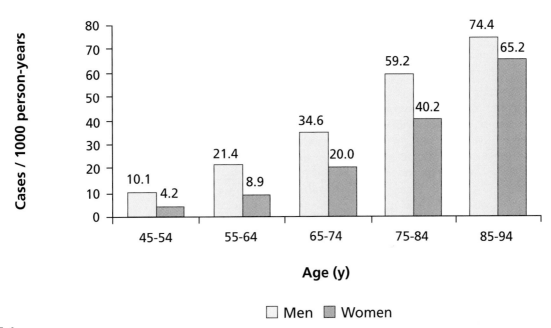

FIGURE 1.
Incidence of Cardiovascular Disease by Age and Sex.
Cardiovascular disease consists of coronary artery disease, heart failure, cerebrovascular accident, or intermittent claudication. Framingham Heart Study 1980-2003.

Data from National Heart, Lung, and Blood Institute. Incidence and Prevalence: 2006 Chartbook on Cardiovascular and Lung Diseases. www.nhlbi.nih.gov/resources/docs/cht-book_ip.htm. Published May, 2006. Accessed February 2, 2009. Chart 2-1.

- More women than men die of cardiovascular disease each year, and the number of women dying of cardiovascular disease has not decreased over time.

Ethnicity and Cardiovascular Disease

In 2005 in the United States, the prevalence of myocardial infarction or coronary heart disease/angina was approximately 5% for Asians, 6% for whites and blacks, 7% for Hispanics, and 11% for American Indian/Alaskan natives. This variable prevalence is largely attributable to the presence of risk factors in these ethnic groups: two or more risk factors for heart disease and stroke are found in nearly 50% of blacks and American Indian/Alaskan natives but in 25% of Asian adults. The prevalence of hypertension and stroke also has significant ethnic variability. Approximately 30% of the adult American population have high blood pressure: 16% of Asians, 19% of Hispanics or Latinos, 32% of whites, and 41% of blacks. The prevalence in American blacks is among the highest in the world. Compared with whites, blacks develop high blood pressure at a younger age, have higher average blood pressure measurements, and carry a much greater risk of end-organ complications such as stroke and end-stage kidney disease.

Diabetes Mellitus and Cardiovascular Disease

Approximately 10% of the U.S. adult population has diabetes mellitus, 95% of whom have type 2 diabetes. Since 1990, the prevalence of diabetes has increased 61%. The prevalence is approximately 1.5- to 2-fold higher in blacks, Hispanic Americans, and American Indian/native Alaskan adults than in whites. Diabetes is a risk factor for coronary artery disease, heart failure, and stroke, and adults with diabetes are 2 to 4 times more likely to have heart disease or experience a stroke than persons without diabetes. In 2000, the prevalence of any self-reported cardiovascular condition among persons with diabetes older than 35 years was greater than 30%. At least 65% of people with diabetes eventually die of cardiovascular disease, which is the leading cause of premature death among patients with diabetes. Although the cardiovascular disease mortality rate has declined in the United States, the relative reduction in mortality is much lower in persons with diabetes than in those without.

Among persons with diabetes, the presence of microalbuminuria is strongly associated with coronary artery disease, left ventricular hypertrophy, and peripheral vascular disease. Microalbuminuria is an adverse prognostic indicator for cardiovascular disease outcomes and all-cause mortality in persons with diabetes.

- The prevalence of cardiovascular disease and the death rate due to cardiovascular disease are 2 to 4 times higher among persons with diabetes than those without diabetes.
- Microalbuminuria in persons with diabetes is strongly associated with cardiovascular disease and poorer cardiovascular disease outcomes.

Metabolic Syndrome and Cardiovascular Disease

The term *metabolic syndrome* refers to the clustering of risk factors for cardiovascular disease and type 2 diabetes. The most commonly utilized definition in the United States is the presence of at least three of the following five risk factors:

1. Fasting plasma glucose level ≥110 mg/dL (6.11 mmol/L)
2. HDL cholesterol level <40 mg/dL (1.0 mmol/L) in men or <50 mg/dL (1.3 mmol/L) in women
3. Triglyceride level ≥150 mg/dL (1.7 mmol/L)
4. Waist circumference ≥102 cm (40 in) in men or ≥88 cm (35 in) in women
5. Blood pressure ≥130 mm Hg systolic or ≥85 mm Hg diastolic or drug treatment for hypertension

An estimated 47 million U.S. residents have metabolic syndrome, with the highest prevalence in Mexican Americans (32%) and the lowest prevalence in whites (24%). Persons with metabolic syndrome have a higher risk of developing diabetes and cardiovascular disease and have a higher risk of death from cardiovascular disease.

Cancer and Cardiovascular Disease

Radiation therapy or chemotherapy for cancer may predispose the patient to cardiovascular disease. In a recent study of long-term survivors of childhood cancer, nearly 75% of patients had at least one long-term adverse event as a result of therapy for their primary malignancy, including 175 cardiovascular events among 1362 patients (predominantly cardiomyopathy). Radiation therapy was associated with the highest risk of adverse event, and patients treated with mediastinal radiation for lymphoma were predisposed to coronary artery disease, thickening and fibrosis of the aortic and mitral valve leaflets resulting in stenosis or regurgitation, pericardial adhesions and constriction, conduction defects, and ventricular diastolic dysfunction due to myocardial fibrosis. Radiation therapy also increases the procedural complexity and potentially affects the results of cardiac surgery for these patients.

Specific types of cardiovascular disease associated with previous radiation therapy are more likely to develop or manifest at certain time intervals from the exposure. In a study of

415 patients treated with radiation therapy for Hodgkin lymphoma, 10.4% of patients developed coronary artery disease at a median of 9 years after treatment, 7.4% developed carotid and/or subclavian artery disease at a median of 17 years, and 6.2% developed clinically significant valvular dysfunction (most commonly, aortic stenosis) at a median of 22 years. The observed-to-expected ratios for interventions for these valvular and coronary lesions were increased, particularly for valve surgery.

Previous chemotherapy, most notably with anthracyclines such as doxorubicin, is associated with an increased risk of cardiomyopathy. These agents are used for the treatment of acute leukemia, Hodgkin and non-Hodgkin lymphoma, and breast cancer. The overall incidence of cardiomyopathy in patients who have been treated with doxorubicin is estimated to be 1.7%. The strongest risk factor for the development of cardiomyopathy is the cumulative dosage administered—among patients who receive greater than 500 mg/m^2, the risk of cardiomyopathy is more than 18%. Other risk factors for doxorubicin cardiomyopathy include peak serum levels of the drug; very young or very advanced age; mediastinal radiotherapy; treatment with other cardiotoxic chemotherapy, such as cyclophosphamide; and a history of other cardiovascular disease, including hypertension. The onset of cardiomyopathy may occur as early as 30 days after last administration of the drug, and the mortality rate is nearly 50%. In long-term survivors of childhood cancer (mostly leukemia), anthracycline cardiotoxicity occurs in approximately 5%. Risk factors include younger age at treatment, female sex, and repeat treatment for secondary malignancies. It appears that the dose limit for cardiotoxicity is lower in children. Trastuzumab, a monoclonal antibody against the HER2 receptor protein on breast cancer cells, has been associated with an up to 28% incidence of cardiac dysfunction. Age and concomitant anthracycline therapy have been associated with developing cardiotoxicity with trastuzumab.

KEY POINTS

- Patients treated with radiation therapy have higher than expected rates of valvular and coronary artery disease.

- Cardiomyopathy occurs in approximately 2% of patients treated with anthracyclines; it is directly related to the cumulative dose and is associated with a mortality rate of nearly 50%.

- Trastuzumab is associated with a high risk of cardiotoxicity, and cardiac function should be closely monitored during and after treatment.

Systemic Inflammatory Conditions and Cardiovascular Disease

Patients with systemic inflammatory conditions are at greater risk of coronary artery disease, pericarditis, myocarditis or myocardial fibrosis, endocardial involvement causing valvular dysfunction or thrombus formation, coronary arteritis, pulmonary arterial hypertension, conduction abnormalities, and systemic hypertension (**Table 1**). These complications may result from organ-specific effects of these diseases on heart and vascular structures as well as from a less direct effect of chronic systemic inflammation. For example, patients with rheumatoid arthritis have a 2- to 3-fold increased risk of coronary artery disease and those with systemic lupus

TABLE 1 Systemic Inflammatory Conditions and Associated Cardiovascular Diseases	
Systemic Inflammatory Condition	**Cardiac Involvement and Prevalence**
Systemic lupus erythematosus	Pericarditis (25%-50%), noninfective endocarditis (22%-61%), moderate or severe valvular regurgitation (up to 20%), premature coronary artery disease
Rheumatoid arthritis	Pericardial effusion (30%-40%), coronary artery disease, leaflet fibrosis (up to 30%), left ventricular diastolic dysfunction (up to 15%)
Ankylosing spondylitis	Proximal aortitis/valvulitis (25%-60%), moderate or severe aortic regurgitation (up to 40%), conduction system disease (2%-20%), left ventricular diastolic dysfunction
Systemic sclerosis	Systemic hypertension, including scleroderma renal crisis; pulmonary arterial hypertension; myocardial fibrosis; pericardial disease
Takayasu arteritis	Arteritis, predominantly aortic (aneurysms, stenosis, occlusion); coronary arteritis (15%-25%); aortic regurgitation; pulmonary artery stenosis or aneurysm; malignant hypertension due to renovascular involvement
Giant cell arteritis	Peripheral artery disease, stroke, myocardial infarction
Polyarteritis nodosa	Cardiomyopathy
Kawasaki disease	Coronary artery aneurysms, occlusion
Behçet disease	Aortic valve regurgitation, myocarditis, pericarditis, conduction abnormalities
Sarcoidosis	Cardiomyopathy (dilated or restrictive); conduction abnormalities; ventricular arrhythmias, including sudden death

erythematosus may have up to a 50-fold increased risk of myocardial infarction.

Lifestyle Factors and Cardiovascular Disease

Approximately 41% of the adult U.S. population has a history of smoking cigarettes, and nearly 22% currently smoke. Cigarette smoking is a risk factor for coronary artery disease, myocardial infarction, stroke, and peripheral artery disease. A dose-response relationship between cigarettes smoked and cardiovascular disease risk has been established, with heavy smokers having a relative risk of nearly 5.5 for fatal cardiovascular disease events compared with nonsmokers. Notably, the risk of cardiovascular events decreases rapidly after cessation of smoking, with previous smokers having the same risk as persons who never smoked at 5 to 10 years after stopping smoking.

Although moderate alcohol consumption (approximately one to three drinks daily) is associated with a lower risk of coronary artery disease, excessive alcohol intake accounts for approximately 4% of cases of dilated cardiomyopathy. The level of ingestion has been estimated to be 8 to 21 drinks per day for at least 5 years before abnormalities in cardiac structure and function occur.

Cocaine use is associated with chest pain, myocardial infarction, left ventricular hypertrophy, cardiomyopathy, aortic dissection, and cardiac arrhythmias. The adverse cardiac effects of cocaine seem to be exacerbated by concomitant use of tobacco or alcohol. The use of methamphetamine has been associated with cardiovascular complications similar to those associated with cocaine use.

For physically inactive adults, the relative risk of a cardiovascular event is 1.5 to 2.4, an increase in risk comparable to other major risk factors such as smoking, high blood pressure, or high cholesterol levels. Only about 60% of adults report engaging in at least some physical activity for 10 minutes or longer per session, and this percentage decreases with older age.

The intravenous injection of any illicit drug is associated with a risk of infective endocarditis, particularly *Staphylococcus aureus* infection of the tricuspid valve resulting in tricuspid valve regurgitation. Although infection of the tricuspid valve is the most common site of involvement for endocarditis associated with injection drug use, infection of the mitral and aortic valves has been reported in 32% and 19%, respectively, of cases.

Bibliography

Geenen MM, Cardous-Ubbink MC, Kremer LC, et al. Medical assessment of adverse health outcomes in long-term survivors of childhood cancer. JAMA. 2007;297(24):2705-2715. [PMID: 17595271]

Hull MC, Morris CG, Pepine CJ, Mendenhall NP. Valvular dysfunction and carotid, subclavian, and coronary artery disease in survivors of Hodgkin lymphoma treated with radiation therapy. JAMA. 2003;290(21):2831-2837. [PMID: 14657067]

Kenfield SA, Stampfer MJ, Rosner BA, Colditz GA. Smoking and smoking cessation in relation to mortality in women. JAMA. 2008;299(17):2037-2047. [PMID: 18460664]

Knockaert DC. Cardiac involvement in systemic inflammatory diseases. Eur Heart J. 2007;28(15):1797-1804. [PMID: 17562669]

Lange RA, Hillis LD. Cardiovascular complications of cocaine use [erratum in N Engl J Med. 2001;345(19):1432.]. N Engl J Med. 2001;345(5):351-358. [PMID: 11484693]

Mathew J, Addai T, Anand A, Morrobel A, Maheshwari P, Freels S. Clinical features, site of involvement, bacteriologic findings, and outcome of infective endocarditis in intravenous drug users. Arch Intern Med. 1995;155(15):1641-1648. [PMID: 7618988]

Rosamond W, Flegal K, Furie K, et al. Heart disease and stroke statistics—2008 update: a report from the American Heart Association Statistics Committee and Stroke Statistics Subcommittee. Circulation. 2008;117(4):e25-146. [PMID: 18086926]

Sarnak MJ, Levey AS, Schoolwerth AC, et al. Kidney disease as a risk factor for development of cardiovascular disease: a statement from the American Heart Association Councils on Kidney in Cardiovascular Disease, High Blood Pressure Research, Clinical Cardiology, and Epidemiology and Prevention. Circulation. 2003;108(17):2154-2169. [PMID: 14581387]

Takemura G, Fujiwara H. Doxorubicin-induced cardiomyopathy from the cardiotoxic mechanisms to management. Progress in Cardiovascular Diseases. 2007;49(5):330-352. [PMID: 17329180]

Telli ML, Hunt SA, Carlson RW, Guardino AE. Trastuzumab-related cardiotoxicity: calling into question the concept of reversibility. J Clin Oncol. 2007;25(23):3525-3533. [PMID: 17687157]

Extensions of the Physical Examination

Introduction

Although a clinical history and physical examination are essential for identification of cardiac disease, additional diagnostic testing is needed in most patients. An overview of the available diagnostic modalities is presented here. The appropriate diagnostic sequence in various clinical situations is presented in other sections.

Structural Heart Disease

Structural heart disease is defined as any anatomic abnormality of the heart other than coronary artery disease. It usually is suspected based on clinical history or physical examination findings of a murmur or of heart failure. In adults with a murmur, cardiac auscultation is not sufficiently reliable to be the sole diagnostic modality for identifying the cause of a murmur, and it rarely provides information on disease severity. Electronic stethoscopes provide better sound quality than acoustic models and also allow recording and visual displays of the audio data, thus serving as a useful teaching tool. However, agreement among physicians for the identification of cardiac murmurs by auscultation is low and is not improved by either the use of an electronic stethoscope or clinical experience. Whereas a completely normal cardiac examination is reassuring and, conversely, a very loud murmur is clearly abnormal, the reliability of other findings is low for detection of structural heart disease.

Transthoracic echocardiography typically is the initial diagnostic test in patients who present with evidence of a structural abnormality, such as a pathologic heart murmur or evidence of heart failure (**Table 2**). This test provides detailed information on left and right ventricular size and systolic function, valve anatomy and function, pulmonary pressures, the presence of pericardial disease, and the proximal great vessels. Transthoracic echocardiography is indicated for the following murmurs:

TABLE 2 Diagnostic Tests for Suspected or Known Structural Heart Disease			
Diagnostic Test	**Major Indications**	**Advantages**	**Limitations**
Transthoracic echocardiography	Heart failure Cardiomyopathy Valve disease Congenital heart disease Pulmonary hypertension Aortic disease Pericardial disease	Accurate diagnosis of the presence and severity of structural heart disease Quantitation of left ventricular size and function, pulmonary pressures, valvular stenosis and regurgitation, and intracardiac shunts No known adverse effects Widely available, portable, fast	Operator-dependent data acquisition Interpretation requires expertise Variability in instrumentation Image quality limits diagnosis in some patients
Transesophageal echocardiography	Endocarditis Prosthetic valve dysfunction Aortic disease Left atrial thrombus	High-quality images, especially of posterior cardiac structures Most accurate test for evaluation of endocarditis, prosthetic valves, and left atrial thrombus	Requires esophageal intubation, typically with conscious sedation
Radionuclide angiography	Evaluation of left ventricular systolic function	Quantitative ejection fraction measurements	Less accurate with atrial fibrillation Radiation exposure No data on other cardiac structures
Cardiac catheterization	Congenital heart disease Coronary angiography for coronary disease (see Table 3)	Direct measurement of intracardiac pressures Contrast angiography provides visualization of complex cardiac anatomy Allows percutaneous intervention for structural heart disease, often with intracardiac echocardiographic guidance	Invasive Radiation exposure Images are not tomographic, limiting evaluation of complex 3-D anatomy
CMR imaging	Congenital heart disease Aortic disease Myocardial viability Myocardial disease (infiltrative, myocarditis, hypertrophic cardiomyopathy) Right ventricular cardiomyopathy (ARVC) Quantitation of left ventricular mass and function	High-resolution tomographic imaging and blood-flow data Quantitative right ventricular volumes and ejection fraction No ionizing radiation or contrast Enables 3-D reconstruction of aortic and coronary anatomy	Limited availability and expertise Some patients experience claustrophobia May not be appropriate for patients with pacemaker, ICD, or other implanted devices
Chest CT	Aortic disease Coronary disease (see Table 3) Cardiac masses Pericardial disease	High-resolution tomographic images Enables 3-D reconstructions of aortic and coronary anatomy	Contrast injection Radiation exposure

ARVC = arrhythmogenic right ventricular cardiomyopathy; CMR = cardiac magnetic resonance; ICD = implantable cardioverter-defibrillator.

- Any diastolic murmur
- A systolic murmur grade 3/6 or louder
- A murmur of any grade if associated with possible cardiac symptoms or a history of cardiac disease

A normal flow murmur occurs with increased cardiac output, for example, in a patient with fever or anemia. A flow murmur also is present in more than 80% of normal pregnant women. Echocardiography is not needed for evaluation of these soft midsystolic murmurs in the absence of symptoms or other signs of cardiac disease. In addition, current guidelines do not recommend endocarditis prophylaxis in patients with native cardiac valve disease; therefore, even if mild valve disease were present, echocardiography would not change clinical management.

In patients with heart failure symptoms, some physical examination findings are useful when present; for example, an S_3 has a 95% specificity for a left-ventricular ejection fraction below 50% or a filling pressure greater than 15 mm Hg. However, heart failure cannot be excluded in the absence of an S_3 because sensitivity is only 30% to 50%. In addition, physical examination does not provide quantitative measures of ventricular function. In contrast, echocardiography provides quantitation of ventricular systolic function, assessment of other hemodynamic consequences (such as mitral regurgitation and pulmonary hypertension), and often provides clues to the cause of heart failure.

Smaller, hand-held echocardiographic instruments can be used for limited bedside imaging in patients with chest pain, dyspnea, or other cardiac symptoms. This approach can assist in triage; for example, differentiating the chest pain patient with a large anterior myocardial infarction from the one with a pericardial effusion. However, these instruments must be used by trained providers and in appropriate clinical situations. When in doubt, a standard echocardiographic study should be requested as well.

Transesophageal echocardiography is appropriate when transthoracic images are nondiagnostic and as the initial imaging test in some clinical situations, such as detection of left atrial thrombus, evaluation of prosthetic mitral valve dysfunction, evaluation of suspected aortic dissection, and in patients with a moderate to high pretest probability of endocarditis. Advanced cardiac imaging procedures for structural heart disease include radionuclide angiography, cardiac catheterization, CT scanning, and cardiac magnetic resonance (CMR) imaging (see Table 2). Typically, these tests are considered only after echocardiographic evaluation and in consultation with a cardiologist.

KEY POINTS

- Transthoracic echocardiography is the initial diagnostic test for suspected or known structural heart disease.
- Hand-held echocardiographic instruments may be helpful for triage when used by an appropriately trained and experienced individual.

Coronary Artery Disease

The goals of physical examination in patients with suspected or known coronary artery disease (CAD) are to exclude noncoronary causes of chest pain, including aortic stenosis, hypertrophic cardiomyopathy, and aortic dissection; and to detect any signs of heart failure. Then, the most appropriate diagnostic test (**Table 3**) depends on the pretest probability of disease, estimated from the description of symptoms, age, and sex.

The standard diagnostic approach in patients with suspected or known coronary artery disease continues to be history and physical examination followed by stress testing when appropriate. Exercise stress testing is preferred because it provides an objective measure of functional status in addition to detection of ischemia. In patients who cannot exercise, stress testing with pharmacologic agents that increase the heart rate–blood pressure product (such as dobutamine) or result in relative inequality in myocardial blood flow (such as adenosine) are appropriate. Exercise electrocardiographic (ECG) stress testing with ECG monitoring alone is appropriate when the resting ECG is normal. Any resting ST-segment changes reduce diagnostic accuracy, and ECG stress testing is not useful with conditions such as pre-excitation (Wolff-Parkinson-White syndrome), greater than 1-mm ST-segment depression, and left bundle branch block. Following an abnormal resting ECG or with pharmacologic stress testing, echocardiographic or nuclear imaging is needed. Based on a recent meta-analysis, echocardiographic and nuclear stress imaging are equivalent for the diagnosis of ischemia with a negative predictive value of 98% for adverse cardiovascular outcomes over the next 3 years.

Coronary angiography is appropriate when the stress test is consistent with CAD, particularly if there is a large area of myocardium at risk. In patients with a very high pretest probability of disease, coronary angiography is an appropriate initial diagnostic test.

Newer diagnostic approaches for coronary disease include CT imaging, CMR imaging, and positron emission tomography (PET). CT can be used for measuring coronary artery calcium (CAC) and for noninvasive coronary angiographic imaging. CAC scores are measured from noncontrast CT images, whereas CT coronary angiography requires a radiocontrast agent and use of a high-resolution scanner, necessitating a higher radiation dose to the patient.

The CAC score correlates with cardiovascular risk but is not a direct measure of the severity of luminal coronary disease, and CAC scores are not indicated for routine screening. CAC measurement may be considered in *asymptomatic* patients with an intermediate risk of CAD (10%-20% 10-year risk), because a high CAC score (>400) is an indication for more intensive preventive medical treatment. However, a low CAC score (score = 0) should not change intensity of treatment for cardiac risk factors. CAC scoring is not recommended in patients with low CAD risk (<10% 10-year risk of coronary events). In addition, CAC scores are not recommended in asymptomatic patients at high risk for CAD; these patients should receive appropriate risk factor reduction therapy.

In *symptomatic* patients, CAC testing has a high negative predictive value (96%-100%); therefore, a patient with a CAC score of zero is highly unlikely to have obstructive CAD. A CAC score below 100 confers a low probability of abnormal perfusion (<2%) or significant obstruction (<3%). CAC testing, therefore, may benefit patients with atypical cardiac symptoms to help rule out obstructive CAD, although there are no direct comparisons to other diagnostic approaches in this clinical setting.

CT or CMR coronary angiography is appropriate for identification of anomalous coronary arteries. CT coronary angiography also is appropriate to evaluate coronary anatomy in a patient with new-onset heart failure and in patients with acute chest pain syndromes when the risk of CAD is intermediate but cardiac enzyme results are negative. CT coronary angiography or CMR pharmacologic stress testing may be considered in symptomatic patients with an intermediate probability of CAD when the ECG is abnormal at baseline, the patient is unable to exercise, or previous test results are equivocal. During CT angiography, additional noncardiac structures are also imaged, and significant noncardiac findings (for example, lung nodules and infiltrates, pulmonary embolism, hiatal hernia, and aortic dissection) are present in approximately 20% of patients. PET scanning has several advantages compared with conventional pharmacologic nuclear perfusion imaging using single-photon emission computed tomography (SPECT). Compared with SPECT, a PET study is shorter for the patient (45-90 minutes), results in a lower radiation dose, provides evaluation of both myocardial perfusion and function, and reduces interpretive uncertainty, particularly in obese patients. In addition, PET provides the option of quantification of absolute myocardial blood flow and can be combined with CAC scoring. Guidelines for diagnostic use of PET have not yet been established, but it is a reasonable option when other tests are not diagnostic.

The risks in diagnostic evaluation for CAD include exposure to radiation (angiography, CT, and nuclear imaging) and to radiocontrast agents (angiography and CT imaging). The major risk of radiocontrast exposure is acute renal failure, which occurs in approximately 3% of patients undergoing coronary interventions but up to 25% of those with a baseline serum creatinine concentration greater than 2.0 mg/dL.

Radiation exposure depends on patient body habitus, operator technique, procedure length, and the imaging system. Relative radiation exposure for coronary diagnostic imaging procedures is shown in **Table 4**. It is likely that radiation exposure with CT coronary angiography will decrease substantially with refinements in instrumentation and imaging protocols.

KEY POINTS

- The appropriate diagnostic test for coronary artery disease is based on symptoms and an estimate of cardiovascular risk.

- Exercise and pharmacologic stress testing, using electrocardiography, echocardiography, or radionuclide myocardial perfusion imaging, remains the standard initial approach when coronary artery disease is suspected.

- Coronary angiography provides a definitive diagnosis of coronary artery disease severity and allows simultaneous intervention.

Cardiac Arrhythmias

In a patient with palpitations, dizziness, syncope, or a known arrhythmia, clinical history is the primary determinant of the diagnostic approach. Physical examination is directed toward detection of underlying structural heart disease. For patients whose history suggests a cardiac cause of syncope, after echocardiography is performed to evaluate for underlying structural heart disease, the key diagnostic test is an ECG recorded during the clinical event. In most patients, a resting ECG is not helpful; however, there are exceptions, such as the presence of a delta wave or a long QT interval. There are several approaches to recording an intermittent arrhythmia; the most appropriate test is based on the frequency and duration of symptoms (**Table 5**, page 10). For infrequent arrhythmias that are brief or that prevent the patient from activating the monitoring device (such as syncope), a loop recorder is helpful. Some loop recorders can be set to save data based on heart rate parameters.

If an arrhythmia cannot be captured on ECG during an event using standard event monitors or loop recorders, an implantable recorder can be used. This small device is surgically placed subcutaneously, similarly to a pacemaker, but there are no leads in the heart chambers. Recording parameters are set based on heart rate and QRS width, and, like a pacemaker, the device can be interrogated noninvasively.

KEY POINTS

- The key to diagnosis of a cardiac arrhythmia is an ECG recorded during the event.

- Event monitors allow recording of infrequent but symptomatic arrhythmias.

- Syncope due to a cardiac arrhythmia is best evaluated with a loop recorder.

- Asymptomatic arrhythmias are best evaluated with a continuously monitored ECG, such as a 24-hour ambulatory ECG (frequent arrhythmias) or an implanted recorder (infrequent arrhythmias).

TABLE 3 Diagnostic Tests for Suspected or Known Coronary Artery Disease

Diagnostic Test	Utility	Advantages	Limitations
Exercise Testing			
ECG	Initial test in most patients with suspected coronary disease	Exercise testing provides data on exercise capacity, blood pressure and heart rate response, and possible provoked symptoms	Not useful when the baseline ECG is abnormal Accuracy depends on pretest probability of disease
Echocardiography	Recommended when baseline ECG is abnormal or when information on the area of myocardium at risk is needed	Exercise data are acquired along with imaging for wall motion abnormalities that indicate ischemia Entire study is complete in <1 hour	Image quality is suboptimal in some patients but can be improved by use of echo-contrast
Nuclear myocardial perfusion	Recommended when baseline ECG is abnormal or when information on the area of myocardium at risk is needed	Technetium scanning provides improved specificity compared with thallium scanning Dual isotope studies can be completed in about 3 hours	Attenuation artifacts due to breast or diaphragm Radiation exposure Repeat imaging after several hours is needed for most nuclear perfusion studies unless a dual isotope protocol is used
Pharmacologic Stress Testing			
Dobutamine echocardiography	Recommended in patients who cannot exercise (e.g., due to arthritis, pulmonary disease)	Images are acquired continuously, allowing the test to be stopped as soon as ischemia is evident by echocardiography	Contraindications to dobutamine stress are severe baseline hypertension and history of arrhythmias ß-Blockers must be withheld before the test
Dobutamine nuclear perfusion	Recommended in patients who cannot exercise	Diagnostic accuracy equivalent to echocardiography Nuclear perfusion preferred when echo image quality is suboptimal	Contraindications to dobutamine stress are severe baseline hypertension and history of arrhythmias ß-Blockers must be withheld before the test
Adenosine or dipyridamole nuclear perfusion	Recommended in patients who cannot exercise and have contraindications to dobutamine	Late reperfusion imaging allows evaluation of myocardial viability	Contraindications include bronchospastic airway disease and theophylline use Caffeine must be withheld before the test Baseline 2nd-degree heart block is a contraindication to adenosine
Adenosine positron emission tomography	Provide best perfusion images in larger patients Provides data on myocardial perfusion and function	Study duration is shorter and radiation dose is lower than conventional nuclear perfusion imaging Absolute myocardial blood flow can be measured Can be combined with coronary calcium scoring	Not widely available More expensive Pharmacologic stress only (no exercise)
Other Tests			
Coronary angiography	Definitive diagnosis of the presence and severity of CAD	Percutaneous revascularization can be performed following the diagnostic study	Invasive Radiation exposure Risks of contrast dye (renal dysfunction, allergy)
CAC testing	CAC testing is reasonable in asymptomatic patients at intermediate risk of CAD	CAC scores are predictive of cardiovascular risk	Radiation exposure Does not provide data on coronary luminal narrowing

(Continued on next page)

TABLE 3 Diagnostic Tests for Suspected or Known Coronary Artery Disease *(continued)*

Diagnostic Test	Utility	Advantages	Limitations
Other Tests (continued)			
Coronary CT imaging	Identifies anomalous coronary arteries Useful in selected patients with an intermediate risk of CAD	Coronary artery vessel lumen and atherosclerotic lesions can be visualized in detail	Radiation exposure Risks of contrast agent Requires high-resolution (64-slice) CT instruments Does not provide detailed images of distal vessel anatomy Catheterization still needed for intervention when disease is present
CMR imaging	Gadolinium-enhanced images accurately identify viable and infarcted myocardium Identification of anomalous coronary arteries	More accurate test for myocardial viability	Some patients experience claustrophobia May not be appropriate for patients with pacemaker, ICD, or other implanted devices

CAC = coronary artery calcium; CAD = coronary artery disease; CMR = cardiac magnetic resonance; ECG = electrocardiography; ICD = implantable cardioverter-defibrillator.

TABLE 4 Relative Radiation Exposure for Diagnostic Imaging for Coronary Artery Disease

Procedure	Relative Exposure[a]
Stress echocardiography	0
Cardiac magnetic resonance coronary angiography	0
Coronary artery calcium score	20-40
Coronary angiography (diagnostic)	200-500
Nuclear perfusion imaging	100-500
Positron emission tomographic perfusion imaging	100-400
CT coronary angiography	700-2100

[a]Compared with the exposure with a chest radiograph (set at 1).

Bibliography

Douglas PS, Khandheria B, Stainback RF, et al. ACCF/ASE/ACEP/ASNC/SCAI/SCCT/SCMR 2007 appropriateness criteria for transthoracic and transesophageal echocardiography: a report of the American College of Cardiology Foundation Quality Strategic Directions Committee Appropriateness Criteria Working Group, American Society of Echocardiography, American College of Emergency Physicians, American Society of Nuclear Cardiology, Society for Cardiovascular Angiography and Interventions, Society of Cardiovascular Computed Tomography, and the Society for Cardiovascular Magnetic Resonance endorsed by the American College of Chest Physicians and the Society of Critical Care Medicine. J Am Coll Cardiol. 2007;50(2):187-204. [PMID: 17616306]

Greenland P, Bonow RO, Brundage BH, et al. ACCF/AHA 2007 clinical expert consensus document on coronary artery calcium scoring by computed tomography in global cardiovascular risk assessment and in evaluation of patients with chest pain: a report of the American College of Cardiology Foundation Clinical Expert Consensus Task Force (ACCF/AHA Writing Committee to Update the 2000 Expert Consensus Document on Electron Beam Computed Tomography) developed in collaboration with the Society of Atherosclerosis Imaging and Prevention and the Society of Cardiovascular Computed Tomography. J Am Coll Cardiol. 2007;49(3):378-402. [PMID: 17239724]

Hellmann DB, Whiting-O'Keefe Q, Shapiro EP, Martin LD, Martire C, Ziegelstein RC. The rate at which residents learn to use hand-held echocardiography at the bedside. Am J Med. 2005;118(9):1010-1018. [PMID: 16164888]

Hendel RC, Patel MR, Kramer CM, et al. ACCF/ACR/SCCT/SCMR/ASNC/NASCI/SCAI/SIR 2006 appropriateness criteria for cardiac computed tomography and cardiac magnetic resonance imaging: a report of the American College of Cardiology Foundation Quality Strategic Directions Committee Appropriateness Criteria Working Group, American College of Radiology, Society of Cardiovascular Computed Tomography, Society for Cardiovascular Magnetic Resonance, American Society of Nuclear Cardiology, North American Society for Cardiac Imaging, Society for Cardiovascular Angiography and Interventions, and Society of Interventional Radiology. J Am Coll Cardiol. 2006;48(7):1475-1497. [PMID: 17010819]

Iversen K, Greibe R, Timm HB, et al. A randomized trial comparing electronic and conventional stethoscopes. Am J Med. 2005;118(11):1289. [PMID: 16271920]

Metz LD, Beattie M, Hom R, Redberg RF, Grady D, Fleischmann KE. The prognostic value of normal exercise myocardial perfusion imaging and exercise echocardiography: a meta-analysis. J Am Coll Cardiol. 2007;49(2):227-237. [PMID: 17222734]

Tavel ME. Cardiac auscultation: a glorious past—and it does have a future! Circulation. 2006;113(9):1255-1259. [PMID: 16520426]

Vignon P, Dugard A, Abraham J, et al. Focused training for goal-oriented hand-held echocardiography performed by noncardiologist residents in the intensive care unit. Intensive Care Med. 2007;33(10): 1795-1799. [PMID: 17572874]

TABLE 5 Diagnostic Tests for Suspected or Known Cardiac Arrhythmias

Diagnostic Test	Utility	Advantages	Limitations
Resting ECG	Initial diagnostic test in all patients	12-lead ECG recorded during the arrhythmia often identifies the specific arrhythmia	Most arrhythmias are intermittent and not recorded on a resting ECG
Ambulatory (24-hour) ECG	Frequent (at least daily) asymptomatic or symptomatic arrhythmias	Records every heart beat during a 24-hour period for later analysis Patient log allows correlation with symptoms	Not helpful when arrhythmia occurs less frequently ECG leads limit patient activities
Exercise ECG	Arrhythmias provoked by exercise	Allows diagnosis of exercise-related arrhythmias Allows correlation with exercise response	Physician supervision needed in case a serious arrhythmia occurs Most arrhythmias are not exercise related
Event monitor	Infrequent symptomatic arrhythmias that last more than 1-2 minutes	Small, pocket-sized recorder is held to the chest when symptoms are present Recorded data are sent by phone to physician's office	Only useful for symptomatic arrhythmias that persist long enough for patient to activate the device Arrhythmia onset not recorded Not useful for syncope
Loop recorder	Infrequent symptomatic brief arrhythmias Syncope	Continuous ECG signal is recorded with the previous 30 seconds to 2 minutes saved when the patient activates the recording mode Arrhythmia onset is recorded	ECG leads limit patient activities Device records only when activated by patient
Implanted recorder	Infrequent asymptomatic or symptomatic arrhythmias	Long-term continuous ECG monitoring Specific heart rate or QRS parameters can be set to initiate recording of data	Invasive procedure with some risk Device must be explanted later
Electrophysiology study	Primarily used for treatment (e.g. catheter ablation), not for diagnosis	The origin and mechanism of an arrhythmia can be precisely defined	Invasive procedure with some risk Time consuming and expensive

ECG = electrocardiogram.

Coronary Artery Disease

Risk Factors for Coronary Artery Disease

Between 1980 and 2000, the age-adjusted death rate for coronary artery disease (CAD) decreased, and based on changes in mortality and estimated treatment effects, approximately 44% of this decrease was attributed to changes in risk factors.

Conventional Risk Factors

The Framingham risk score was derived from a 30-year prospective, population-based study of 5209 men and women who were between 30 and 59 years of age at study entry. This study found that the risk of developing CAD is associated with older age, male sex, elevated blood pressure, high serum cholesterol levels, cigarette smoking, and diabetes mellitus. One or more of these risk factors is present in more than 90% of persons who experience a coronary disease event. This risk score was modified by the National Cholesterol Education Program Expert Panel on Detection, Evaluation, and Treatment of High Blood Cholesterol in Adults (ATP III) by defining diabetes, atherosclerosis in other vascular beds, or prior stroke as CAD equivalents, rather than risk factors. The updated score encompasses a greater age range (20-79 years) than the original Framingham score and incorporates smoking and total serum cholesterol levels as well as treatment for hypertension. A Framingham risk calculator can be accessed at the National Cholesterol Education Program web site (http://hp2010.nhlbihin.net/atpiii/calculator .asp?usertype=prof). A family history of premature CAD (defined as CAD in a first-degree male relative <55 years of age or female relative <65 years of age) augments the risk of these other factors.

The Framingham risk score was derived in a predominantly white cohort, and thus may not extrapolate to other populations. For some sex-age groups in the Framingham study, the number of events was low, resulting in imprecise estimation of risk in those groups. The risk score estimates the probability of developing CAD within a 10-year period but may not accurately reflect the long-term risk of disease in young patients. The Framingham/ATP III score also has limited predictive accuracy for patients with chronic kidney disease, and the American Heart Association has proposed that patients with estimated glomerular filtration rate below 60 mL/min/1.73 m^2 or any proteinuria detected by dipstick be considered among the highest risk groups for cardiovascular disease.

The metabolic syndrome, which consists of insulin resistance, hypertension, elevated triglycerides, low HDL cholesterol, and obesity, has been found to confer an approximately two-fold greater risk of CAD—even in persons without diabetes—and emphasizes the detrimental effects of obesity on CAD risk. However, it appears that the metabolic syndrome in itself does not confer an independent risk beyond that associated with the specific individual risk factors that comprise this syndrome.

Conditional Risk Factors

Factors that have an association with an increased risk of CAD but have not been confirmed to be causative or independent have been termed *emerging* or *conditional* risk factors and are broadly characterized as potential promoters of atherosclerosis, arterial vessel injury, and thrombosis. One conditional risk factor is homocysteine, an intermediate amino acid in methionine metabolism, which may be elevated owing to genetic variation in metabolic enzymes. Although studies have found an association between serum homocysteine level and risk of CAD, large randomized studies of folic acid supplementation, which can reduce homocysteine levels, have not demonstrated a reduction in CAD events. Lipoprotein(a) [Lp(a)] is a circulating lipoprotein that resembles LDL cholesterol with the addition of a glycoprotein, apolipoprotein A. Plasma Lp(a) levels vary widely in the general population and have been associated with an increased risk of CAD in many observational studies. However, measurement of Lp(a) is not standardized, few pharmacologic agents lower its level, and no outcome studies have shown that lowering Lp(a) level reduces risk of CAD events.

The use of conditional risk factors for risk assessment is currently based on clinical judgment rather than validated risk estimates and includes markers of inflammation and LDL cholesterol particle size. The most widely studied inflammatory marker is C-reactive protein (CRP), an acute-phase reactant that is present in low concentrations in healthy persons. Cohort studies of healthy persons have shown that the concentration of CRP measured by high-sensitivity assay (hs-CRP) directly correlates with future risk of CAD independent of conventional risk factors (low risk <0.1 mg/dL [1.0 mg/L];

average risk 0.1-0.3 mg/dL [1.0-3.0 mg/L]; high risk >0.3 mg/dL [3.0 mg/L]). Recent studies suggest that patients with high hs-CRP levels have only a modestly increased risk for CAD events after adjusting for multiple other risk factors. The American Heart Association and Centers for Disease Control and Prevention do not recommend routine measurement of hs-CRP. It may help to guide primary preventive interventions in patients with an intermediate (10%-20%) risk of future CAD events based on the Framingham risk score. Measurement of hs-CRP has been found to reclassify up to 30% of intermediate-risk patients as either low- or high-risk.

In JUPITER, a primary prevention study, patients with hs-CRP greater than or equal to 0.2 mg/dL (2.0 mg/L) but LDL cholesterol below 130 mg/dL (3.4 mmol/L) and few other CAD risk factors (for example, diabetes was an exclusion criterion) were randomized to high-dose rosuvastatin therapy. The median age of the study population was 66 years. After less than 2 years, the results demonstrated a significant reduction in first cardiovascular events in the statin arm (hazard ratio for rosuvastatin, 0.56). However, because an elevated hs-CRP level was the main inclusion criterion, this study did not evaluate whether routine evaluation of hs-CRP level improved outcome.

Increased LDL cholesterol levels are an accepted risk factor for CAD, with an approximate 2% to 3% increase in risk for CAD events for every 1% increase in LDL cholesterol level. Working from the hypothesis that direct measurement of the total number of atherogenic particles may be superior to LDL cholesterol level alone for assessing risk, a study by Ingelsson and colleagues found that measurement of apolipoprotein B did not improve prediction of CAD compared with measurement of LDL cholesterol.

Retrospective studies have reported an association between smaller LDL particle size and risk of CAD, but the association is weaker after adjustment for other lipoprotein levels. Treatment with fibrates and niacin increases LDL particle size, whereas statins lower the number of LDL particles. Additional studies are required to determine whether LDL particle size determination consistently improves risk stratification and whether increasing particle size results in fewer CAD events.

Multiple randomized studies of antioxidant therapies, including vitamin E, vitamin C, and β-carotene, in patients after myocardial infarction or at high risk of cardiovascular disease, have found no benefit for lowering the risk of cardiovascular disease morbidity or mortality. Therefore, the use of these supplements for the prevention of cardiovascular disease is not recommended. Increased intake of omega-3 fatty acids, found in fish, has been found to be associated with lower risk of cardiovascular disease in observational cohorts (primary prevention), but the effect of supplemental intake is not well defined. Although fish or fish oil consumption is recommended as part of a "heart healthy" diet, the benefit of supplementation has not been clearly shown.

Cardiovascular Risk Reduction

The U.S. Preventive Services Task Force recommends that aspirin therapy be considered in men ages 45-79 years for primary prevention of cardiovascular disease if the benefits of therapy outweigh the risks of gastrointestinal bleeding. Other therapies to reduce risk include control of hypertension (see MKSAP 15 Nephrology) and treatment of hyperlipidemia (see MKSAP 15 General Internal Medicine).

Although treatment of cardiovascular risk factors has resulted in a substantial reduction in the death rate from CAD, lack of physical activity and increases in BMI on a population level have attenuated this benefit. Lifestyle factors such as smoking cessation, a healthy diet, regular exercise, and weight loss (to BMI <25) are important interventions for reducing the risk of CAD events. A recent study of more than 54,000 persons found that the presence of behavioral lifestyle risk factors contribute to the risk of acute coronary syndromes in an additive manner.

Cardiovascular Disease and Depression

The prevalence of depression is substantially increased in persons with cardiovascular disease, and the presence of depression is independently associated with worse outcomes. All CAD patients should be periodically screened for depression with a simple two-item screening test: *Over the past 2 weeks, have you been bothered by any of the following problems? (1) Little interest or pleasure in doing things; (2) Feeling down, depressed, or hopeless.* If the answer is "yes" to either question, the patient should be referred for more comprehensive clinical evaluation for depression. Selective serotonin reuptake inhibitors are safe and effective in patients with depression and

CAD; however, whether treatment of depression in CAD reduces cardiovascular events or mortality is unknown.

KEY POINTS

- Risk factors for developing coronary artery disease include older age, male sex, elevated blood pressure, high serum cholesterol, cigarette smoking, and diabetes mellitus.
- The Framingham risk score is useful to evaluate whether a patient is at low, intermediate, or high risk of a coronary artery disease event in a 10-year period (http://hp2010.nhlbihin.net/atpiii/calculator.asp?usertype=prof).
- The benefit of assessing conditional risk factors for coronary artery disease (CAD), such as high-sensitivity C-reactive protein level, LDL particle size, lipoprotein(a), and homocysteine level in risk evaluation, has not been determined, and these tests are not recommended for routine screening for determining CAD risk.

Chronic Stable Coronary Artery Disease

Diagnosis of Coronary Artery Disease

A variety of noninvasive stress tests are available to determine whether a patient with cardiovascular symptoms has CAD. The decision to order a specific stress test is based upon: (1) the pretest probability of CAD; (2) the ability of the patient to exercise; (3) findings on the resting electrocardiogram (ECG); and (4) the presence of comorbid conditions such as reactive airways disease (**Figure 2**). The pretest probability of CAD can be estimated using an approach that incorporates the patient's age, sex, and description of the chest pain (**Table 6**). For patients with a low pretest probability of CAD,

TABLE 6 Clinical Assessment of Pretest Probability of Coronary Artery Disease				
		Pretest Probability		
Age (years)	Sex	Typical Chest Pain[a]	Atypical Chest Pain[b]	Nonanginal Chest Pain[c]
30-39	Male	Intermediate	Intermediate	Low
	Female	Intermediate	Low	Low
40-49	Male	High	Intermediate	Intermediate
	Female	Intermediate	Low	Low
50-59	Male	High	Intermediate	Intermediate
	Female	Intermediate	Intermediate	Low
60-69	Male	High	Intermediate	Intermediate
	Female	High	Intermediate	Intermediate

[a]Typical chest pain has three components: (1) substernal chest pain or discomfort; (2) provoked by exertion or emotional stress; (3) relieved by rest and/or nitroglycerin.

[b]Atypical chest pain has two of the above three components for typical chest pain.

[c]Nonanginal chest pain has none of the above components for typical chest pain.

Data from Diamond GA, Forrester JS. Analysis of probability as an aid in the clinical diagnosis of coronary-artery disease. N Engl J Med. 1979;300(24):1350-1358. [PMID: 440357]

[handwritten notes: male >40 or female >60 c typical CP = High Risk (Pre-Test Prob); Low → ∅ stress; Inter → stress; High → Meds +/- stress ?cath]

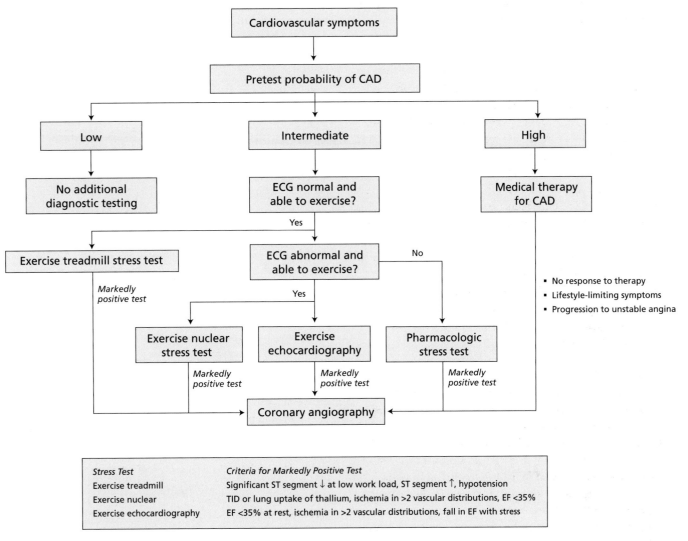

FIGURE 2.
Diagnosis of Coronary Artery Disease.

CAD = coronary artery disease; ECG = electrocardiogram; EF = ejection fraction; TID = transient ischemic dilation.

diagnostic stress testing is not useful; noninvasive stress testing provides the most useful information for patients with an intermediate pretest probability of CAD.

Exercise testing is preferred over pharmacologic stress testing. Absolute contraindications to exercise stress testing include recent myocardial infarction or unstable angina (within 48 hours), uncontrolled arrhythmias, symptomatic severe aortic stenosis, decompensated heart failure, acute pulmonary embolism, and acute aortic dissection. In addition, patients unable to exercise because of physical limitations such as arthritis, severe pulmonary disease, or physical deconditioning may undergo pharmacologic stress testing. Pharmacologic stress agents include dobutamine, dipyridamole, and adenosine (see Extensions of the Physical Examination). Patients with a markedly abnormal stress test (see Figure 2) have a higher incidence of multivessel and left main arterial disease, and should therefore be referred for coronary angiography.

Patients with a high pretest probability of CAD should begin empiric medical therapy. Stress testing in these patients may be useful to establish the effectiveness of current medical therapy, to obtain an objective measure of exercise capacity, and to evaluate the extent and severity of ischemia. Stress testing also has a role in selected patients to aid in preoperative risk assessment prior to noncardiac surgery.

Coronary angiography should be reserved for patients with chronic CAD who have lifestyle-limiting angina despite medical therapy, markedly positive results on noninvasive stress testing, successful resuscitation from sudden cardiac death, or documented ventricular tachycardia. Coronary angiography can also be considered in patients with nonspecific chest pain who have had recurrent hospitalizations, in order to completely exclude CAD as a cause for the current symptoms.

Coronary calcium testing may be considered in asymptomatic persons with a 10% to 20% Framingham 10-year risk category (moderately high risk) and in young persons with a strong family history of premature cardiovascular disease.

The diagnostic accuracy of CT angiography to detect obstructive CAD is approximately 90%; accuracy is reduced with distal lesions. Given that CT angiography provides no functional information (that is, the extent of ischemia), a markedly abnormal study should be followed by referral to coronary angiography or stress testing to determine the ischemic burden. Recent consensus guidelines suggest that the benefits of CT angiography are greatest in symptomatic patients with an intermediate pretest probability of CAD.

KEY POINTS

- Noninvasive stress testing is most useful in patients with an intermediate pretest probability of coronary artery disease as determined by the patient's age, sex, and description of the chest pain.
- Exercise electrocardiogram (ECG) is the preferred noninvasive test for patients who can exercise and have a normal resting ECG (that is, absence of left bundle branch block, <1 mm ST-segment depression, and no evidence of preexcitation).

Medical Treatment of Chronic Stable Coronary Artery Disease

Medical therapy remains the cornerstone of long-term treatment for patients with chronic stable angina regardless of whether coronary artery revascularization is performed (**Figure 3**). Medical therapy for chronic stable CAD can be classified as antianginal or vascular protective. Antianginal medications improve exercise duration until the onset of angina; reduce the severity and frequency of anginal episodes; and improve objective measures of ischemia, such as time to the onset of exercise-induced ST-segment depression. Vascular-protective medications may reduce the progression of atherosclerosis and may also potentially stabilize coronary plaques, thereby reducing plaque rupture and subsequent cardiovascular events.

Antianginal Medications

β-Blockers

β-Blockers are first-line therapy in patients with chronic stable angina. For patients with a history of myocardial infarction, even if they do not have angina or have undergone coronary artery revascularization, β-blockers reduce mortality by approximately 20%. Despite concerns about the use of cardioselective β-blockers in patients with reactive airways disease, peripheral vascular disease, and diabetes mellitus, these agents are well tolerated in most patients. Absolute contraindications to β-blockers include severe bradycardia, advanced atrioventricular block, decompensated heart failure, severe depression, and severe reactive airways disease. Potential side effects of β-blockers include impaired sexual function, reduced exercise capacity, bradycardia, and generalized fatigue.

Calcium Channel Blockers

For patients with absolute contraindications to β-blockers, a calcium channel blocker should be initiated as first-line therapy. Patients with chronic stable angina can be treated with calcium channel blockers if they are unable to tolerate β-blockers or if symptoms are inadequately controlled with β-blockers. Side effects of calcium channel blockers include peripheral edema, dizziness, headache, and constipation. Bradycardia and heart block can occur in patients with significant conduction system disease. In those with severe systolic dysfunction, calcium channel blockers can worsen or precipitate heart failure. Short-acting preparations of calcium channel blockers have been associated with an increased risk of myocardial infarction and perhaps mortality. Nondihydropyridine agents, such as verapamil and diltiazem, have a greater effect on myocardial contractility and conduction; dihydropyridine agents, such as nifedipine, amlodipine, felodipine, and isradipine, exert relatively more effect on vasodilation.

Nitrates

Chronic nitrate therapy must be administered in such a manner as to avoid nitrate tolerance, which is defined as the loss of the hemodynamic and antianginal effects that occurs during prolonged nitrate therapy. The only accepted method to prevent nitrate tolerance is to include a "nitrate-free" period, with nitrates not used for 8 to 12 hours once each day, typically during the overnight period. All patients with chronic stable angina should carry either sublingual or a spray form of nitroglycerin for emergency use. Contraindications to the routine use of nitroglycerin are severe symptomatic aortic stenosis and hypertrophic cardiomyopathy.

Phosphodiesterase type 5 (PDE-5) inhibitors used for erectile dysfunction (tadalafil, vardenafil HCl, sildenafil citrate) relax vascular smooth muscle cells and potentiate the hypotensive effects of nitrates. For patients using nitrates in any form, either on a daily basis or intermittently, PDE-5 inhibitors are therefore contraindicated.

Ranolazine

Ranolazine is a novel antianginal agent that causes selective inhibition of the late sodium channel and was recently approved for the treatment of chronic stable angina. In randomized studies of patients with continued angina despite optimal doses of conventional agents, ranolazine reduced both the frequency of angina and the use of nitroglycerin.

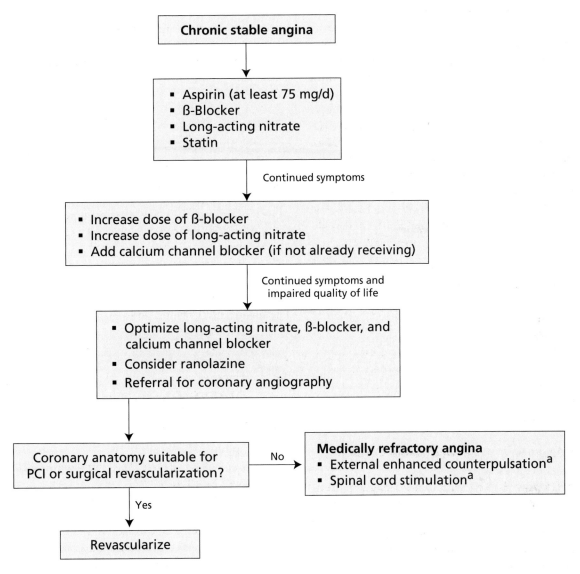

FIGURE 3.
Management of Chronic Stable Angina.

PCI = percutaneous coronary intervention.

[a]Not recommended by current guidelines.

Ranolazine should be considered in patients who remain symptomatic despite optimal doses of β-blockers, calcium channel blockers, and nitrates. Common side effects of ranolazine include dizziness, headache, constipation, and nausea. Ranolazine is metabolized in the liver by the cytochrome P-450 system and its use is therefore contraindicated in patients with hepatic impairment, those with baseline prolongation of the QT interval, and those taking other drugs that inhibit the cytochrome P-450 system. Diltiazem and verapamil increase serum levels of ranolazine, and combined use of ranolazine with either of these agents is contraindicated.

Vascular-Protective Medications

Aspirin

Meta-analyses of patients with chronic stable angina have shown that the use of aspirin reduces the risk of stroke, myocardial infarction, sudden death, and vascular death by 33%. In the chronic setting, the appropriate dose of aspirin for secondary prevention should be at least 75 mg/d.

Clopidogrel

Although clopidogrel is beneficial in patients with acute coronary syndromes, its role in the long-term management of patients with chronic stable angina is less clear. The

Clopidogrel versus Aspirin in Patients at Risk of Ischemic Events (CAPRIE) trial included a proportion of patients with chronic stable angina and found clopidogrel to be superior to aspirin alone in reducing the composite end point of stroke, myocardial infarction, or vascular death. However, the recently reported Clopidogrel for High Atherothrombotic Risk and Ischemic Stabilization, Management and Avoidance (CHARISMA) trial found only a possible benefit of clopidogrel in reducing myocardial infarction, stroke, and cardiovascular death in patients with chronic stable angina. Given that the clinical benefit was small and bleeding events were increased, the routine use of clopidogrel in patients with chronic stable angina remains controversial.

Angiotensin-Converting Enzyme Inhibitors

For patients with CAD and preserved left ventricular systolic function (normal ejection fraction), angiotensin-converting enzyme (ACE) inhibitors have been found to reduce cardiovascular mortality and all-cause mortality by 17% and 13%, respectively. The same meta-analysis found that nonfatal myocardial infarction and revascularization rates were reduced by 16% and 7%, respectively. These findings translate into the need to treat 100 patients for approximately 4 years to prevent one cardiovascular event (death, nonfatal myocardial infarction, or coronary revascularization procedure). For patients with reduced left ventricular systolic function, ACE inhibitors provide a more substantial benefit and reduce death or myocardial infarction and all-cause mortality by 23% and 20%, respectively. To avoid one death, 15 patients would need to be treated for approximately 2.5 years.

Contraindications to ACE inhibitors include pregnancy, a history of angioedema or anuric renal failure during previous exposure to an ACE inhibitor, and severe hypotension. A baseline serum creatinine level above 2.5 mg/dL (191 µmol/L) should be considered a relative contraindication to use of an ACE inhibitor. A nonproductive cough is the most common side effect of an ACE inhibitor and occasionally requires substituting an angiotensin receptor blocker.

Statins

In patients with established CAD, statins reduce future cardiovascular events, including myocardial infarction and death, by approximately 25% to 30%. The benefits of statins are proportional to the level of LDL cholesterol reduction. Current guidelines specify an LDL cholesterol target level of less than 100 mg/dL (2.6 mmol/L) for patients with CAD or CAD-equivalent disease, with an optional goal of less than 70 mg/dL (1.8 mmol/L) for patients at very high risk.

Statins are generally well tolerated but require monitoring of liver enzyme levels at the initiation of therapy and with any change in dose. A moderate elevation in liver enzyme values (>3 times the normal level) occurs in approximately 3% of patients treated with high-dose statins (for example, atorvastatin, 80 mg/d). Decisions regarding stopping a statin and switching to another agent are based on expert opinion and clinical circumstances. Serious side effects, such as myositis and rhabdomyolysis, are extremely rare.

KEY POINTS

- β-Blockers are first-line therapy for patients with chronic stable angina as well as those with a history of myocardial infarction.
- Patients with chronic stable coronary artery disease and without contraindications should take aspirin.
- Patients with reduced left ventricular ejection fraction (<35%) should be treated with an angiotensin-converting enzyme inhibitor.
- Statins should be given to most patients with established coronary artery disease.

Coronary Revascularization

Percutaneous Coronary Intervention

Although percutaneous coronary intervention (PCI) reduces both the frequency and severity of angina and improves overall quality of life in patients with chronic stable CAD, it does not reduce future cardiovascular events nor does it improve survival. The Clinical Outcomes Utilizing Revascularization and Aggressive Drug Evaluation (COURAGE) trial found that PCI combined with aggressive medical therapy was not superior to aggressive medical therapy alone. PCI should, therefore, be reserved for patients who remain symptomatic despite optimal medical therapy. One exception to this approach may be in patients with significant silent ischemia diagnosed by noninvasive stress testing. The Swiss Interventional Study on Silent Ischemia Type II (SWISS II) randomized patients with a recent myocardial infarction or silent myocardial ischemia on stress imaging and one- or two-vessel CAD by coronary angiography to receive either medical therapy or PCI. Although the PCI group received balloon angioplasty only (no coronary stents), there was a significant reduction in long-term major cardiac events (10-year follow-up) and an improvement in left ventricular function compared with those who received medical therapy.

Coronary Artery Bypass Grafting

Surgical revascularization is indicated for patients with left main CAD and multivessel disease (two- or three-vessel) with involvement of the left anterior descending coronary artery and reduced systolic function (**Table 7**). Patients with diabetes who have multivessel CAD have a mortality benefit from surgery compared with PCI when they receive a left internal mammary artery bypass graft.

In about 10% of patients, traditional coronary artery bypass surgery with median sternotomy and use of a cardiopulmonary bypass machine results in excessive pain, prolonged hospital stay, or postoperative neurologic dysfunction. For patients with significant comorbid conditions, off-pump and minimally invasive surgery may reduce operative risk and improve

TABLE 7 Class I Indications for CABG in Patients with Stable Angina[a]

CABG is recommended in patients who have:
Significant left main coronary artery stenosis
Left main coronary artery equivalent disease: ≥70% stenosis of proximal LAD and proximal left circumflex artery
Three-vessel disease
Two-vessel disease with significant proximal LAD stenosis and either ejection fraction <50% or demonstrable ischemia on noninvasive testing
CABG is beneficial in patients who have:
One- or two-vessel disease without significant proximal LAD stenosis but with a large area of viable myocardium and high-risk criteria on noninvasive testing
Developed disabling angina despite maximal noninvasive therapy, when surgery can be performed with acceptable risk (if angina is not typical, objective evidence of ischemia should be obtained)

CABG = coronary artery bypass grafting; LAD = left anterior descending coronary artery.

[a]Class I indications: Conditions for which there is evidence and/or general agreement that a given procedure or treatment is beneficial, useful, and effective.

Recommendations from Eagle KA, Guyton RA, Davidoff R, et al. ACC/AHA 2004 guideline update for coronary artery bypass graft surgery: a report of the American College of Cardiology/American Heart Association Task Force on Practice Guidelines (Committee to Update the 1999 Guidelines for Coronary Artery Bypass Graft Surgery) [published errata appears in Circulation. 2005;111(15):2014.]. Circulation. 2004;110(15):e340-437. [PMID: 15466654]

recovery times. Hybrid coronary revascularization refers to the combination of minimally invasive surgery and PCI and attempts to further reduce operative risk by taking advantage of both surgical and interventional techniques.

KEY POINTS

- Percutaneous coronary intervention reduces the frequency and severity of angina but not future cardiovascular events; it should be reserved for patients with continued symptoms despite optimal medical therapy.

- Surgical revascularization is indicated for left main coronary artery disease and multivessel coronary artery disease with involvement of the left anterior descending coronary artery and reduced ejection fraction.

Medically Refractory Angina

A small proportion of patients with chronic stable angina have progressive angina despite optimal doses of antianginal and vascular-protective medications and after achieving complete percutaneous or surgical revascularization. Several alternative therapies have been proposed for medically refractory angina, although none are recommended by current guidelines. External enhanced counterpulsation uses three sets of pneumatic cuffs wrapped around the lower extremities to achieve a hemodynamic effect similar to an intra-aortic balloon pump. Typically, patients undergo this therapy daily for a period of 4 to 6 weeks. The treatment is associated with an improvement in angina and exercise capacity that can persist for up to 2 years. The mechanism for this improvement is unknown. External enhanced counterpulsation does not decrease mortality.

Stimulation of the spinal cord region that receives the cardiac nerve fibers was shown in a placebo-controlled trial to reduce angina and improve functional status.

KEY POINT

- Patients with medically refractory angina may benefit from external enhanced counterpulsation or spinal cord stimulation.

Follow-Up Care

Routine stress testing for asymptomatic patients with known CAD or following successful PCI is not advocated by current practice guidelines. Routine, periodic resting ECGs should not be performed in the absence of changes in medications, symptoms, or physical examination findings.

Restenosis following successful PCI, which usually presents as recurrent angina approximately 6 to 9 months after the index procedure, has been dramatically reduced with the use of drug-eluting stents. Clopidogrel should be continued without interruption for a minimum of 1 year following placement of a drug-eluting stent and for a minimum of 1 month with a bare metal stent. Consideration for extended use of clopidogrel (beyond 1 year) should be individualized and take into account the overall risk profile (extent and severity of CAD) and underlying bleeding risk. Aspirin should be continued at 325 mg/d during clopidogrel therapy unless bleeding events occur. The risk of stent thrombosis is approximately 0.7% and is increased with the premature discontinuation of dual antiplatelet therapy (aspirin and clopidogrel). Stent thrombosis is associated with a short-term mortality rate of 40%.

Elective noncardiac surgery should be delayed for at least 6 weeks following placement of a bare metal stent and for at least 1 year following a drug-eluting stent to allow for completion of the patient's dual antiplatelet regimen. For emergency or urgent surgery that cannot be delayed in order to complete the required dual antiplatelet course of therapy, a guideline of the American College of Cardiology and the American Heart Association (ACC/AHA) has suggested continuing aspirin during the perioperative period, if at all possible, and restarting clopidogrel as soon as possible following the procedure.

KEY POINTS

- Clopidogrel should be continued for a minimum of 1 year following drug-eluting stent placement and for a minimum of 1 month following bare metal stent placement.

- The risk of coronary stent thrombosis is approximately 0.7% and is increased with the premature discontinuation of dual antiplatelet therapy (aspirin and clopidogrel).

- Patients who must undergo noncardiac surgery that cannot be delayed to allow completion of dual antiplatelet therapy should continue aspirin during the perioperative period and restart clopidogrel as soon as possible following the procedure.

Acute Coronary Syndromes

Clinical Presentation and Classification

Acute coronary syndrome (ACS) refers to a spectrum of diseases ranging from unstable angina, to non–ST-elevation myocardial infarction (NSTEMI), to ST-elevation myocardial infarction (STEMI). Patients who present with presumed ischemic chest pain can initially be classified based on the ECG and the results of assays for the serum biomarkers troponin and creatine kinase (**Figure 4**).

Although the initial ECG is nondiagnostic in up to 50% of patients presenting with chest pain, it is a critical part of the evaluation. A simplified approach to initiating therapy is based on making the distinction early between STEMI and NSTEMI or unstable angina. Patients with a STEMI benefit from reperfusion therapy—either thrombolytic therapy or primary angioplasty. Patients with a NSTEMI or unstable angina require risk stratification to determine their risk for death or nonfatal myocardial infarction prior to initiating therapy (**Figure 5**). Patients with unstable angina may have similar ECG findings to those with a NSTEMI, but can be differentiated by the absence of elevated serum biomarkers.

The pain of an acute myocardial infarction is usually retrosternal in location, may radiate to the shoulders or arms, and may be associated with nausea and vomiting (more commonly associated with an inferior STEMI), diaphoresis, or shortness of breath. Elderly patients and those with diabetes mellitus may present with atypical symptoms such as shortness of breath in the absence of pain, heart failure, or confusion. Myocardial ischemia is associated with the classic symptoms of severe retrosternal chest pressure in only about 25% of patients. Twenty-five percent of patients have chest discomfort that mimics heartburn pain, and another 25% have ischemia that is clinically silent. The remaining 25% complain of stabbing or sharp chest pain; chest pain reproducible by palpation; or jaw, neck, back, and left arm discomfort. Women, persons with diabetes, and the elderly more commonly have atypical chest pain or shortness of breath rather than ischemic-type chest pain.

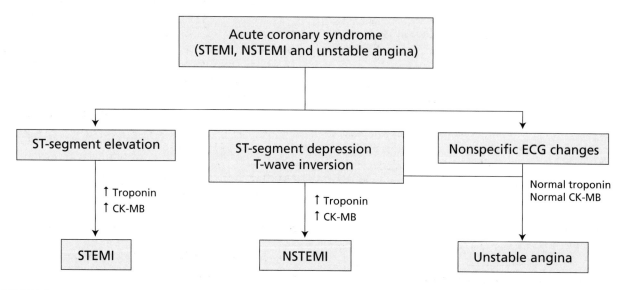

FIGURE 4.
Diagnosis of Acute Coronary Syndromes.

CK-MB = creatine kinase MB; NSTEMI = non–ST-elevation myocardial infarction; STEMI = ST-elevation myocardial infarction.

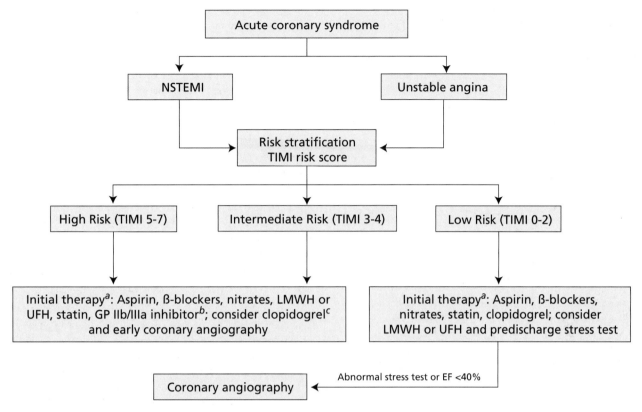

FIGURE 5.
Initial Management of Unstable Angina/Non–ST-Elevation Myocardial Infarction.

EF = ejection fraction; GP = glycoprotein; LMWH = low-molecular-weight heparin; NSTEMI = non–ST-elevation myocardial infarction; UFH = unfractionated heparin.

[a]For patients with continued symptoms despite initial medical therapy, consider GP IIb/IIIa inhibitor and emergent coronary angiography.

[b]Indications for GP IIb/IIIa inhibitor include ongoing chest pain, dynamic electrocardiographic changes, elevated troponin on presentation, heart failure, and diabetes mellitus.

[c]Clopidogrel can be given prior to coronary angiography. If coronary artery bypass grafting is required, clopidogrel should be stopped and surgery delayed for at least 5 days.

The physical examination should focus on conditions that can mimic a STEMI such as aortic dissection and pericarditis, potential contraindications to thrombolytic therapy, and conditions, such as heart failure, that influence prognosis and treatment decisions.

Initial Medical Treatment of Acute Coronary Syndromes

Unless there are compelling contraindications, all patients presenting with ischemic chest pain and a presumed ACS should be treated with aspirin (162 to 325 mg/d), β-blockers, and nitrates (see Figure 5). Patients should chew the aspirin tablet in order to quickly achieve therapeutic blood levels.

β-Blockers should be given to all patients except those with decompensated heart failure, systolic blood pressure below 90 mm Hg, bradycardia with a heart rate below 50/min, or second-degree atrioventricular block. For patients with unstable angina or NSTEMI, oral β-blockers are typically used. Intravenous β-blockers can be considered, but caution should be used in patients with heart failure, hypotension, or hemodynamic instability. Calcium channel blockers, with the exception of nifedipine, can be used in patients with contraindications to β-blockers and in those with continued angina despite optimal doses of β-blockers and nitrates. For STEMI patients, intravenous β-blockers are commonly given. β-Blockers should not be used in patients with STEMI precipitated by cocaine use because of the risk of potentiating coronary artery spasm. Sublingual nitroglycerin should be given to all patients except those with an inferior STEMI and presumed right ventricular infarction. Following sublingual nitroglycerin and in the absence of hypotension, intravenous nitroglycerin should be initiated for patients with continued chest pain. Transdermal or oral nitrates should be used for unstable angina and NSTEMI patients with recent episodes of chest pain but no active symptoms at presentation.

Non–ST-Elevation Myocardial Infarction and Unstable Angina

Risk Stratification

The short-term (14-day) risk for death and nonfatal myocardial infarction in patients presenting with unstable angina and

NSTEMI can be estimated using the Thrombolysis in Myocardial Infarction (TIMI) risk score (**Table 8**). A TIMI risk score of 0 to 2 is associated with an 8% rate of recurrent myocardial infarction or death, compared with an event rate of approximately 31% associated with a risk score of 6 to 7. The TIMI risk score also identifies which patients will derive the greatest benefit from aggressive medical therapy with glycoprotein IIb/IIIa inhibitors and an early invasive treatment approach.

Invasive versus Conservative Management

Following initiation of medical therapy, management options for patients presenting with unstable angina or NSTEMI include either a conservative approach, with continued medical therapy and noninvasive stress testing prior to hospital discharge, or an early invasive approach, with coronary angiography and subsequent revascularization (PCI or surgical revascularization). Several large randomized trials have largely favored an early invasive approach. These trials have used aggressive anticoagulation and antiplatelet therapy (low-molecular-weight heparin, glycoprotein IIb/IIIa inhibitors, and clopidogrel) not available previously as well as use of coronary stents, including drug-eluting stents, and adjustment of anticoagulation during PCI. Based on these results, a conservative approach may be considered for stable patients with a TIMI risk score of 0 to 2, whereas those with TIMI risk scores of 3 or more would benefit from an early invasive approach.

Medical Therapy

After the initiation of standard antianginal therapy (aspirin, β-blockers, nitrates, and possibly calcium channel blockers), patients should be classified as low, intermediate, or high risk using the TIMI risk score and additional therapy initiated based upon patient risk.

Antiplatelet Medications

For patients who subsequently go on to an invasive strategy and undergo placement of a coronary stent, aspirin should be increased to 325 mg/d and continued for at least 1 month for a bare metal stent, with a 1-year course if tolerated, and for at least 1 year following placement of a drug-eluting stent. In patients who are unable to tolerate aspirin, clopidogrel should be initiated on hospital presentation.

Clopidogrel should be added to background aspirin therapy in all patients regardless of their TIMI risk score unless there is an elevated risk of bleeding, such as recent gastrointestinal bleeding or newly diagnosed anemia. Patients with coronary stents should receive dual antiplatelet therapy (see Chronic Stable Coronary Artery Disease). For patients undergoing coronary angiography who are found to have multivessel CAD requiring surgical revascularization, clopidogrel must be stopped and surgery delayed for 5 days to avoid excessive postoperative bleeding. Aspirin should be continued. If coronary artery bypass surgery is deemed to be urgent or emergent, it may be necessary to perform surgery without allowing for a full 5-day clopidogrel cessation period. In patients with a low TIMI risk score who receive a conservative treatment approach, clopidogrel should be continued for at least 1 year.

Glycoprotein IIb/IIIa inhibitors act by occupying platelet receptors that would otherwise bind with fibrinogen. This blocking of fibrinogen binding serves to prevent platelet aggregation. The glycoprotein IIb/IIIa inhibitors that are currently approved for patients with unstable angina or NSTEMI are tirofiban, eptifibatide, and abciximab. The main adverse effect of these agents is increased bleeding events, which usually occur at the site of vascular access (in patients undergoing coronary angiography) or at mucocutaneous locations (for example, gingival bleeding).

Patients with an intermediate or high TIMI risk score derive the most benefit from glycoprotein IIb/IIIa inhibitors, along with patients who are managed with an early invasive approach and undergo PCI. Glycoprotein IIb/IIIa inhibitors may also be considered in patients who have ongoing symptoms after the initiation of standard medical therapy and those with dynamic ECG changes, diabetes mellitus, or heart failure. The benefit for glycoprotein IIb/IIIa inhibitors in patients who receive conservative medical therapy is less clear, and most physicians would only choose these agents in the setting of an intermediate or high TIMI risk score in a patient with a low risk of bleeding who is not deemed to be a candidate for early angiography because of a comorbid condition (such as malignancy) or patient preference.

TABLE 8 TIMI Risk Score for Unstable Angina/Non–ST-Elevation Myocardial Infarction
Prognostic Variables
Age ≥65 years
≥3 traditional CAD risk factors[a]
Documented CAD with ≥50% diameter stenosis
ST-segment deviation
≥2 anginal episodes in the past 24 hours
Aspirin use in the past week
Elevated cardiac biomarkers (creatine kinase MB or troponin)
TIMI Risk Score (Sum of Prognostic Variables)
0–2 Low risk
3–4 Intermediate risk
5–7 High risk

CAD = coronary artery disease.

[a]Family history of CAD, hypertension, hypercholesterolemia, diabetes, being a current smoker.

Adapted from Antman EM, Cohen M, Bernink PJ, et al. The TIMI risk score for unstable angina/non-ST elevation MI: a method for prognostication and therapeutic decision making. JAMA. 2000;284(7):835-842. [PMID: 10938172]

Anticoagulant Medications

Anticoagulants used for the treatment of unstable angina and NSTEMI include unfractionated heparin, low-molecular-weight heparin, and, more recently, the direct thrombin inhibitor bivalirudin. The decision to use a particular agent is based upon the TIMI risk score, whether a patient undergoes an early invasive or conservative treatment approach, and consideration of the bleeding risk. Unfractionated or low-molecular-weight heparin can be considered in low-risk patients but provides more benefit to those in the intermediate- and high-risk TIMI groups (see Figure 5).

Unfractionated heparin was the initial anticoagulant used in the treatment of unstable angina and NSTEMI and reduces early ischemic events by approximately 50%. Uninterrupted therapy should be continued for at least 2 days with an activated partial thromboplastin time (aPTT) goal of between 60 and 80 seconds. Disadvantages of unfractionated heparin include difficulty achieving stable therapeutic levels, the need for frequent laboratory monitoring, and the potential for heparin-induced thrombocytopenia. These factors have led to the use of newer anticoagulants such as low-molecular-weight heparin. For certain patients, however, including those being considered for an early invasive approach, those with an increased bleeding risk, and those with renal insufficiency, unfractionated heparin may be preferable to low-molecular-weight heparin because of its reversibility, shorter half-life, and ease of use in the catheterization laboratory.

Low-molecular-weight heparin has been compared with unfractionated heparin in several trials, including ESSENCE and TIMI 11B. Both of these trials showed a reduction in cardiovascular events (death, myocardial infarction, and recurrent angina) with low-molecular-weight heparin without an increase in bleeding events. Advantages of low-molecular-weight heparin include twice daily subcutaneous administration and achievement of predictable levels of anticoagulation without the need for laboratory monitoring.

Bivalirudin is a synthetic direct thrombin inhibitor that has been adopted for use in patients undergoing elective PCI, but its role in patients with unstable angina or NSTEMI who undergo an early invasive approach remains unclear.

Lipid-Lowering Medications

The MIRACL and PROVE IT trials found that high-dose statin therapy initiated soon after an ACS reduced cardiovascular events at 18 months and 2 years, respectively. Current consensus in patients with unstable angina or NSTEMI favors early treatment with high-dose statins to achieve a target LDL cholesterol level of less than 100 mg/dL (2.6 mmol/L), with less than 70 mg/dL (1.8 mmol/L) considered a reasonable optional goal.

KEY POINTS

- All unstable angina/non–ST-elevation myocardial infarction patients without contraindications should be treated initially with aspirin, β-blockers, and nitrates.
- Unstable angina or non–ST-elevation myocardial infarction patients with TIMI risk scores of 3 or more generally benefit from an early invasive approach.
- All unstable angina/non–ST-elevation myocardial infarction patients without contraindications should be given antiplatelet therapy with aspirin and clopidogrel.
- Unstable angina/non–ST-elevation myocardial infarction patients should receive early treatment with high-dose statins to achieve a target LDL cholesterol of less than 100 mg/dL (2.6 mmol/L) (optional goal <70 mg/dL [1.8 mmol/L]).

ST-Elevation Myocardial Infarction

Recognition of ST-Elevation Myocardial Infarction

Optimal management of patients with STEMI relies heavily upon timely recognition and rapid initiation of reperfusion therapy, either thrombolytic therapy or PCI. The differential diagnosis of a patient with a presumed STEMI includes pericarditis, pulmonary embolism, and aortic dissection. An acute type A aortic dissection will occasionally present as an inferior wall STEMI if the dissection plane extends into the origin of the right coronary artery. High risk STEMI subgroups include those presenting with a new or presumed new left bundle branch block, anterior wall myocardial infarction, cardiogenic shock, heart failure, ventricular arrhythmias, and elderly age (>75 years).

Reperfusion Therapy

The two initial reperfusion strategies for patients with a STEMI are thrombolytic therapy and primary PCI (**Figure 6**). The decision to use one strategy over the other is based on time from onset of symptoms, the presence of high-risk features, any contraindications (absolute or relative) to thrombolytic therapy (**Table 9**), and the anticipated time to achieve balloon inflation with PCI.

For patients with absolute contraindications to thrombolytic therapy, PCI should be performed. In the setting of relative contraindications to thrombolytic therapy and in the absence of significant delays, most physicians would advocate the use of primary PCI. Elderly patients represent a unique high-risk subgroup with an increased risk for bleeding complications with thrombolytic therapy, and care must be individualized.

The time to achieve balloon inflation is a major determinant of the benefits of PCI over thrombolytic therapy. Current guidelines recommend a door-to-balloon time of 90

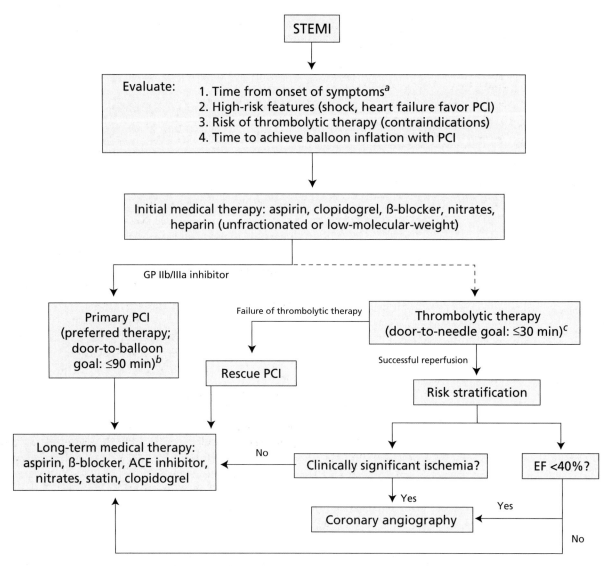

FIGURE 6.
Management of ST-Elevation Myocardial Infarction.

ACE = angiotensin-converting enzyme; EF = ejection fraction; GP = glycoprotein; PCI = percutaneous coronary intervention; STEMI = ST-elevation myocardial infarction.

[a]If 3 or more hours have elapsed since symptom onset, PCI is preferred.

[b]STEMI patients presenting to a hospital with PCI capability should be treated with primary PCI within 90 minutes of first medical contact ("door-to-balloon time") as a systems goal.

[c]STEMI patients presenting to a hospital without PCI capability and who cannot be transferred to a PCI center and undergo PCI within 90 minutes of first medical contact should be treated with thrombolytic therapy within 30 minutes of hospital presentation ("door-to-needle time") as a systems goal unless thrombolytic therapy is contraindicated.

minutes or less. If inherent delays in performing PCI are present, thrombolytic therapy should be considered. Randomized trials indicate a benefit of transfer for primary PCI compared with onsite thrombolytic therapy, despite transfer delays in some studies exceeding 1 hour. However, observational data from community hospitals within the United States document that fewer than 4% of patients achieve the guideline-suggested door-to-balloon time of less than 120 minutes. Recent position papers advocate the development of "STEMI receiving centers" with comprehensive and efficient protocols to minimize transfer delays and improve access to primary PCI.

Approximately 70% of STEMI patients in the United States present to hospitals without onsite PCI capabilities, and thrombolytic therapy is therefore the predominant method of reperfusion used. Characteristics of three commonly used thrombolytic agents are shown in **Table 10**.

In the presence of high-risk features such as cardiogenic shock or heart failure, or if a diagnosis of STEMI is in doubt, onsite PCI or transfer to a PCI facility is preferred over

TABLE 9 Contraindications to Thrombolytic Therapy for ST-Elevation Myocardial Infarction

Absolute Contraindications

Any prior intracerebral hemorrhage

Known cerebrovascular lesion (e.g., arteriovenous malformation)

Ischemic stroke within 3 months

Suspected aortic dissection

Active bleeding or bleeding diathesis (excluding menses)

Significant closed head or facial trauma within 3 months

Relative Contraindications

History of chronic, severe, poorly controlled hypertension

Severe uncontrolled hypertension on presentation (SBP >180 mm Hg or DBP >110 mm Hg)[a]

History of prior ischemic stroke >3 months, dementia, or known intracranial pathology

Traumatic or prolonged (>10 minutes) CPR or major surgery (<3 weeks)

Recent (within 2-4 weeks) internal bleeding

Noncompressible vascular puncture site

For streptokinase/anistreplase: prior exposure (>5 days) or prior allergic reaction to these agents

Pregnancy

Active peptic ulcer disease

Current use of anticoagulants: the higher the INR, the higher the bleeding risk

CPR = cardiopulmonary resuscitation; DBP = diastolic blood pressure; SBP = systolic blood pressure.

[a]Thrombolytic therapy can be considered if SBP can be reduced to <140 mm Hg and DBP to <90 mm Hg with initial medical therapy.

thrombolytic therapy. For patients with cardiogenic shock who present to facilities without onsite PCI, thrombolytic therapy, placement of an intra-aortic balloon pump and emergent transfer to a PCI facility may be superior to direct transfer for PCI.

Rescue PCI refers to PCI that occurs in the setting of failed thrombolytic therapy and provides a benefit over conservative medical therapy or the repeat administration of thrombolytics.

Initial Medical Therapy

In addition to prompt reperfusion, initial medical therapy for STEMI includes aspirin, analgesics, nitrates, and oxygen; therapy to reduce infarct size; antithrombotic agents; and antiplatelet therapy. Control of chest pain with analgesics such as morphine sulfate suppresses the heightened sympathetic response that occurs during a STEMI. Nitrates reduce preload by increasing venous capacitance and improve coronary blood flow by coronary vasodilation. Although it is common practice to give supplemental oxygen to all patients, the main benefit is seen in those with arterial hypoxemia.

Therapy to Reduce Infarct Size

Intravenous β-blockers should be given to all patients without contraindications. Metoprolol is commonly given as three consecutive 5-mg intravenous bolus doses, each dose given over 3 to 5 minutes. If systolic blood pressure remains above 90 mm Hg, metoprolol, 25 mg or 50 mg orally every 6 hours, should be given. For patients with relative contraindications to β-blockers, such as reactive airways disease, a short-acting intravenous agent such as esmolol can be considered.

TABLE 10 Thrombolytic Agents Commonly Used in the Treatment of ST-Elevation Myocardial Infarction

Thrombolytic Agent	Alteplase	Reteplase	Tenecteplase
Dose	Up to 100 mg in 90 min[a]	10 U × 2 (30 min apart); each 2-min duration	30-50 mg[a]
Bolus administration	No	Yes	Yes
Allergic reaction on repeat exposure possible	No	No	No
TIMI flow grade 2/3[b]	~75%	~83%	~83%
Rate of intracerebral hemorrhage	~0.4%-0.7%	~0.8%	~0.9%
Fibrin specificity	+++	+	++++
Need for unfractionated or low-molecular-weight heparin	Yes	Yes	Yes

[a]Based on body weight.

[b]*TIMI flow grade 2/3* refers to mildly impaired flow through the coronary artery involved in the myocardial infarction. The higher the percentage of TIMI 2/3 flow, the more effective the thrombolytic agent.

Adapted from Boden WE, Eagle K, Granger CB. Reperfusion strategies in acute ST-segment elevation myocardial infarction: a comprehensive review of contemporary management options. J Am Coll Cardiol. 2007;50(10):917-929. [PMID: 17765117] Copyright 2007 American College of Cardiology Foundation, with permission from Elsevier.

ACE inhibitors are beneficial in patients with reduced left ventricular function and no heart failure as well as those with clinical evidence of heart failure following a myocardial infarction. These agents inhibit postinfarction remodeling, allowing subsequent preservation of ventricular function. Early initiation (within 24 hours) of an ACE inhibitor in patients with a systolic blood pressure above 100 mm Hg and in the absence of clinically significant renal failure provides the most benefit. For patients intolerant of an ACE inhibitor or in those with contraindications (bilateral renal artery stenosis), an angiotensin receptor blocker can be considered.

Antithrombotic Therapy

For patients receiving thrombolytic therapy with fibrin-specific agents such as reteplase and tenecteplase, unfractionated heparin is thought to prevent reocclusion of the infarct-related artery. More recently, low-molecular-weight heparin has been used in combination with thrombolytic agents and appears to yield improved outcomes compared with unfractionated heparin. For patients undergoing primary PCI, unfractionated heparin is preferable to low-molecular-weight heparin because of the ease to which the degree of anticoagulation can be assessed with the activated clotting time during PCI.

Antiplatelet Therapy

Recent trials have found that clopidogrel added to standard medical and thrombolytic therapy further reduces cardiovascular events without a significant increase in bleeding. For patients undergoing primary PCI, clopidogrel should be given on hospital presentation because the majority of patients will subsequently receive a coronary stent during PCI, and there appears to be a benefit of pretreatment.

Glycoprotein IIb/IIIa inhibitors are beneficial in patients undergoing primary PCI, and early administration in the emergency department improves coronary patency.

Early Complications

The main adverse effect of thrombolytic therapy during the early management period (within several hours of hospital presentation) is bleeding complications. Intracerebral hemorrhage occurs in less than 1% of patients but is associated with a mortality rate of 50% to 65%. Risk factors for intracerebral hemorrhage include older age, lower body weight, female sex, previous stroke, and systolic blood pressure above 160 mm Hg on presentation. Streptokinase has the lowest rate of intracerebral hemorrhage among the available thrombolytic agents. Additional bleeding complications include bruising at venipuncture sites, hematuria, and gastrointestinal bleeding. For life-threatening bleeding events, blood transfusions, cryoprecipitate, and fresh frozen plasma may be required.

Despite significant advances in the treatment of STEMI patients, the diagnosis of thrombolytic therapy failure remains difficult. Resolution of chest pain, improvement in ST-segment elevation, and the presence of reperfusion arrhythmias (most commonly idioventricular rhythms) indicate successful thrombolysis. Complete ST-segment elevation resolution is associated with coronary patency; however, complete resolution occurs in only a minority of patients. Improvement in ST-segment elevation greater than 50% on an ECG obtained 60 minutes after the administration of thrombolytic therapy is the most commonly used criterion to indicate successful reperfusion. Continued chest pain, lack of improvement in ST-segment elevation, hemodynamic instability, or the presence of ventricular arrhythmias most likely indicates failure of thrombolytic therapy. Accelerated idioventricular rhythms are the most common reperfusion arrhythmia.

In the setting of an inferior STEMI with successful reperfusion, sinus bradycardia and hypotension may occur. Other arrhythmias that may indicate successful reperfusion are accelerated idioventricular rhythm and nonsustained ventricular tachycardia.

With increased myocardial injury (larger infarct size), the likelihood of left ventricular dysfunction and heart failure increases. The severity of left ventricular dysfunction is directly related to mortality. Heart failure after myocardial infarction is managed using standard medical therapy (see Heart Failure). For patients with progressive symptoms despite aggressive medical care, invasive hemodynamic monitoring with a pulmonary artery catheter may be useful.

Late Complications

Complications that may occur in the first several days include cardiogenic shock, ventricular septal defect, papillary muscle rupture with secondary severe mitral regurgitation, free wall rupture, and left ventricular thrombus. The in-hospital mortality rate for cardiogenic shock approaches 50%, with half of the deaths occurring in the first 48 hours of hospitalization. The loss of myocardial contractility that occurs with a large myocardial infarction was previously thought to be the fundamental basis for cardiogenic shock. However, recent studies indicate that a systemic inflammatory process may also be involved. Therapy for cardiogenic shock includes early revascularization with PCI or coronary artery bypass surgery in an attempt to limit the degree of myocardial damage. Inotropic agents including dopamine and dobutamine, vasopressor agents at moderate to high doses, mechanical ventilation, and an intra-aortic balloon pump are often required.

Right ventricular infarction should be considered in the setting of an inferior wall infarction complicated by hypotension. Occlusion of the right coronary artery proximal to the origin of the acute marginal vessels results in ischemia to the right ventricle. Right ventricular ischemia impairs the systolic function of the right ventricle, causing limited filling to the left ventricle, which results in the clinical triad of hypotension, clear lung fields, and jugular venous distention.

The diagnosis can be made with a right-sided ECG that shows ST-segment elevation in leads V_3R and V_4R. Echocardiography can confirm the diagnosis with findings of hypokinesis and dilation of the right ventricle. Echocardiography can help exclude other causes of cardiogenic shock, such as ischemic mitral regurgitation or a ventricular septal defect.

Treatment of right ventricular infarction includes early revascularization (PCI or thrombolytic therapy) to restore blood flow to the ischemic right ventricle, aggressive volume loading to increase filling to the left ventricle, and inotropic support with dopamine or dobutamine if hypotension persists after achieving a pulmonary capillary wedge pressure of greater than 18 mm Hg. Even with successful revascularization, it can take up to 3 days for right ventricular function to return to normal.

A ventricular septal defect typically occurs within a thin and akinetic segment of the ventricular septum and presents as hemodynamic compromise with a new systolic murmur. A thrill along the left sternal border may also be present. Echocardiography is the most reliable and rapid tool for establishing the diagnosis. Treatment includes stabilization with an intra-aortic balloon pump and vasopressor agents prior to urgent surgical repair. The surgical mortality rate is extremely high (>50%), but the mortality rate with medical therapy alone approaches 95%. Percutaneous devices for the repair of a ventricular septal defect have been reported in recent years and may be a useful option for nonsurgical candidates.

Mechanisms of mitral regurgitation following a myocardial infarction include severe left ventricular dysfunction with annular dilation, worsening of pre-existing mitral regurgitation, and rupture of a papillary muscle or chordae tendineae. Papillary muscle rupture presents with acute pulmonary edema, a loud systolic murmur in the absence of a thrill, and rapid progression to cardiogenic shock. Echocardiography should be used to establish the diagnosis and can accurately differentiate between a ruptured papillary muscle and a ventricular septal defect. Treatment includes stabilization with an intra-aortic balloon pump, afterload reduction with sodium nitroprusside, diuretics, and urgent surgical intervention.

Rupture of the left ventricular free wall presents as hemopericardium with electromechanical dissociation and death. Risk factors include elderly age, female sex, first myocardial infarction, and anterior location of the infarction. Mortality is uniformly high, but salvage is possible with early recognition and emergent pericardiocentesis.

Left ventricular thrombus may occur following a STEMI because of impaired contractility of a myocardial segment resulting in blood stasis, endocardial tissue injury, and a possible hypercoagulable state. Prior to the era of early revascularization with PCI and thrombolytic therapy, a left ventricular thrombus was present in up to 60% of patients with a large anterior STEMI. Despite these advances, however, the risk for development of a left ventricular thrombus following an anterior STEMI remains 10% to 20%. The most common location for a thrombus is in the apex of the left ventricle. The diagnosis is made by the echocardiographic finding of an echodense structure within the left ventricle adjacent to an area of the myocardium with impaired contractility. Anticoagulation with warfarin for 3 to 6 months should be initiated once the diagnosis is made to reduce the risk of systemic arterial embolization.

Long-Term Medical Therapy

Aspirin should be continued indefinitely. In patients without coronary stents, the dose should be reduced to 75 mg/d after approximately 1 month. Clopidogrel should be continued for at least 1 year for patients who receive thrombolytic therapy in the absence of bleeding events. Patients with coronary stents should receive dual antiplatelet therapy (see Chronic Stable Coronary Artery Disease). β-Blockers should be continued indefinitely in patients without contraindications. ACE inhibitors should be continued indefinitely and can be changed to an angiotensin receptor blocker in those who are intolerant. Statins should be used to achieve a serum LDL cholesterol level below 100 mg/dL (2.6 mmol/L), with an optional goal of below 70 mg/dL (1.8 mmol/L), and should be continued indefinitely.

Risk Stratification

Patients undergoing primary PCI are essentially risk stratified by the coronary angiogram—that is, the coronary anatomy is defined and treatment is based upon the extent and severity of disease. In contrast, patients who receive thrombolytic therapy with successful reperfusion require risk stratification prior to hospital discharge. The purpose of risk stratification is to identify high-risk patients (left main or three-vessel disease) that may benefit from revascularization. Left ventricular function should be assessed by either echocardiography or nuclear imaging, and those with an ejection fraction below 40% should be referred for coronary angiography to identify patients who would benefit from revascularization. Episodes of chest pain during the index hospitalization, clinically significant heart failure, and ventricular arrhythmias also indicate the need for coronary angiography.

In all other patients, a functional evaluation is required prior to hospital discharge with either a symptom-limited exercise ECG, exercise nuclear perfusion testing or exercise echocardiography, or a pharmacologic stress test for those unable to exercise. Clinically significant ischemia on noninvasive testing mandates referral for coronary angiography. In the absence of clinically significant ischemia, medical therapy can be continued.

- ST-elevation myocardial infarction patients presenting to a hospital with percutaneous coronary intervention (PCI) capability should be treated with primary PCI within 90 minutes of first medical contact; those presenting to a hospital without PCI capability and who cannot be transferred to a PCI center and undergo PCI within 90 minutes should be treated with fibrinolytic therapy.

- Initial medical therapy for ST-elevation myocardial infarction includes general treatment measures (aspirin, analgesics, nitrates, and oxygen), therapy to reduce infarct size (β-blockers and angiotensin-converting enzyme inhibitors), antithrombotic therapy (unfractionated or low-molecular-weight heparin), and antiplatelet therapy (clopidogrel and glycoprotein IIb/IIIa inhibitors).

- Clopidogrel should be added to standard medical and thrombolytic therapy, as it further reduces cardiovascular events without a significant increase in bleeding.

- Early complications after ST-elevation myocardial infarction include failure of thrombolytic therapy.

Coronary Artery Disease in Women

Presentation and Evaluation

CAD in women is a leading cause of mortality and disability, and important differences exist in symptoms, diagnostic test characteristics, and outcome compared with men. The diagnosis of CAD in women occurs, on average, approximately 10 years later than in men, possibly related to later onset of disease and/or delayed presentation and diagnostic testing.

As a result of the older age at diagnosis, women with unstable angina or NSTEMI are more likely to have comorbid conditions such as hypertension, diabetes mellitus, and heart failure with preserved left ventricular systolic function compared with men. Women have a higher frequency of angina/chest pain than men but have a lower prevalence of obstructive CAD compared with men with similar symptoms. In the Coronary Artery Surgery Study, CAD was diagnosed by catheterization in 63% of women with definite angina, 40% of women with probable angina, and 4% of women with nonischemic pain. Other potential causes of chest pain in women include an increased prevalence of vasospasm and noncoronary chest pain syndromes. In addition, women with CAD are more likely to have atypical symptoms or angina equivalents, including dyspnea, palpitations, and presyncope.

Owing to the higher frequency of chest pain and atypical symptoms in women, as well as the lower prevalence of obstructive CAD, results of noninvasive diagnostic testing have lower specificity compared with men. ECG treadmill exercise testing in women has a false-positive rate of 38% to

67%, compared with 7% to 44% in men. The false-negative rate is low, however, and ECG exercise testing remains a reliable diagnostic test. Approximately 70% of women will have the diagnosis of CAD confirmed or excluded on the basis of this test, with the remainder referred for additional testing. Therefore, although some experts have proposed the routine use of imaging with stress testing in women to improve specificity, current guidelines recommend similar diagnostic approaches among women and men with suspected CAD.

Women have a poorer prognosis than men after myocardial infarction. In addition to the older age of presentation for women who experience a myocardial infarction, a higher prevalence of comorbid conditions, including hypertension and diabetes mellitus, negatively impacts survival. Women also have a delayed presentation and time to treatment after symptom onset and have more hemodynamic instability and cardiogenic shock compared with men.

Medical Treatment

Women have the same benefit as men from pharmacologic treatment with aspirin, clopidogrel, anticoagulants, β-blockers, ACE inhibitors, and statins, but are prescribed aspirin and anticoagulants less frequently than men. Women with myocardial infarction have a higher rate of complications associated with anticoagulation therapies. Women with STEMI treated with fibrinolytic agents are 2 to 3 times more likely to experience hemorrhagic stroke than men, and female sex has been found to be independently associated with intracranial hemorrhage after adjustment for other differences. In NSTEMI, women have a higher rate of major bleeding complications compared with men, particularly with the use of glycoprotein IIb/IIIa inhibitors. Excessive dosing of antiplatelet and antithrombotic agents accounts for a significant percentage of this increased bleeding risk, and factors such as female sex and characteristics more prevalent in women with myocardial infarction (such as reduced creatinine clearance, advanced age, and diabetes) are independently associated with excessive dosing of these medications. It is important, therefore, that the dosing of these medications in women be based on the estimated glomerular filtration rate and patient weight.

Oral hormone replacement therapy with estrogen alone or a combination of estrogen and progesterone has been evaluated in multiple randomized, placebo-controlled clinical trials in postmenopausal women with and without a history of CAD. These studies have uniformly shown no relative risk reduction in all-cause mortality, nonfatal acute myocardial infarction, or death due to CAD, regardless of age (younger versus older than 65 years) in women taking these agents. In addition, adverse events of venous thromboembolism and stroke were higher in women treated with hormone replacement therapy.

Women who are taking hormone replacement therapy when an acute coronary syndrome occurs generally should not continue taking these medications. Women who have taken these agents for more than 1 to 2 years and who wish to continue taking hormone replacement therapy for a compelling condition should understand the relative benefits and risks, including an increased risk of cardiovascular events and stroke. These medications should not be used for primary or secondary prevention of cardiac events.

Invasive Treatment

PCI in the setting of an acute STEMI has been shown to have a lower risk of intracranial hemorrhage compared with fibrinolytic therapy. In women with acute coronary syndromes with high-risk features, including elevated cardiac enzymes, an early invasive strategy reduces major adverse cardiac events. For women with low-risk features, however, there may be an early excess risk associated with an early invasive approach. Recent single center experience has found that women and men had similar short- and long-term survival after PCI. Long-term results of revascularization, including both PCI and coronary artery bypass grafting, are comparable for women and men.

KEY POINTS

- Treadmill exercise electrocardiographic testing has a higher false-positive rate in women than men but remains the first-line noninvasive test for women with suspected coronary artery disease because of the low false-negative rate.
- Women with myocardial infarction treated with fibrinolytic, antiplatelet, and/or antithrombotic therapies have a higher rate of bleeding complications compared with men, and appropriate dosing of these medications should be based on patient weight and estimated glomerular filtration rate.
- An early invasive strategy in women with unstable angina or non–ST-elevation myocardial infarction and high-risk features reduces major adverse cardiac events, but this approach in women with low risk features may be associated with an early excess risk.

Coronary Artery Disease in Patients with Diabetes Mellitus

Prevention of Cardiovascular Complications

Persons with diabetes mellitus have a 2- to 8-times increased prevalence of, incidence of, and mortality from cardiovascular diseases. Achieving treatment goals for patients with diabetes results in reduction of cardiovascular risk. These goals include optimized glycemic control, control of hypertension and hyperlipidemia, and daily aspirin for those older than 40 years or with additional cardiovascular risk factors. A large randomized trial of clopidogrel found no additional benefit over aspirin alone for the primary prevention of cardiovascular events, even among patients with diabetes or multiple CAD risk factors.

Diagnosis of Coronary Artery Disease in Patients with Diabetes

Patients with diabetes and CAD often have atypical or blunted CAD symptoms. This attenuation of symptoms is thought to result from autonomic neuropathy (damaged afferent sympathetic fibers), a common complication of diabetes. Thus, typical angina occurs less frequently, whereas atypical symptoms of myocardial ischemia, including dyspnea, nausea, vomiting, unexplained fatigue, diaphoresis, and fluctuations in plasma glucose level, may predominate. Moreover, silent ischemia, characterized by the absence of angina despite an abnormal ECG, noninvasive study, or coronary angiography, occurs more frequently in patients with diabetes versus those without diabetes.

In patients with diabetes who experience angina, exercise ECG testing has similar diagnostic sensitivity (approximately 50%) and specificity (approximately 80%) as for nondiabetic patients. In addition to the prognostic value of the magnitude of ST-segment depression during exercise testing, exercise capacity and heart rate recovery offer significant prognostic information.

The addition of myocardial imaging increases the sensitivity and diagnostic accuracy above that of exercise ECG testing alone. Stress nuclear testing, the most extensively studied stress imaging modality in diabetic patients, has a sensitivity of approximately 88% and specificity of approximately 74% for the detection of CAD confirmed angiographically. In addition, the number of ischemic (fixed) segments seen on myocardial imaging is directly correlated with worse cardiovascular outcomes. Similarly, stress echocardiography has a higher diagnostic accuracy for CAD in diabetic patients in comparison to exercise ECG testing alone, and the assessment of left ventricular function at rest and exercise-induced wall motion abnormalities has significant prognostic implications. Either of these imaging modalities may be useful in patients with diabetes and suspected CAD who have an abnormal baseline ECG or inability to exercise.

Although patients with diabetes are more likely to have silent ischemia, which has important prognostic implications, outcome data to support routine stress testing in asymptomatic diabetic patients do not exist. Noninvasive testing for asymptomatic CAD, therefore, is currently not recommended for patients with diabetes. Likewise, before initiating an exercise program, routine screening for asymptomatic CAD is not recommended.

Pharmacologic Treatment and Secondary Prevention

Recommendations for pharmacologic therapy for acute treatment and secondary prevention of cardiovascular events in patients with diabetes and stable angina or acute coronary syndromes are the same as recommendations for nondiabetic patients. Although β-blockers are prescribed in a much lower percentage of diabetic patients after myocardial infarction compared with those without diabetes, randomized, controlled trials have shown that the magnitude of mortality reduction with β-blockers among those with diabetes is substantially greater than that among those without. Similarly, aspirin therapy should be used for secondary prevention. In patients who are intolerant or have contraindications to aspirin, other antiplatelet agents may be reasonable alternatives. Lipid-lowering therapy with a statin reduces the risk of cardiovascular events and mortality in persons with diabetes regardless of the presence of known heart disease. Intensive glycemic control is recommended in the setting of acute coronary syndromes, with goal plasma glucose measurements below 150 mg/dL (8.33 mmol/L) in the initial days of hospitalization, and subsequent preprandial glucose levels below 110 mg/dL (6.11 mmol/L) during hospitalization.

Invasive Approaches in Patients with Diabetes

The invasive evaluation of CAD in patients with diabetes should be performed with an understanding of the angiographic features in these patients. Diabetic patients typically have more severe coronary artery disease, more extensive coronary calcifications, a higher prevalence of left main CAD, and impaired collateral artery recruitment. In addition, diabetic patients have reduced arterial dimensions; for any given amount of plaque deposition in the arterial wall, therefore, the diabetic patient develops a greater degree of luminal obstruction.

Invasive management of CAD in diabetic patients should be guided by evidence of ischemia and by risk stratification. In patients with stable angina, the recent COURAGE trial included more than 2200 diabetic patients with stable angina randomized to either an initial invasive approach of PCI or medical therapy, with the primary endpoints of death from any cause or nonfatal myocardial infarction. Although the event rate in both arms was higher for patients with diabetes than for those without, there was no difference in event rates between the treatment arms at 3 years' follow-up, although there was substantial cross-over from initial medical therapy to revascularization. Therefore, medical therapy for patients with diabetes and stable angina is a safe initial approach before proceeding to PCI for refractory symptoms.

In diabetic patients with acute coronary syndromes, patients at higher risk of a poor outcome (that is, biomarker positive) benefit from a routine invasive treatment strategy. In diabetic patients with single-vessel CAD and inducible ischemia, PCI is a reasonable treatment option. In those with multivessel disease, coronary artery bypass grafting with an internal mammary graft may be beneficial compared with PCI.

> **KEY POINTS**
>
> - In patients with diabetes who experience angina, exercise electrocardiographic testing has similar diagnostic sensitivity and specificity as for nondiabetic patients.
>
> - Although patients with diabetes mellitus are more likely to have coronary artery disease without symptoms (silent ischemia), outcome data do not support routine stress testing in asymptomatic patients.

Bibliography

Alexander KP, Chen AY, Newby LK, et al. Sex differences in major bleeding with glycoprotein IIb/IIIa inhibitors: results from the CRUSADE (Can Rapid risk stratification of Unstable angina patients Suppress ADverse outcomes with Early implementation of the ACC/AHA guidelines) initiative. Circulation. 2006;114(13):1380-1387. [PMID: 16982940]

Al-Mallah MH, Tleyjeh IM, Abdel-Latif AA, Weaver WD. Angiotensin-converting enzyme inhibitors in coronary artery disease and preserved left ventricular systolic function: a systematic review and meta-analysis of randomized controlled trials. J Am Coll Cardiol. 2006; 47(8):1576-1583. [PMID: 16630993]

American Diabetes Association. Standards of medical care in diabetes—2008. Diabetes Care. 2008;31 Suppl 1:S12-54. [PMID: 18165335]

Anderson JL, Adams CD, Antman EM, et al. ACC/AHA 2007 guidelines for the management of patients with unstable angina/non ST-elevation myocardial infarction: a report of the American College of Cardiology/American Heart Association Task Force on Practice Guidelines (Writing Committee to Revise the 2002 Guidelines for the Management of Patients With Unstable Angina/Non ST-Elevation Myocardial Infarction): developed in collaboration with the American College of Emergency Physicians, the Society for Cardiovascular Angiography and Interventions, and the Society of Thoracic Surgeons: endorsed by the American Association of Cardiovascular and Pulmonary Rehabilitation and the Society for Academic Emergency Medicine. Circulation. 2007;116(7):e148-304. [PMID: 17679616]

Antman EM, Hand M, Armstrong PW, et al. 2007 Focused update of the ACC/AHA 2004 guidelines for the management of patients with ST-elevation myocardial infarction: a report of the American College of Cardiology/American Heart Association Task Force on Practice Guidelines: developed in collaboration with the Canadian Cardiovascular Society endorsed by the American Academy of Family Physicians. Circulation. 2008;117(2):296-329 [erratum in: Circulation. 2008 Feb 12;117(6):e162.]. [PMID: 18071078]

Bhatt DL, Fox KA, Hacke W, et al; CHARISMA Investigators. Clopidogrel and aspirin versus aspirin alone for the prevention of atherothrombotic events. N Engl J Med. 2006;354(16):1706-1717. [PMID: 16531616]

Bluemke DA, Achenbach S, Budoff M, et al. Noninvasive coronary artery imaging: magnetic resonance angiography and multidetector computed tomography angiography: a scientific statement from the American Heart Association committee on cardiovascular imaging and intervention of the council on cardiovascular radiology and intervention, and the councils on clinical cardiology and cardiovascular disease in the young. Circulation. 2008;118(5):586-606. [PMID: 18586979]

Boden WE, O'Rourke RA, Teo KK, et al; COURAGE Trial Research Group. Optimal medical therapy with or without PCI for stable coronary disease. N Engl J Med. 2007;356(15):1503-1516. [PMID: 17387127]

Bravata DM, Gienger AL, McDonald KM, et al. Systematic review: the comparative effectiveness of percutaneous coronary interventions and coronary artery bypass graft surgery. Ann Intern Med. 2007; 147(10):703-716. [PMID: 17938385]

Erne P, Schoenenberger AW, Burckhardt D, et al. Effects of percutaneous coronary interventions in silent ischemia after myocardial infarction: the SWISSI II randomized controlled trial. JAMA. 2007;297(18):1985-1991. [PMID: 17488963]

Fraker TD Jr, Fihn SD, Gibbons RJ, et al. 2007 chronic angina focused update of the ACC/AHA 2002 guidelines for the management of patients with chronic stable angina: a report of the American College of Cardiology/American Heart Association Task Force on Practice Guidelines Writing Group to Develop the Focused Update of the 2002 guidelines for the management of patients with chronic stable angina [erratum in Circulation. 2007;116(23):e558.]. Circulation. 2007;116(23):2762-2772. [PMID: 17998462]

Grines CL, Bonow RO, Casey DE Jr, et al. Prevention of premature discontinuation of dual antiplatelet therapy in patients with coronary artery stents: a science advisory from the American Heart Association, American College of Cardiology, Society for Cardiovascular Angiography and Interventions, American College of Surgeons, and American Dental Association, with representation from the American College of Physicians. Circulation. 2007;115(6): 813-818. [PMID 17224480]

Ingelsson E, Schaefer EJ, Contois JH, et al. Clinical utility of different lipid measures for prediction of coronary heart disease in men and women. JAMA. 2007;298(7):776-785. [PMID: 17699011]

Jacobs AK. Regional systems of care for patients with ST-elevation myocardial infarction: being at the right place at the right time. Circulation. 2007;116(7):689-692. [PMID: 17679610]

Jensen MK, Chiuve SE, Rimm EB, et al. Obesity, behavioral lifestyle factors, and risk of acute coronary events. Circulation. 2008;117(24): 3062-3069. [PMID: 18541738]

Lichtman JH Bigger JT Jr, Blumenthal JA, et al. Depression and coronary heart disease: recommendations for screening, referral, and treatment: a science advisory from the American Heart Association Prevention Committee of the Council on Cardiovascular Nursing, Council on Clinical Cardiology, Council on Epidemiology and Prevention, and Interdisciplinary Council on Quality of Care and Outcomes Research: endorsed by the American Psychiatric Association. Circulation. 2008;118(17):1768-1776. [PMID: 18824640]

Mosca L, Banka CL, Benjamin EJ, et al. Evidence-based guidelines for cardiovascular disease prevention in women: 2007 update. Circulation. 2007;115(11):1481-1501. [PMID: 17309915]

Ridker PM, Danielson E, Fonseca FA, et al; JUPITER Study Group. Rosuvastatin to prevent vascular events in men and women with elevated C-reactive protein. N Engl J Med. 2008;359(21):2195-2207. [PMID: 18997196]

Sarnak MJ, Levey AS, Schoolwerth AC, et al. Kidney disease as a risk factor for development of cardiovascular disease: a statement from the American Heart Association Councils on Kidney in Cardiovascular Disease, High Blood Pressure Research, Clinical Cardiology, and Epidemiology and Prevention. Circulation. 2003;108(17):2154-2169. [PMID: 14581387]

Weiner DE, Tighiouart H, Elsayed EF, et al. The Framingham predictive instrument in chronic kidney disease. J Am Coll Cardiol. 2007;50(3):217-224. [PMID: 17631213]

Heart Failure

Diagnosis and Evaluation of Heart Failure

Clinical Evaluation

The initial evaluation of a patient with suspected heart failure should focus on possible causes of heart failure, assessing current clinical status, and identifying any comorbidities that may exacerbate the heart failure. Determining the cause of heart failure may lead to treatment of potentially reversible causes such as ischemia or certain metabolic or toxic causes. Among patients presenting to the emergency department with dyspnea, several signs and symptoms influence the likelihood of heart failure. Features that increase the likelihood of heart failure include the presence of paroxysmal nocturnal dyspnea (greater than 2-fold likelihood) and the presence of an S_3 (11 times greater likelihood). The likelihood of heart failure is halved by the absence of dyspnea on exertion and by the absence of crackles on pulmonary auscultation. However,

patients frequently do not present with classic, easily identifiable physical examination findings, especially if heart failure has been present chronically or has developed gradually. Also, inter- and intra-observer variability and clinical experience affect the reliability of physical examination findings; for example, the overall accuracy of assessing central venous pressure by determining jugular venous pressure is only slightly above 50%.

Diagnostic Testing

Because symptoms and physical examination findings have limited accuracy for the diagnosis of heart failure, additional diagnostic testing is needed to assess the cause and severity of disease.

Echocardiography

Echocardiography is an essential part of the initial evaluation of heart failure and should be performed in all patients with newly diagnosed or suspected heart failure. Echocardiography can help identify specific causes of heart failure, including hypertensive heart disease, ischemic disease, hypertrophic or infiltrative cardiomyopathy or primary valvular heart disease.

Echocardiography is necessary for distinguishing systolic heart failure from heart failure with preserved systolic function. Heart failure with preserved systolic function is generally diagnosed when signs and symptoms of systolic heart failure are present, but an echocardiogram reveals a normal left ventricular ejection fraction and the absence of significant valvular or pericardial abnormalities that would account for heart failure signs and symptoms. As many as 50% of patients with symptoms of heart failure have heart failure with preserved systolic function, although the estimated prevalence varies widely because of heterogeneous diagnostic criteria. Doppler techniques can assist in assessing more subtle measures of diastolic function and estimated hemodynamics.

Electrocardiography

The electrocardiogram (ECG) provides evidence for prior myocardial infarction (suggesting an ischemic cause of heart failure), atrial enlargement or ventricular hypertrophy, arrhythmia, and conduction abnormalities. In addition, the ECG may be used in decision making regarding cardiac resynchronization therapy.

Laboratory Evaluation

Routine laboratory studies obtained during initial evaluation of the patient with heart failure should include assessment of electrolytes, renal and hepatic function, blood counts, and, if clinically indicated, assessment for specific causes of heart failure, such as thyroid abnormalities or hemochromatosis (see Specific Cardiomyopathies, below).

B-type natriuretic peptide (BNP) may be helpful for differentiating heart failure from noncardiac causes of shortness of breath in the acute setting. Patients presenting to the emergency department with acute dyspnea and a serum BNP concentration below 100 pg/mL are unlikely to have acute heart failure. In the Breathing Not Properly study, a BNP cutoff of 100 pg/mL alone had a sensitivity of 90% and specificity of 73% to diagnose heart failure in the emergency department, and improved accuracy of diagnosis compared with clinical judgment alone.

BNP levels may be helpful in nonacute settings if additional evidence is needed to support a clinical assessment of volume status; however, caution should be used in interpreting BNP levels outside of the acute setting. In stable outpatients with chronic heart failure, BNP levels can vary considerably. Patients with chronic heart failure may have very low BNP levels, even below 100 pg/mL. In patients with severe heart failure, BNP may correlate poorly with invasive measurements of volume status. BNP cannot be used to differentiate between systolic heart failure and heart failure with preserved systolic function because, when decompensated, both conditions have increased ventricular wall stress, which triggers the release of BNP. In addition, causes of increased wall stress other than heart failure, such as acute myocardial infarction and pulmonary embolism, can also raise BNP levels. Factors other than ventricular wall stress that influence BNP levels include renal failure, older age, and female sex, all of which increase BNP; and obesity, which reduces BNP. Interpretation of BNP results should take these factors into account.

Evaluation for Ischemia

Ischemia is a significant cause of ventricular dysfunction, either as a primary cause or an exacerbating factor. In appropriate patients, revascularization can result in major benefits, including improved ventricular function, reduced symptoms, and increased survival. Evaluation for the presence of ischemia is, therefore, a necessary part of almost all initial evaluations of new-onset or worsening heart failure unless the clinical evidence strongly suggests a cause other than ischemia.

The American College of Cardiology/American Heart Association (ACC/AHA) heart failure guidelines recommend coronary angiography for those patients with new-onset heart failure who have angina or significant ischemia and are potential candidates for revascularization. There is conflicting evidence regarding appropriateness of coronary angiography for other subgroups of patients with new-onset heart failure. Of note, these recommendations for evaluation of ischemia (with coronary angiography or noninvasive testing) are applicable only to those patients who do not have contraindications to coronary revascularization. In general, the weight of evidence and expert opinion favor performing coronary angiography for patients who have chest pain and unknown coronary anatomy and for patients who have known or suspected coronary artery disease. For patients with known coronary disease who present with heart failure, noninvasive imaging to assess for myocardial ischemia and viability is also reasonable.

Other Diagnostic Testing

Other testing may be considered if standard clinical data are ambiguous with regard to current disease status or when advanced therapies such as cardiac transplantation are being considered. If volume status is not clear based on physical examination or laboratory evaluation, evaluation of the inferior vena cava by hand-held ultrasonography may be a useful adjunct to improve accuracy in assessing right atrial (and thus central venous) pressure. Assessment of central venous pressure in this manner should be performed with awareness of factors other than volume overload that may raise central venous pressure, such as lung hyperinflation associated with chronic obstructive pulmonary disease or cardiac tamponade. In critically ill cardiac patients for whom additional hemodynamic information is needed for management, right heart catheterization is useful for clarifying volume status as well as cardiac output if either or both factors are unclear based on usual clinical data alone; for example, in the setting of low blood pressure, elevated serum creatinine level, and symptoms of shock, in which empiric diuresis would be limited by blood pressure and renal function. Cardiopulmonary exercise testing is helpful in differentiating cardiac from noncardiac causes of exercise intolerance and also provides an objective assessment of functional capacity. Cardiopulmonary exercise testing is an essential part of the evaluation for cardiac transplantation, as functional capacity is strongly correlated with prognosis in heart failure.

Endomyocardial biopsy is rarely diagnostic owing to the heterogeneous disease involvement of the myocardium. Biopsy is indicated in patients with unexplained new-onset heart failure and cardiogenic shock. In addition, biopsy is recommended in patients with new-onset heart failure (2 weeks' to 3 months' duration) associated with dilation of the left ventricle and new ventricular arrhythmias, second- or third-degree atrioventricular heart block, or failure to respond to usual care within 1 to 2 weeks. Biopsy may be considered if there is a reasonable clinical suspicion of a specific cause of cardiomyopathy that may be revealed on biopsy, if evaluation prior to biopsy has been nondiagnostic, and if establishing a specific diagnosis would impact management. In heart transplant recipients, endomyocardial biopsies are performed for routine surveillance for rejection because most patients with rejection are asymptomatic.

Nuclear medicine studies, such as a radionuclide ventriculogram, can provide information on ventricular size and systolic function; however, a radionuclide ventriculogram is not recommended for the initial evaluation of heart failure because it provides only an ejection fraction with no additional significant information on cardiac structure. Cardiac MRI can be useful in diagnosing inflammatory or infiltrative cardiomyopathies such as sarcoidosis or arrhythmogenic right ventricular dysplasia. (See Extensions of the Physical Examination for specific indications for these tests.)

If clinically indicated, evaluation for sleep apnea may be helpful in uncovering a cause or exacerbating factor of heart failure.

- Echocardiography is an essential part of the initial evaluation of heart failure.
- Patients presenting to the emergency department with acute dyspnea and a B-type natriuretic peptide concentration below 100 pg/mL are unlikely to have acute heart failure.
- B-type natriuretic peptide is not a reliable measure of severity of chronic heart failure.
- Evaluation for ischemia should be part of the initial evaluation for most patients with new-onset or worsening heart failure.

Therapeutic Options for Heart Failure

Classification systems have been developed for the purposes of grading disease severity, guiding management, and estimating prognosis. The most commonly used currently are the New York Heart Association (NYHA) functional classification and the system developed by the American College of Cardiology and the American Heart Association (ACC/AHA) (**Table 11**). The primary difference between these two classification systems is that the NYHA classification is based on symptoms, whereas the ACC/AHA classification is based on the presence of or potential to develop structural heart disease. Although the NYHA classification system is ultimately subjective in nature, it has consistently proved to have prognostic value in heart failure.

Initiation of therapy in patients with newly diagnosed heart failure can be prioritized based on the patient's NYHA functional class and volume status (**Table 12**). Specific medications and doses from the drug classes discussed below are shown in **Table 13**.

Initiation and Titration of Medical Therapy

Angiotensin-Converting Enzyme Inhibitors and Angiotensin Receptor Blockers

Angiotensin-converting enzyme (ACE) inhibitors are indicated for treatment of any and all NYHA functional class systolic heart failure, including asymptomatic (NYHA class I) patients. ACE inhibitors reduce mortality and morbidity in asymptomatic and symptomatic patients and delay the onset of clinical heart failure in patients with asymptomatic left ventricular dysfunction. Overall, ACE inhibitor therapy reduces mortality by about 20%, risk for myocardial infarction by about 20%, and hospitalization for heart failure by 30% to 40%. ACE inhibitors increase concentrations of bradykinin, which, in addition to beneficial cardiovascular effects, causes a side effect of cough in some patients.

Angiotensin receptor blockers (ARBs) also reduce mortality and morbidity in patients with systolic heart failure. The primary reason to use an ARB instead of an ACE inhibitor is to avoid the side effect of cough. In general, there is a lower incidence of hyperkalemia and no significant difference with regard to the incidence of renal insufficiency with ARB treatment. Angioedema is a very rare but potentially

TABLE 11 Clinical Stages of Chronic Heart Failure		
ACC/AHA Stage	**NYHA Functional Class**	**Estimated 1-Year Mortality**
A At risk; no structural disease or symptoms	—	*See note*
B Structural disease but no symptoms	**I** Asymptomatic	5%–10%
C Structural disease with prior or current symptoms	**II** Symptomatic; slight limitation of physical activity	15%–30%
	III[a] Symptomatic; marked limitation of physical activity	15%–30%
D Refractory disease	**III**[a] Symptomatic; marked limitation of physical activity	15%–30%
	IV Inability to perform any physical activity without symptoms	50%–60%

ACC/AHA = American College of Cardiology/American Heart Association; NYHA = New York Heart Association.

[a]NYHA class III overlaps with ACC/AHA stages C and D.

Note: Mortality in Stage A is that associated with any existing comorbid conditions.

Adapted with permission from Givertz MM, Colucci WS, Braunwald E. Clinical Aspects of Heart Failure; Pulmonary Edema, High-Output Failure. In: Zipes DP, Libby P, Bonow RO, Braunwald E, eds. Heart disease: a textbook of cardiovascular medicine. 7th ed. Philadelphia, PA: WB Saunders; 2005:552. Copyright 2005, Elsevier.

TABLE 12 Medical Therapy for Systolic Heart Failure by Functional Status

Initial Therapy

All NYHA classes (I-IV):

ACE inhibitor (if ACE inhibitor is not tolerated because of cough, an ARB can be used; if ACE inhibitor is contraindicated because of hyperkalemia or renal insufficiency, hydralazine/isosorbide dinitrate can be used)

β-Blocker

Additional Therapy

NYHA class I-II (asymptomatic or mild symptoms):

Diuretic as needed to maintain euvolemia

NYHA class III-IV (moderate to severe symptoms):

Spironolactone (if bothersome side effect of gynecomastia occurs, eplerenone can be used)

For black patients, hydralazine/isosorbide dinitrate

Digoxin

Diuretic as needed to maintain euvolemia

ACE = angiotensin-converting enzyme; ARB = angiotensin receptor blocker; NYHA = New York Heart Association.

TABLE 13 Oral Medications Commonly Used for Treatment of Heart Failure

Drug	Initial Dose	Maximum Dose
ACE inhibitors		
Captopril	6.25 mg TID	50 mg TID
Enalapril	2.5 mg BID	10-20 mg BID
Fosinopril	5-10 mg once daily	40 mg once daily
Lisinopril	2.5-5.0 mg once daily	20-40 mg once daily
Quinapril	5 mg BID	20 mg BID
Ramipril	1.25-2.5 mg once daily	10 mg once daily
Trandolapril	1 mg once daily	4 mg once daily
ARBs		
Candesartan	4-8 mg once daily	32 mg once daily
Losartan[a]	25-50 mg once daily (may divide dose to twice daily)	50-100 mg once daily
Valsartan	20-40 mg BID	160 mg BID
β-Blockers		
Bisoprolol[a]	1.25 mg once daily	10 mg once daily[b]
Carvedilol	3.125 mg BID	25 mg BID; 50 mg BID for >85 kg[b]
Metoprolol succinate	12.5-25.0 mg daily	200 mg once daily[b]
Loop diuretics[c]		
Bumetanide	0.5-1.0 mg once or twice daily	Up to 10 mg daily[d]
Furosemide	20-40 mg once or twice daily	Up to 600 mg daily[d]
Torsemide	10-20 mg once daily	Up to 200 mg daily[d]
Digitalis		
Digoxin	0.125-0.250 mg once daily	0.125-0.250 mg once daily
Aldosterone antagonists		
Spironolactone	12.5 to 25.0 mg once daily	50 mg once daily
Eplerenone	25 mg once daily	50 mg once daily

ACE = angiotensin-converting enzyme; ARB = angiotensin receptor blocker; BID = twice daily; TID = three times daily.

[a]Off-label use.

[b]Target dose.

[c]Thiazide diuretics are not listed but may be appropriate for patients with mild heart failure or associated hypertension or as a second diuretic in patients refractory to loop diuretics alone.

[d]Titrate to achieve dry weight.

Information from Hunt SA, Abraham WT, Chin MH, et al. ACC/AHA 2005 Guideline Update for the Diagnosis and Management of Chronic Heart Failure in the Adult: a report of the American College of Cardiology/American Heart Association Task Force on Practice Guidelines (Writing Committee to Update the 2001 Guidelines for the Evaluation and Management of Heart Failure): developed in collaboration with the American College of Chest Physicians and the International Society for Heart and Lung Transplantation: endorsed by the Heart Rhythm Society. Circulation. 2005;112(12):e154-e235. [PMID: 16160202] life-threatening side effect of ACE inhibitor therapy, and patients who experience angioedema should avoid both ACE inhibitors and ARBs. Combined treatment with an ACE inhibitor and ARB is generally not recommended, as concurrent therapy is significantly associated with increased risk of medication nonadherence and adverse effects, including worsening renal function and symptomatic hypotension, whereas the additional benefit of using these two medications together is not well established. ACE inhibitors are currently preferred over ARBs for most patients because there is more clinical experience with these agents.

Initiation of vasodilators such as ACE inhibitors, ARBs, or hydralazine should be avoided in the setting of hypovolemia because the risk of hypotension is increased if the patient is not volume replete. If contraindications such as renal failure or hyperkalemia are present, hydralazine/isosorbide dinitrate combination is a suitable alternative to an ACE inhibitor or ARB.

The relative benefit of high- versus low-dose ACE inhibitors is minor; there may be fewer hospitalizations with higher dosages, but no survival benefit has been demonstrated. Follow-up blood work after initiation of an ACE inhibitor should include serum potassium and creatinine levels within 1 or 2 weeks after starting. Abrupt withdrawal of an ACE inhibitor should be avoided because it can result in rapid clinical deterioration.

β-Blockers

As with ACE inhibitors, β-blockers are indicated for treatment of systolic heart failure of any NYHA functional class, including asymptomatic (NYHA class I) and severe (NYHA class IV) patients. Treatment with a β-blocker is consistently associated with a roughly 30% reduction in total mortality. Both sudden death and death due to pump failure are reduced. In the United States, carvedilol and extended-release metoprolol (metoprolol succinate) are currently approved for the treatment of heart failure. The issue of which β-blocker is better is still controversial. Although a large randomized trial compared carvedilol with short-acting metoprolol (metoprolol tartrate), there has not been a direct comparison of carvedilol with extended-release metoprolol.

In general, β-blockers should not be initiated when a patient is acutely decompensated (hypotensive or volume overloaded), as initiation of therapy is associated with a transient decline in cardiac output. β-Blockers can be initiated and tolerated once euvolemia or near-euvolemia has been established, even prior to hospital discharge. Even patients with severe heart failure (symptoms at rest or with minimal exertion; left ventricular ejection fraction <25%) typically can tolerate initiation and maintenance therapy with a β-blocker. Many of the large randomized controlled trials assessing β-blocker therapy excluded patients with systolic blood pressure below 85 mm Hg; thus, a systolic blood pressure of 85 mm Hg or greater is a reasonable range to allow initiation of a β-blocker.

In a small proportion of patients (<1% in some trials), initiation of a β-blocker results in significant fatigue. Fatigue generally resolves over the course of several weeks, but if it is intolerable to the patient, it can be relieved by reducing the dose or discontinuing the medication. Re-initiation of the β-blocker at a later time or with a different agent may be better tolerated.

Hypotension associated with β-blocker use is usually asymptomatic, manifests within 24 to 48 hours of the first dose or increase in dose, and generally diminishes over time. β-Blockers can usually be continued during decompensated states of heart failure if the patient was previously stable while on β-blocker therapy, unless the decompensation is so severe that there is evidence for end-organ hypoperfusion or that intravenous vasoactive medications are needed.

The risk of exacerbating bronchospastic pulmonary disease with β-blockers is low, except in patients with the most refractory pulmonary disease. If reactive airways disease is a concern, more cardioselective (β_1 receptor–selective) agents such as metoprolol should be used. The cardioselective β-blockers do not cause clinically significant respiratory effects in patients with chronic obstructive pulmonary disease or with mild to moderate reactive airways disease.

Initiating Angiotensin-Converting Enzyme Inhibitors and β-Blockers

Factors that help in determining whether to initiate an ACE inhibitor (or ARB), a β-blocker, or both, include blood pressure, serum creatinine and potassium levels, and existence of any potential contraindications to either therapy. If the patient is euvolemic with an acceptable blood pressure and without significantly elevated creatinine or potassium levels, he or she can likely tolerate initiation of both an ACE inhibitor and a β-blocker. Although it would be ideal to attain the same doses of ACE inhibitors used in clinical trials, given the minor benefit with higher doses versus the significant reduction in mortality and morbidity with the addition of a β-blocker, it is more beneficial to add a β-blocker than to increase the ACE inhibitor dose. The risk of hypotension can be minimized by staggering the timing of β-blocker and ACE inhibitor dosing with other agents that can lower blood pressure.

Diuretics

Diuretics are used for the management of volume overload and typically are needed acutely to achieve euvolemia before starting β-blocker therapy and on a long-term basis to prevent recurrent volume overload. Spironolactone is the only diuretic that has been shown to improve survival in heart failure (for NYHA class III-IV patients); at the doses typically used for heart failure treatment, however, the diuretic effect is weak. In general, loop diuretics, such as furosemide, bumetanide, and torsemide, are used for volume management in heart failure because of their superior natriuretic effects compared with other classes of diuretics.

Management of diuretic resistance includes restriction of fluid and sodium intake, changing the route or timing of administration of the diuretic, and combining diuretics. Although specific practices vary among centers and practitioners, a general guideline for sodium restriction is a daily intake of less than 2000 mg, and for fluid restriction, a daily intake of no more than 2 L, with adjustments made according to the patient's clinical status. Diuretic resistance that occurs because of poor absorption due to gut edema can be addressed by switching to a diuretic with greater bioavailability (bumetanide or torsemide) or switching to the intravenous route of administration. Apparent diuretic resistance may also occur because of inadequate dosing. If increased urine output does not occur within approximately 1 hour of taking the diuretic dose, the dosage is inadequate and should be doubled. If the urine output is adequate after each dose, greater diuresis can be achieved by increasing the number of doses per day. Greater diuresis can also be achieved by adding a synergistic diuretic agent, most commonly a thiazide diuretic (hydrochlorothiazide and metolazone are frequently used). For hospitalized patients, if maximal doses of intermittent intravenous diuretics are not effective for volume overload, a continuous infusion of a loop diuretic can be used.

Digoxin

The role of digoxin in treating heart failure patients in sinus rhythm is primarily for symptom control rather than improving survival. Treatment with digoxin has not been shown to affect mortality but has been shown to reduce hospitalizations. Digoxin can be added to other therapy in patients with NYHA class III or IV heart failure for symptom control. Maintaining lower serum concentrations of digoxin is as effective as maintaining higher concentrations, and potential toxicities are avoided. Higher digoxin levels ($\geq$1.2 ng/mL [1.5 nmol/L] versus 0.5–0.8 ng/mL [0.64–1.02 nmol/L]) appear to be associated with higher mortality.

Spironolactone

In NYHA class III-IV heart failure, spironolactone is recommended in addition to ACE inhibitor and β-blocker therapy. Spironolactone further blocks the actions of aldosterone, which is not completely suppressed by chronic ACE inhibitor therapy; aldosterone has adverse effects of sodium retention, potassium wasting, and myocardial fibrosis. The RALES trial demonstrated a 30% reduction in risk of death and 35% reduction in risk of hospitalization for heart failure in patients with severe heart failure treated with spironolactone versus placebo. The incidence of serious hyperkalemia was low (2%) in the treatment group, although outside of the environment of a controlled clinical trial, appropriate prescription practices and close laboratory monitoring are necessary to avoid problems associated with hyperkalemia.

The ACC/AHA 2005 heart failure guidelines include several measures to reduce the risk of hyperkalemia in patients taking aldosterone antagonists. Impaired renal function is a risk factor for hyperkalemia, with risk increasing progressively when the serum creatinine level exceeds 1.6 mg/dL (122.1 µmol/L) or the glomerular filtration rate drops to 30 mL/min/1.73 m^2 or less. In addition, the risk of hyperkalemia increases with concurrent use of higher doses of ACE inhibitors (captopril $\geq$75 mg/d; enalapril or lisinopril $\geq$10 mg/d). Serum potassium levels and renal function should be monitored closely in all patients: values should be checked 3 days and 1 week after initiation of therapy and at least monthly for the first 3 months. In general, if the baseline serum potassium level is greater than 5.0 meq/L (5.0 mmol/L), aldosterone antagonists should not be given. To reduce the risk of hyperkalemia, NSAIDs and cyclooxygenase 2 (COX-2) inhibitors should be avoided, and potassium supplements should be avoided or reduced.

The selective aldosterone blocker eplerenone has been shown to reduce mortality risk by 15% among patients with left ventricular dysfunction after acute myocardial infarction. In the United States, eplerenone is currently approved for treatment of patients with left ventricular dysfunction after myocardial infarction as well as for hypertension. Eplerenone can be used in place of spironolactone if spironolactone is not tolerated because of gynecomastia.

Hydralazine and Isosorbide Dinitrate

The African-American Heart Failure trial (AAHeFT) demonstrated that black patients with severe heart failure (NYHA class III-IV) had a significant reduction in mortality (approximately 40% reduction) with the addition of hydralazine and isosorbide dinitrate to standard heart failure therapy (including ACE inhibitor or ARB, β-blocker, spironolactone, digoxin, and diuretics as determined appropriate by the patient's physician). As with initiation of other vasodilators, blood pressure should be checked prior to starting hydralazine and isosorbide dinitrate. Most patients with severe heart failure tolerate the addition of hydralazine and isosorbide dinitrate without hypotension problems because the additional vasodilation usually increases cardiac output.

Calcium Channel Blockers

First-generation calcium channel blockers (such as nifedipine) have been shown to increase the risk of heart failure decompensation and hospitalization; however, second-generation dihydropyridine calcium channel blockers do not appear to increase the risk of heart failure decompensation or adversely affect mortality. These agents can be used in patients with heart failure for the management of hypertension or angina not adequately controlled with other agents such as ACE inhibitors or β-blockers. Amlodipine and felodipine are the only calcium channel blockers with demonstrated neutral effects on mortality in patients with heart failure in large-scale randomized controlled trials.

KEY POINTS

- Angiotensin-converting enzyme inhibitors (or angiotensin receptor blockers) and β-blockers are indicated for treatment of any New York Heart Association class of systolic heart failure, including asymptomatic patients.

- Spironolactone is indicated for New York Heart Association class III-IV heart failure patients with acceptable serum creatinine and potassium levels.

- In black patients with New York Heart Association class III-IV heart failure, hydralazine/isosorbide dinitrate should be added to standard therapy.

- Diuretic resistance can be treated by restriction of fluid and sodium intake, changes in route of administration and timing of diuretic medication, and use of diuretic combinations.

Treatment of Heart Failure with Preserved Systolic Function

Treatment of heart failure with preserved systolic function focuses on controlling exacerbating factors, including ischemia, hypertension, and tachycardia, and also managing symptoms of pulmonary and peripheral congestion. Unlike for systolic heart failure, few large clinical trials have been published to determine optimal therapy for heart failure with preserved systolic function, although one large trial (CHARM-Preserved) does suggest that treatment with the ARB candesartan may reduce hospitalizations.

Device Therapy

The primary areas to assess when determining whether a heart failure patient might benefit from implantable cardioverter-defibrillator (ICD) or biventricular pacemaker placement are ejection fraction for ICD implantation, and functional status and evidence of ventricular dyssynchrony for cardiac resynchronization therapy (CRT). The most common cause of sudden death in patients with heart failure is arrhythmia, including both ventricular tachyarrhythmia and bradyarrhythmia. This section discusses the ICDs for primary prevention (no history of resuscitation from sudden cardiac death) in patients with systolic heart failure. See Arrhythmias for further discussion of secondary prevention of sudden cardiac death and ICD implantation. Indications for device therapy are listed in **Table 14**.

Implantable Cardioverter-Defibrillator Placement for Primary Prevention of Sudden Cardiac Death

In patients with left ventricular dysfunction and hemodynamically significant ventricular tachycardia or who were resuscitated after sudden cardiac death, ICD implantation has

TABLE 14 Indications for Device Therapy in Heart Failure

Implantable Cardioverter-Defibrillator
NYHA class II or III while on optimal medical therapy *and*
Expectation of survival >1 year *and*
Either of the following:
Ischemic or nonischemic cardiomyopathy with ejection fraction ≤35% (primary prevention)
History of hemodynamically significant ventricular arrhythmia or cardiac arrest (secondary prevention)

Cardiac Resynchronization Therapy
All of the following:
NYHA class III or IV
Ejection fraction ≤35%
Ventricular dyssynchrony (QRS >120 msec, left bundle branch block)

NYHA = New York Heart Association.

Recommendations from Epstein AE, Dimarco JP, Ellenbogen KA, et al; American College of Cardiology; American Heart Association Task Force on Practice Guidelines; American Association for Thoracic Surgery; Society of Thoracic Surgeons. ACC/AHA/HRS 2008 Guidelines for device-based therapy of cardiac rhythm abnormalities. Heart Rhythm. 2008;5(6):e1-62. [PMID: 18534360]

been shown to improve survival. The primary eligibility criterion for ICD implantation for primary prevention of sudden cardiac death in the setting of heart failure is left ventricular ejection fraction, regardless of the presence or absence of coronary disease or the occurrence of non–hemodynamically significant arrhythmia. The eligibility criteria include the presence of NYHA class II or III symptoms; however, there are less data to guide the use of ICDs in patients with NYHA class I or IV symptoms.

Cardiac Resynchronization Therapy

Interventricular conduction delay is common in patients with heart failure and results in poor coordination of ventricular contraction, which contributes to the hemodynamic consequences of chronic left ventricular systolic dysfunction. A biventricular pacemaker includes three leads: one lead located in and pacing the right ventricle, one lead in the coronary sinus to pace the left ventricle, and one lead in the right atrium to sense intrinsic rhythm to ensure an appropriate atrioventricular timing interval. Patients with heart failure frequently have indications for both a biventricular pacemaker and an ICD; both functions can be governed with a single pulse generator.

CRT improves quality of life, reduces symptoms, and increases exercise capacity. In addition, a meta-analysis found a 37% reduction in hospitalizations and a 22% reduction in all-cause mortality in patients with left ventricular systolic dysfunction, prolonged QRS duration, and NYHA class III or IV symptoms who received CRT. Current standard criteria for biventricular pacing clearly need improvement, however, as up to one-third of patients meeting these criteria do not demonstrate the expected clinical benefit, and research aimed at refining the selection criteria is ongoing. CRT is not currently standard therapy for NYHA class I or II heart failure, but studies are ongoing to assess this area.

Management of Chronic Heart Failure

Disease Management Team Approach

Follow-up for patients with chronic heart failure is facilitated by a multidisciplinary heart failure clinic with nurses playing a major role. The role of the heart failure nurse is central to monitoring and managing patient symptoms, laboratory evaluations, medication titration, and continued reinforcement of appropriate lifestyle modifications such as sodium restriction. This oversight allows a degree of intensity that is not possible in most clinics that do not specialize in chronic disease management. Such a multidisciplinary approach has been shown to reduce recurrent heart failure hospitalizations. However, a randomized controlled trial of 1023 patients (COACH) found only a nonsignificant trend toward improved survival with heart failure nurse management.

Serial Assessment

Serial assessment of chronic heart failure includes determination of volume status and functional status and, when appropriate, assessment of prognosis. Functional status is most commonly and easily assessed by NYHA classification, which is ascertained by subjective patient report. An easily performed, more objective measure of functional capacity is the 6-minute walk test. An inability to walk more than 300 meters in a 6-minute walk test is associated with a 3- to 4-fold higher risk of death. If more specific information is required for functional status assessment, cardiopulmonary exercise testing can also be performed. Volume status can be assessed by physical examination and change in weight. In selected patients, hand-held ultrasonography to assess inferior vena cava size—and thus volume status—may be useful.

Serial laboratory assessment primarily focuses on electrolytes and renal function, as both are affected by many medicines used in the treatment of heart failure. Changes in cardiac function and the state of disease compensation may also affect these values. Increased serum creatinine or hepatic aminotransferase levels may indicate a decline in systemic perfusion due to reduced cardiac output or increased congestion due to high venous filling pressures associated with volume overload.

Ongoing assessment should look for potential factors that may exacerbate heart failure (see Acute Exacerbation of Chronic Heart Failure, below). The risk of coronary artery disease, which may worsen heart failure, is reduced by properly managing dyslipidemia, diabetes, and hypertension, as well as by smoking cessation.

Serial B-Type Natriuretic Peptide Measurement

In the context of management of chronic heart failure, measurement of BNP level may be helpful if the patient's volume status is not clear by physical examination and routine laboratory studies. Otherwise, there are no robust data to support routine serial measurements of BNP levels in the management of chronic heart failure, although this is an area of ongoing research. High BNP level at time of hospital discharge is associated with higher risk of subsequent death and re-hospitalization, with progressively increasing risk with higher BNP levels. One study found a 5-fold risk of death or readmission if the discharge BNP level was between 350 and 700 pg/mL, and a 15-fold risk of death or readmission if the BNP levels were greater than 700 pg/mL (compared with BNP <350 pg/mL).

Although levels of BNP correlate with severity of heart failure symptoms and prognosis, large-scale prospective randomized trials of clinical care guided by BNP levels have not demonstrated reduction in hard endpoints such as mortality; clinical benefits such as reduced hospitalization have primarily been associated with more intensive titration of medical therapy such as ACE inhibitors and β-blockers. In the multi-center TIME-CHF trial, compared to symptom-guided therapy, BNP-guided therapy did not improve quality of life or 18-month survival free of any hospitalization. Of note, many patients taking optimal regimens of medications and who are clinically compensated have chronically elevated BNP levels, whereas some patients who are clinically decompensated have relatively lower BNP levels. Interpretation of the significance of BNP findings should be made in the context of the clinical scenario and with the knowledge of factors independent of heart failure status that affect BNP results (see Laboratory Evaluation, above).

Echocardiography in Chronic Heart Failure

Reassessment of ejection fraction with echocardiography is most useful when there is a notable change in clinical status rather than at regular or arbitrary intervals. Changes in ejection fraction should be considered in the context of the patient's clinical status and are frequently in concordance with the patient's physical examination or interval history. Rarely should clinical management be guided solely by changes in ejection fraction alone in the absence of other concurrent clinical data. Improvement may indicate response to medical therapy or recovery from a prior event, such as myocarditis, whereas deterioration may indicate disease progression or an intervening event such as myocardial infarction. Ejection fraction and valvular regurgitation (in particular, mitral and tricuspid valves) may be worsened in decompensated, volume-overloaded states and frequently improve once euvolemia is restored.

KEY POINTS

- An inability to walk more than 300 meters in a 6-minute walk test is associated with a 3- to 4-fold increased risk of death in chronic heart failure patients.

- Ongoing assessment of chronic heart failure patients should look for potential factors that may exacerbate heart failure, such as hypertension, ischemia, arrhythmia, obesity, medications, and medication or lifestyle noncompliance.

- Reassessment of ejection fraction with echocardiography is most useful when there is a change in clinical status rather than at regular or arbitrary intervals.

Assessing Prognosis

Various models have been developed to help assess prognosis in chronic heart failure. Of note, these models predict survival for populations and can at best provide only an approximation of risk on an individual level. A more recently developed tool, the Seattle Heart Failure Model, provides an individualized risk assessment for ambulatory patients with systolic heart failure based on several predictors of survival, including age and sex, cause of ischemia, NYHA class, ejection fraction, systolic blood pressure, medication use, current device modalities, and other biomarkers of risk. These easily assessed factors are combined in a predictive model that yields estimated survival at 1, 2, and 5 years. In addition, the effect of various interventions (for example, adding an ACE inhibitor or implanting an ICD) on estimated survival can be calculated. Knowledge of prognosis can assist the clinician in discussion of appropriate management, including referral for hospice services, with patients and their families. The Seattle Heart Failure Model can be accessed online at www.Seattle HeartFailureModel.org.

KEY POINT

- The Seattle Heart Failure Model provides an individualized risk assessment for ambulatory patients with systolic heart failure, with estimated survival at 1, 2, and 5 years based on several easily assessed predictors of survival.

Acute Exacerbation of Chronic Heart Failure

Decompensation of chronic heart failure should trigger a diligent search for initiating factors. Estimates vary significantly, but preventable precipitating factors, such as dietary or medication noncompliance, may account for 25% to 50% of hospital admissions for heart failure decompensation. Arrhythmias and superimposed illness such as infection account for approximately 20% to 30%, and hypertension and myocardial ischemia account for approximately 10% each. Other precipitating factors include obesity, deleterious medications (such as NSAIDs), and drug use (alcohol, stimulants).

In patients with severe heart failure, decompensation may be caused by volume overload, low cardiac output, or a combination of both. Low cardiac output, which may be due to a fluctuation in disease severity, disease progression, or a superimposed stressor (such as another illness or negative inotropic medication), causes systemic hypoperfusion. Patients with low output typically present with general symptoms that overlap with those of volume overload, including fatigue and dyspnea.

Evaluation of the patient with acute exacerbation of chronic heart failure focuses on identifying any precipitating factors and assessing the patient's clinical status with regard to volume and perfusion status. A careful history may reveal evidence for dietary or medication noncompliance or use of inappropriate medications or toxic substances. Most patients with decompensated heart failure have physical signs of volume overload or low cardiac output. However, it is not uncommon for patients with long-standing heart failure, particularly if it is severe, to have unrevealing or confusing physical examination findings (such as the absence of pulmonary crackles) despite actual decompensation.

Cardiogenic Shock

Most patients with acute exacerbation of chronic heart failure can be managed by treatment of the exacerbating factors along with diuresis and reinstitution of afterload reduction. However, if cardiac output is decreased (in the absence of hypovolemia) to such a degree as to cause tissue and end-organ hypoperfusion, then cardiogenic shock is present. Clinically, the patient manifests evidence of hypoperfusion, including worsened renal function, decreased mental status, or cool extremities. Extensive myocardial infarction accounts for up to 75% of all cases of cardiogenic shock, with the remainder due to other conditions, including acute myocarditis, end-stage cardiomyopathy, or prolonged cardiopulmonary bypass.

Hemodynamic criteria for the diagnosis of cardiogenic shock include sustained hypotension and reduced cardiac index (<2.2 L/min/m^2) in the setting of elevated pulmonary capillary wedge pressure (>15 mm Hg). A commonly used definition for sustained hypotension is systolic blood pressure less than 90 mm Hg for more than 30 minutes. This definition is reasonable in patients without known prior heart failure; however, given that normal baseline blood pressure can be in this range in patients with chronic moderate to severe heart failure, the cut-off for patients with known heart failure can reasonably be lower, in the range of 80 to 85 mm Hg.

The approach to cardiogenic shock includes treatment of hemodynamic derangements and diagnosis of cause, which may determine the treatment method. ECG and, in most cases, echocardiography, should be performed. Some causes thus revealed require urgent, specific interventions, including revascularization for acute myocardial infarction, surgical repair for ventricular rupture or acute mitral regurgitation, and pericardiocentesis for tamponade. In addition to etiology-specific interventions, treatment goals include correcting

hypotension, optimizing intracardiac filling pressures, and improving end-organ perfusion. **Figure 7** presents a flow chart for assessment and management of the spectrum of exacerbation of heart failure and cardiogenic shock. Continuous intravenous infusion of positive inotropic agents may be indicated for short-term (hours to days) treatment of cardiogenic shock. However, although these agents are useful acutely and improve short-term hemodynamics and symptoms, they increase intermediate- and long-term mortality. Placement of a pulmonary artery catheter in selected patients can assist in addressing hemodynamic derangements, although use of a pulmonary artery catheter does not ultimately appear to affect survival in critically ill patients or those with decompensated heart failure.

If the patient remains refractory or minimally responsive to medical therapy, placement of an intra-aortic balloon

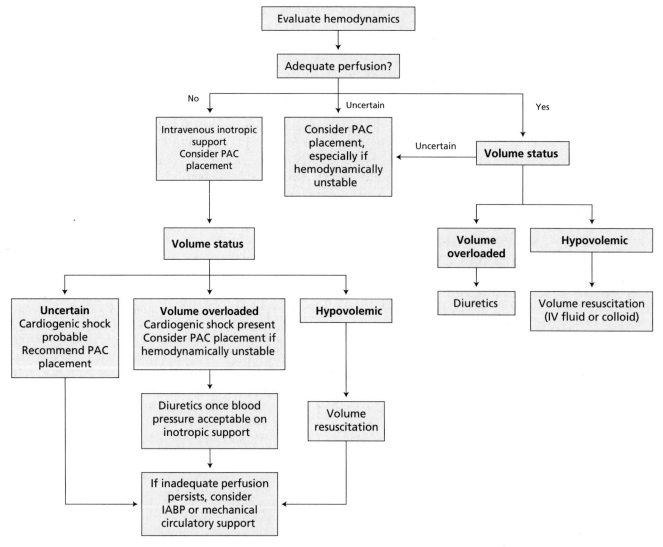

FIGURE 7.
Suggested Management of Hemodynamic Derangements in Decompensated Heart Failure and Cardiogenic Shock.

IABP = intra-aortic balloon pump; PAC = pulmonary artery catheter.

pump is generally indicated. This device inflates during diastole and deflates during systole, thereby improving coronary perfusion and reducing afterload. Finally, if cardiogenic shock is refractory to these measures, ventricular assist device implantation and/or cardiac transplantation can be considered for appropriate candidates.

KEY POINTS

- Common causes of decompensation of chronic heart failure include dietary or medication noncompliance, a new-onset cardiac problem such as atrial fibrillation or ischemia, and intervening medical illness.
- Patients with long-standing heart failure often have unrevealing or confusing physical examination findings, such as the absence of pulmonary crackles, despite actual decompensation.

Advanced Refractory Heart Failure

Prolonged continuous infusion (days to months) of an inotropic agent may be necessary as a bridge to cardiac transplantation or as chronic palliative therapy in end-stage heart failure. In selected patients with severe end-stage heart failure, chronic infusion of inotropic agents improves symptoms and functional status in many patients and may reduce the number of hospitalizations. Mortality is high, however,

ranging from 40% to 95% over a 3- to 6-month period in various series.

For patients with end-stage heart failure refractory to therapy, mechanical circulatory support and cardiac transplantation are potentially lifesaving options. The mechanical circulatory support device most commonly used is the left ventricular assist device (VAD), a surgically implanted pump. Inflow into the VAD is from a cannula in the left ventricular apex, with blood return to the ascending aorta via a second cannula. VADs are used as a bridge to cardiac transplantation, for recovery from severe cardiogenic shock, and as an alternative to medical therapy for patients not eligible for transplantation. Referral for transplantation or VAD implantation should be considered if the patient displays evidence of refractory heart failure, including poor functional status, persistent hypotension, recurrent hospitalizations due to heart failure, or renal failure due to poor perfusion. Although specifics vary by center, general guidelines regarding indications and contraindications to VAD implantation and cardiac transplantation are shown in **Table 15**.

Cardiac transplantation remains the gold standard for treatment of end-stage heart failure, and for appropriate candidates, functional status and survival are improved. However, considerable care must be taken to select appropriate candidates. Patients with comorbidities that would significantly increase the risks of surgery or chronic immunosuppression or would limit potential for rehabilitation after transplantation

TABLE 15 Indications and Contraindications for Cardiac Transplantation or Ventricular Assist Device
Indications (Any of the Following; in the Absence of Contraindications)
Refractory cardiogenic shock
Dependence on intravenous inotropic support to maintain adequate organ perfusion
Severely limited functional capacity despite optimal medical therapy (peak Vo_2 <10-14 mL/kg/min)
Severe ischemia despite optimal medical therapy that consistently limits routine activity and is not amenable to percutaneous or surgical revascularization
Recurrent significant ventricular arrhythmias refractory to optimal therapies
Insufficient Indication Alone
Low ejection fraction
History of New York Heart Association class III or IV symptoms
Potential Contraindications (Center-Specific)
Diabetes with end-organ damage, such as nephropathy or retinopathy
Major chronic disabling illness, such as systemic lupus erythematosus or severe arthritis
Severe pulmonary hypertension
Severe peripheral vascular disease
Active infection
Significant chronic and likely irreversible functional impairment of other vital organs, such as renal failure, cirrhosis, or chronic obstructive pulmonary disease
Active substance abuse, including smoking
Obesity
Current mental or psychosocial instability
Active or recent malignancy

would not be suitable candidates. Candidates listed for cardiac transplantation should have an estimated likelihood of death due to heart failure that is greater than the risk of death or significant morbidity related to undergoing transplantation and chronic immunosuppression.

The international 1-year survival rate following heart transplant is about 85%, with a 3% to 4% annual decline subsequently. Early mortality primarily results from infection or acute graft failure. Later mortality is frequently related to the accelerated coronary disease that is typical of heart transplant patients, characterized by diffuse intimal thickening (transplant vasculopathy). Other problems after transplantation result from immunosuppression (infection and neoplasm) and side effects from medications (renal failure, new or worsened diabetes, hypertension, dyslipidemia).

In patients with end-stage heart failure in whom further active therapies are not options, either due to medical contraindication, futility, or patient desire, end-of-life issues should appropriately be addressed, including advanced directives and hospice care. Hospice care does not preclude the use of intravenous inotropic agents or diuretics for symptom palliation. Deactivation of a patient's ICD also should be considered.

KEY POINT

- Patients with severe heart failure should be considered for referral for cardiac transplantation evaluation or left ventricular assist device implantation if they display evidence of refractory heart failure despite optimal medical and device therapy.

Investigational Therapies for Heart Failure

In patients with heart failure, vasopressin-receptor antagonists result in favorable changes in hemodynamics and urine output and normalization of hyponatremia, without significant changes in blood pressure or heart rate. Short-term mortality and morbidity do not appear adversely affected; long-term effects are still being studied. The vasopressin-receptor antagonist conivaptan is currently approved by the U.S. Food and Drug Administration only for treatment of hyponatremia in euvolemic hospitalized patients and is not approved for treatment of heart failure at this time.

Nesiritide is a recombinant human B-type natriuretic peptide with venous, arterial, and coronary vasodilatory properties without direct inotropic effects. Several short-term trials (mostly of less than 48 hours' treatment duration) examining patients hospitalized with acute heart failure decompensation due to volume overload and low cardiac output demonstrated favorable hemodynamic effects. However, a meta-analysis of nesiritide trials suggested increased short-term mortality after treatment for acutely decompensated heart failure. Current data do not support routine outpatient treatment with intermittent nesiritide infusions.

Anticoagulation is currently recommended only for other conditions often encountered in heart failure patients, such as atrial fibrillation, intracardiac thrombus, and history of thromboembolic disease. Research is ongoing to assess the utility of anticoagulation solely for the treatment of low ejection fraction.

Preliminary studies of ultrafiltration for acute decompensated heart failure due to volume overload suggest that this method may be an effective way to remove fluid. A potential advantage of ultrafiltration over traditional diuretics is restoration of diuretic responsiveness owing to reduced neurohormonal activation. Studies of ultrafiltration have largely involved hospitalized patients with moderate to severe heart failure. Studies are ongoing regarding appropriate selection criteria for treatment as well as long-term effects on morbidity and mortality.

External counterpulsation is a treatment that involves a device with sequentially inflating cuffs around the lower extremities coordinated with the cardiac cycle. This treatment aims to reduce afterload and augment coronary perfusion during diastole and may improve endothelial function of the coronary vasculature. While this therapy has decreased angina in patients with coronary disease, the long-term effects in heart failure are still being studied.

Specific Cardiomyopathies

Specific cardiomyopathies may require specific testing or treatment beyond that generally recommended for systolic heart failure. The distribution of specific cardiomyopathies varies worldwide by region. A large proportion of cardiomyopathy in Africa results from nonischemic causes, including dilated cardiomyopathy, rheumatic heart disease, and peripartum cardiomyopathy, whereas a significant proportion in North America and Europe (50% to 75%) results from coronary artery disease and hypertension.

Takotsubo Cardiomyopathy

Takotsubo cardiomyopathy is a recently described transient form of acute ventricular dysfunction that generally occurs in the setting of intense emotional or physiologic stress (for example, a loved one's death, an argument, or an earthquake). This phenomenon is also called transient left ventricular apical ballooning, stress-induced cardiomyopathy, and, colloquially, "broken heart syndrome." Patients typically present with signs and symptoms mimicking acute myocardial infarction, including chest pain, ST-segment elevation, and elevated cardiac enzyme levels. The vast majority of patients in the published literature are women, with average age in the sixties to seventies. Cardiac imaging reveals dilation and akinesis of the left ventricular apex and mid-ventricle with relatively normal function of the basal segments, in the absence of obstructive epicardial coronary disease on angiography. The etiology of Takotsubo cardiomyopathy is still unknown, although it may be related to microvascular endothelial dysfunction or spasm or catecholamine-induced myocardial damage or stunning. Cardiac dysfunction generally resolves in days to weeks with supportive care. Associated mortality and risk for recurrence appear to be low.

Acute Myocarditis

Acute myocarditis is an inflammation of the heart muscle with a wide range of clinical presentations, from asymptomatic to acute cardiogenic shock. The primary mechanism underlying myocarditis appears to be immunologically mediated damage to the myocardium. Cardiac troponin levels are typically elevated, indicating some degree of myocardial necrosis, and ventricular dysfunction may be global or regional. Therapy generally consists of standard care for heart failure tailored to the severity of the myocarditis. Anti-inflammatory or immune-modulating therapy with corticosteroids or other immunosuppressive agents is controversial.

Tachycardia-Mediated Cardiomyopathy

Tachycardia-mediated cardiomyopathy is myocardial dysfunction caused by structural and cellular changes in the myocardium that develop as a result of chronic tachycardia. The tachycardia is usually supraventricular, but cases associated with ventricular tachycardias have also been described. Regardless of the causative arrhythmia, the primary treatment for tachycardia-mediated cardiomyopathy is to slow or eliminate the arrhythmia using medications for rate or rhythm control or radiofrequency catheter ablation as indicated. In addition, it is important to treat underlying conditions that may be contributing to the tachycardia, such as hyperthyroidism. In true cases of tachycardia-mediated cardiomyopathy, resolution of tachycardia usually results in normalization of myocardial structure and function in weeks to months.

Arrhythmogenic Right Ventricular Dysplasia

Arrhythmogenic right ventricular dysplasia involves a pathologic fibrofatty infiltration of the right ventricle evident on biopsy or by MRI. There is typically significant right ventricular enlargement and dysfunction that is out of proportion to generally preserved left ventricular function. Sudden death may be the initial presentation. Up to 50% to 60% of patients die of progressive heart failure.

Giant Cell Myocarditis

Giant cell myocarditis is a rare disease of uncertain etiology characterized by marked biventricular enlargement and sometimes refractory ventricular arrhythmias, usually in young to middle-aged adults. This disease generally presents as fulminant cardiogenic shock and is usually rapidly fatal, with a 90% short- and intermediate-term mortality rate. Cardiac transplantation is the treatment of choice, although giant cell myocarditis may recur in the transplanted heart.

Bibliography

Binanay C, Califf RM, Hasselblad V, et al. Evaluation study of congestive heart failure and pulmonary artery catheterization effectiveness: the ESCAPE trial. JAMA. 2005;294(13):1625-1633. [PMID: 16204662]

Cooper LT, Baughman KL, Feldman AM, et al. The role of endomyocardial biopsy in the management of cardiovascular disease: a scientific statement from the American Heart Association, the American College of Cardiology, and the European Society of Cardiology. Endorsed by the Heart Failure Society of America and the Heart Failure Association of the European Society of Cardiology. J Am Coll Cardiol. 2007;50(19):1914-31. [PMID: 17980265]

Hunt SA; American College of Cardiology; American Heart Association Task Force on Practice Guidelines (Writing Committee to Update the 2001 Guidelines for the Evaluation and Management of Heart Failure). ACC/AHA 2005 guideline update for the diagnosis and management of chronic heart failure in the adult [erratum in J Am Coll Cardiol. 2006;47(7):1503-1505.]. J Am Coll Cardiol. 2005; 46(6):e1-82. [PMID: 16168273]

Jaarsma T, van der Wal MH, Lesman-Leegte I, et al. Effect of moderate or intensive disease management program on outcome in patients with heart failure: Coordinating Study Evaluating Outcomes of Advising and Counseling in Heart Failure (COACH). Arch Intern Med. 2008;168(3):316-324. [PMID: 18268174]

Jourdain P, Jondeau G, Funck F, et al. Plasma brain natriuretic peptide-guided therapy to improve outcome in heart failure: the STARS-BNP Multicenter Study. J Am Coll Cardiol. 2007;49(16):1733-1739. [PMID: 17448376]

Levy WC, Mozaffarian D, Linker DT, et al. The Seattle Heart Failure Model: prediction of survival in heart failure. Circulation. 2006;113(11):1424-1433. [PMID: 16534009]

McAlister FA, Ezekowitz J, Hooton N, et al. Cardiac resynchronization therapy for patients with left ventricular systolic dysfunction: a systematic review. JAMA. 2007;297(22):2502-2514. [PMID: 17565085]

Pfisterer M, Buser P, Rickli H, et al; TIME-CHF Investigators. BNP-guided vs symptom-guided heart failure therapy. The Trial of Intensified vs Standard Medical Therapy in Elderly Patients With Congestive Heart Failure (TIME-CHF) randomized trial. JAMA. 2009;301(4):382-92. [PMID: 19176440]

Phillips CO, Kashani A, Ko DK, Francis G, Krumholz HM. Adverse effects of combination angiotensin II receptor blockers plus angiotensin-converting enzyme inhibitors for left ventricular dysfunction: a quantitative review of data from randomized clinical trials. Arch Intern Med. 2007;167(18):1930-1936. [PMID: 17923591]

Taylor AL, Ziesche S, Yancy C, et al; African-American Heart Failure Trial Investigators. Combination of isosorbide dinitrate and hydralazine in blacks with heart failure. N Engl J Med. 2004; 351(20):2049-2057. [PMID: 15533851]

Wang CS, FitzGerald JM, Schulzer M, Mak E, Ayas NT. Does this dyspneic patient in the emergency department have congestive heart failure? JAMA. 2005;294(15):1944-1956. [PMID: 16234501]

Myocardial Disease

Restrictive Cardiomyopathy

Restrictive cardiomyopathy is a disease of ventricular myocardium that typically results in delayed diastolic relaxation, decreased compliance, and elevated filling pressures with nondilated ventricles. Systolic function often is preserved. These cardiac changes result in pulmonary venous congestion, pulmonary hypertension, and right-sided heart failure early in the disease. Late in the disease course, systolic dysfunction affecting both ventricles may be seen. Restrictive cardiomyopathy is the least prevalent of all the cardiomyopathies. The differential diagnosis (**Table 16**) is broad but most cases are idiopathic. Amyloidosis is the most common diagnosis when a cause can be identified.

KEY POINT

- Restrictive cardiomyopathy is a disease of ventricular myocardium that typically results in delayed diastolic relaxation, decreased compliance, and elevated filling pressures with nondilated ventricles.

Clinical Presentation and Evaluation

Prominent symptoms include fatigue, weakness, anorexia, and edema. Exercise intolerance, dyspnea, paroxysmal nocturnal dyspnea, and orthopnea also occur. Physical examination may reveal peripheral edema, jugular venous distention, hepatojugular reflux, and Kussmaul sign (an increase in jugular venous distention during inspiration). The apical impulse may be forceful, a loud S_3 is usually present, and regurgitant murmurs are common. Supraventricular tachycardia and conduction disease are frequent complications. As the disease progresses, elevated central venous pressure may lead to hepatomegaly, ascites, and, in advanced cases, anasarca.

Amyloidosis is suggested by neuropathy, marked proteinuria, and hepatomegaly disproportionate to other signs of right-sided heart failure. Characteristic echocardiographic features of amyloidosis include increased ventricular wall thickness, thickened atrioventricular valves, a thickened atrial septum, and pericardial effusion. On electrocardiogram, low voltage, together with thick ventricular walls seen on echocardiography, suggests amyloidosis (or another infiltrative process). Biopsy of noncardiac tissue (abdominal fat pad, rectum, or gingiva) can confirm the diagnosis. Endomyocardial biopsy should be considered only when a definitive diagnosis of cardiac involvement is needed.

Bilateral hilar lymphadenopathy with or without pulmonary reticular opacities and skin, joint, or eye lesions are common presenting signs of sarcoidosis. In patients with sarcoidosis, cardiac involvement is suggested by the presence of arrhythmias, conduction blocks, or heart failure. Cardiac magnetic resonance (CMR) imaging is useful for detection of

TABLE 16 Characteristics of Selected Causes of Restrictive Cardiomyopathy		
Type	**Etiology**	**Notes**
Noninfiltrative Myocardial Conditions		
Idiopathic	Unknown	Diagnosis of exclusion
Scleroderma	Patchy myocardial fibrosis often associated with contraction band necrosis	May result from recurrent vasospasm of small vessels
Infiltrative Myocardial Conditions		
Amyloidosis	Commonly associated with transthyretin gene mutation	Most common identifiable underlying cause of restrictive cardiomyopathy
Sarcoidosis	Noncaseating granulomas, inflammation, and fibrosis	Clinical manifestations uncommon but may include ventricular arrhythmias, conduction block, and sudden death
Hemochromatosis	Iron deposits may be associated with myocardial or endocardial fibrosis	Most often presents as dilated cardiomyopathy but may present as restrictive form
Myocardial Storage Conditions		
Fabry disease	X-linked deficiency of α-galactosidase causing accumulation of globotriaosylceramide	Has some features of hypertrophic cardiomyopathy
Endomyocardial Disorders		
Endomyocardial fibrosis	Unknown cause but may relate to nutritional deficiencies, eosinophilia, or genetics	Endocardial fibrosis of the right and left ventricular apices, occurring mainly in west and central Africa
Eosinophilic cardiomyopathy (Löffler endocarditis)	Hypereosinophilia, organ infiltration, and release of toxic mediators	Fibrosis of the endomyocardium
Toxic effect of anthracycline	Doxorubicin, daunorubicin, idarubicin, epirubicin, and mitoxantrone (an anthraquinone) are the most frequently implicated	Can cause dilated or restrictive disease; risk increases with concomitant irradiation
Radiation	Diffuse fibrosis in the interstitium of the myocardium	May occur years or decades after exposure

localized myocardial high-intensity areas, and when performed with late gadolinium enhancement, has a sensitivity of 100% and specificity of 78% for sarcoidosis. Endomyocardial biopsy specimen showing noncaseating granulomas confirms the diagnosis. However, endomyocardial biopsy is only 20% sensitive for confirming the diagnosis.

Cardiac symptoms are the initial presentation of hemochromatosis in up to 15% of patients. In patients with hemochromatosis and restrictive cardiomyopathy by echocardiography, a presumptive diagnosis of myocardial hemochromatosis is appropriate. If echocardiographic findings are equivocal, CMR imaging may demonstrate very low signal intensity of the myocardium due to the effects of iron deposits. Endomyocardial biopsy may also be useful; however, a normal biopsy does not exclude deposition of myocardial iron because the deposits have a predilection to involve the epicardium.

Differentiating Restrictive Cardiomyopathy from Constrictive Pericarditis

Differentiating restrictive cardiomyopathy and constrictive pericarditis is important because constrictive pericarditis may be effectively treated with pericardiectomy (see Pericardial Disease). Both diseases demonstrate a "restrictive pattern" of early rapid left ventricular filling on Doppler echocardiography. However, restrictive cardiomyopathy is associated with minimal respiratory variation in ventricular filling, whereas patients with constrictive pericarditis have respiratory variation of at least 15% to more than 25%. Constrictive pericarditis is associated with a respiratory variation in ventricular septal motion; restrictive cardiomyopathy lacks this finding.

If echocardiography is equivocal, CMR imaging and cardiac CT can assess pericardial thickness, which is increased in 80% of patients with constrictive pericarditis but is normal in those with restrictive cardiomyopathy.

Hemodynamic cardiac catheterization is warranted when results of noninvasive testing are equivocal. Left and right ventricular diastolic pressures are elevated in both diseases, but are within 5 mm Hg of each other in constrictive pericarditis as compared with the greater difference seen in restrictive cardiomyopathy. Finally, left and right ventricular systolic pressures rise and fall during the respiratory cycle discordantly (in opposite directions) in constrictive pericarditis but concordantly (in the same direction) in restrictive cardiomyopathy.

Plasma B-type natriuretic peptide (BNP) levels are markedly elevated in restrictive cardiomyopathy (mean >800 pg/mL) but only slightly above normal (mean <130 pg/mL) in idiopathic constrictive pericarditis. A low BNP level is useful in ruling out restrictive cardiomyopathy; however, BNP levels may be elevated with some causes of constrictive pericarditis (for example, cardiac surgery, mantle irradiation).

Treatment

General Therapy

There is no specific therapy for most forms of restrictive cardiomyopathy. Treatment is focused on lowering increased intracavitary diastolic pressures and controlling venous and systemic congestion. Loop diuretics are used to treat dyspnea and peripheral edema. However, because ventricular volumes are normal to small, excessive volume reduction can result in reductions in stroke volume and cardiac output, predisposing to orthostatic hypotension and syncope.

β-Blockers and/or nondihydropyridine calcium channel antagonists enhance diastolic function and should be considered if diuretic therapy is not effective or in the presence of atrial tachyarrhythmias. In patients with conduction abnormalities, however, β-blockers and calcium channel blockers can result in third-degree heart block. Angiotensin-converting enzyme inhibitors and angiotensin receptor blockers improve diastolic filling and may be beneficial in patients with diastolic dysfunction.

Because stroke volume is relatively fixed in restrictive cardiomyopathy, bradyarrhythmias can result in a significant decline in cardiac output and heart failure. Pacemaker support may be considered in this situation. Atrial fibrillation, with the associated loss of ventricular filling, can lead to rapid worsening of diastolic function, and attempts should be made to restore sinus rhythm with cardioversion or amiodarone.

Specific Therapies

In addition to general treatment measures, treatment is directed toward specific causes when possible (**Table 17**). Cardiac function may improve with removal of iron by phlebotomy in hereditary forms of hemochromatosis or iron chelation therapy in other iron overload states, such as lifelong transfusion-dependent anemias.

TABLE 17 Treatment Approaches for Specific Causes of Restrictive Cardiomyopathy

Cause	Medical Therapy	Surgical Therapy
Amyloidosis		
Familial/mutant transthyretin	Stem cell transplant	Heart/liver transplant
AL (primary)	Chemotherapy	Heart transplant (controversial)
AA (secondary)	Specific for cause of inflammation or infection	
Granulomatous Disease		
Sarcoidosis	First-line therapy: corticosteroids	
	Second line therapy: chloroquine, hydroxychloroquine, cyclosporine, methotrexate	
Hemochromatosis		
Hereditary	Phlebotomy	Heart transplant
Acquired	Iron chelation	
Endomyocardial Disease		
Endomyocardial fibrosis	Warfarin (for documented cardiac thrombus)	Endomyocardectomy (palliative)
Hypereosinophilic syndrome	First-line therapy: corticosteroids	Endomyocardectomy (palliative)
	Second-line therapy: tyrosine kinase inhibitor, interferon, cyclosporine, chemotherapeutic drugs	Stem cell transplant (for treatment-resistant disease)
	Warfarin (for documented cardiac thrombus)	
Storage Disease		
Fabry disease	α-Galactosidase A replacement	

AA = amyloid-associated; AL = amyloid light chain.

Restrictive cardiomyopathy from mutant-type transthyretin amyloidosis may regress with stem cell transplantation. Cardiac transplantation in patients with amyloid heart disease from AL amyloidosis is controversial, given its high mortality rate and the ongoing systemic nature of the disease that continues after transplantation. However, patients with a mutant-type transthyretin amyloidosis who are candidates for liver transplant should be considered for cardiac transplant if a severe restrictive cardiomyopathy is evident.

Survival of patients with cardiac sarcoidosis may improve with corticosteroid treatment, which is most effective when started before deterioration of the left ventricular ejection fraction. Implantable cardioverter-defibrillators and permanent pacemakers may be justified in patients with cardiac sarcoidosis and recurrent syncope or sustained ventricular tachycardia.

KEY POINTS

- Treatment of restrictive cardiomyopathy is focused on lowering increased intracavitary diastolic pressures and controlling venous and systemic congestion and atrial fibrillation.
- Bradycardia can precipitate heart failure in patients with restrictive cardiomyopathy and may require pacemaker support.

Hypertrophic Cardiomyopathy

Hypertrophic cardiomyopathy is an uncommon inherited disorder that results in diffuse or focal myocardial hypertrophy, diastolic dysfunction, dynamic outflow obstruction, and an increased risk of sudden cardiac death. Inheritance is autosomal dominant; however, only about 50% of patients have a family history of disease, most likely due to variable penetrance and new mutations. Men are affected twice as frequently as women, and blacks twice as frequently as whites.

Clinical Presentation and Evaluation

Most children or adolescents are typically asymptomatic with the diagnosis based on echocardiographic screening prompted by diagnosis in a relative. Affected adults may present with pulmonary congestion, chest pain, fatigue, palpitations, dizziness, or syncope.

Hypertrophic cardiomyopathy is characterized by ventricular hypertrophy, diastolic dysfunction, ischemia, and arrhythmias. Echocardiographic findings include asymmetric hypertrophy of the ventricle with preserved systolic function but abnormal diastolic function. Hypertrophy typically affects the septum most severely, as well as the anterolateral wall and apex (**Figure 8**). However, several patterns of hypertrophy have been described; the only common feature is that the

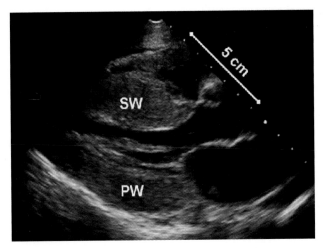

FIGURE 8.
Hypertrophic Cardiomyopathy.
Two-dimensional echocardiography demonstrates marked hypertrophy of the septal wall (SW) and inferolateral wall (PW) from hypertrophic cardiomyopathy.

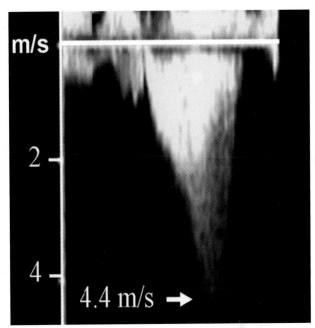

FIGURE 9.
Doppler Flow Image of Hypertrophic Cardiomyopathy.
Continuous-wave Doppler echocardiography demonstrates a high-velocity late-peaking systolic waveform (*arrow*) across the left ventricular outflow tract from a dynamic obstruction in hypertrophic obstructive cardiomyopathy.

basal posterior wall is spared. Apical hypertrophic cardiomyopathy is a specific variant with prominent apical hypertrophy and an absence of outflow obstruction. Intracavitary obstruction may occur in hypertrophic cardiomyopathy in the mid cavity or left ventricular outflow tract and is readily diagnosed with Doppler echocardiography by a characteristic high-velocity late-peaking spectral waveform (**Figure 9**).

The typical pattern of diastolic dysfunction in hypertrophic cardiomyopathy is impaired early diastolic relaxation, but with disease progression, impaired compliance and elevated filling pressures also are evident. In patients with normal ventricular wall thickness, tissue Doppler imaging, which allows measurement of the diastolic velocity of myocardial motion, appears promising for detection of patients with mutations associated with hypertrophic cardiomyopathy who do not yet manifest the phenotypic features. Echocardiography differentiates pathologic hypertrophy from compensatory hypertrophy seen in athletes (**Table 18**).

About 25% of patients also have resting or exercise-induced dynamic outflow obstruction, typically in the subaortic region and predominantly during late systole. The severity of obstruction is more severe with small ventricular volumes, low afterload, and increased contractility. Left ventricular outflow obstruction usually manifests as a midsystolic harsh murmur loudest at the lower left sternal border or between the left sternal border and cardiac apex. The murmur is increased by the strain phase of the Valsalva maneuver or (more reproducibly) by standing and is diminished by handgrip, leg elevation, or squatting. These changes help to distinguish the murmur from that of aortic stenosis or mitral regurgitation.

Electrocardiography in hypertrophic cardiomyopathy typically shows left ventricular hypertrophy and atrial enlargement. Deeply inverted, symmetric anterior T waves are present in the apical hypertrophic form (**Figure 10**), often mimicking ischemia.

If a diagnosis of hypertrophic cardiomyopathy is suspected despite nondiagnostic echocardiography, CMR imaging can detect focal areas of ventricular hypertrophy and small areas of scarring, which would support the diagnosis.

Cardiac catheterization is rarely needed for diagnosis of hypertrophic cardiomyopathy, although pressure tracings are used to monitor catheter-based septal ablation procedures. Pretreatment pressure tracings demonstrate elevated diastolic ventricular and atrial pressure. In the presence of left ventricular outflow obstruction, the left ventricle–to-aortic late-peaking gradient is seen, with the characteristic aortic pressure tracing showing a rapid rise and fall followed by a plateau ("spike and dome" pattern).

Clinical Course

Persons with relatively asymptomatic hypertrophic cardiomyopathy have better prognoses than those with severe symptoms. In 5% to 10% of patients, the disease progresses to dilated cardiomyopathy. Atrial fibrillation occurs commonly and may precipitate heart failure. Studies suggest an improvement in survival in recent years, with an annual mortality rate of 1%. However, many patients are limited by symptoms due to diastolic dysfunction and outflow obstruction.

Arrhythmias are common, including ventricular premature beats; nonsustained ventricular tachycardia; and an increased risk of ventricular tachycardia, ventricular fibrillation,

TABLE 18 Clinical and Echocardiographic Features Differentiating Hypertrophic Cardiomyopathy from Athlete's Heart

Finding	Hypertrophic Cardiomyopathy	Athlete's Heart
Clinical		
Family history of hypertrophic cardiomyopathy	Yes	No
Electrocardiography		
Unusual patterns	Present	Absent
Echocardiography		
Unusual distribution of left ventricular hypertrophy	Present	Absent
Left ventricular diastolic cavity >55 mm (enlarged)	Absent	Present
Left ventricular diastolic cavity <45 mm (normal size)	Present	Absent
Marked left atrial enlargement	Present	Absent
Abnormal left ventricular filling	Present	Absent
Decrease in left ventricular wall thickness with deconditioning	Absent	Present
Metabolic stress test		
Maximal oxygen consumption >45 mL/kg/min or >100% of predicted	No	Yes

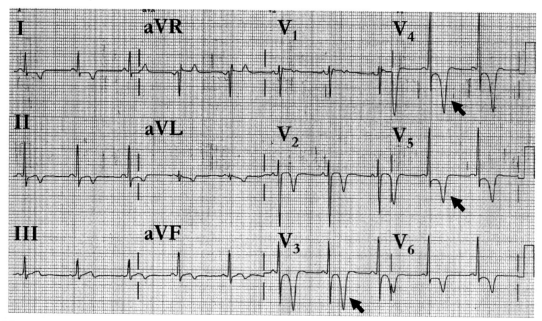

FIGURE 10.
Twelve-Lead Electrocardiography in Marked Apical Hypertrophy.
ST-segment depression and deeply inverted T waves (*arrows*) are seen in the precordial leads. These findings are due to apical hypertrophy, but could be erroneously diagnosed as manifestations of myocardial ischemia and coronary artery disease.

and sudden cardiac death. The overall risk of sudden cardiac death is about 1% over 5 years, but the risk of sudden cardiac death is strongly dependent on the number of risk factors (**Table 19**).

Management

Genetic Testing and Screening
Routine genetic testing is not recommended for persons with hypertrophic cardiomyopathy. Genetic testing may help establish the diagnosis and provide genetic counseling. For this indication, the index adult undergoes genetic screening first. The children then can be screened for the specific gene defect. Children without the genetic defect do not have the disease; children with the defect should be followed carefully.

Echocardiographic screening is recommended for all first-degree relatives of patients with hypertrophic cardiomyopathy, at yearly intervals in adolescents and every 5 years in adults.

TABLE 19 Risk Factors for Sudden Death in Patients with Hypertrophic Cardiomyopathy

Major Risk Factors
Prior cardiac arrest
Sustained ventricular tachycardia
Family history of sudden death (in a first-degree relative younger than 40 years)
Minor Risk Factors
Unexplained syncope (≥2 episodes within 1 year)
Left ventricular septal wall thickness >30 mm in diastole
Abnormal blood pressure on exercise stress testing (systolic decrease or increase of <20 mm Hg)
Nonsustained ventricular tachycardia
Left ventricular outflow obstruction
Microvascular disease
High-risk genetic defect

Adapted with permission from Nishimura RA, Holmes DR Jr. Clinical practice. Hypertrophic obstructive cardiomyopathy [erratum in N Engl J Med. 2004;351(10):1038.]. N Engl J Med. 2004;350(13):1320-1327. [PMID: 15044643] Copyright 2004, Massachusetts Medical Society.

Medical Therapy

Patients with hypertrophic cardiomyopathy should avoid strenuous exercise, competitive sports, and intense isometric exercise such as weight-lifting. However, low- to intermediate-level aerobic activity to maintain physical fitness is reasonable.

In symptomatic patients with preserved left ventricular function, β-blockers can improve diastolic filling. Verapamil and disopyramide are useful second-line agents to improve diastolic function and alleviate symptoms. In symptomatic patients with systolic dysfunction, standard heart failure therapy and consideration for cardiac transplantation are appropriate.

It may be reasonable to treat asymptomatic patients at higher risk for sudden death with β-blockers. Digoxin and vasodilators should be avoided, as either may worsen outflow obstruction. Diuretics may be indicated for patients with persistent heart failure symptoms following treatment with a β-blocker, verapamil, and disopyramide, although hypovolemia should be avoided as it may worsen the severity of outflow obstruction.

Patients with atrial fibrillation should undergo cardioversion, and maintenance of sinus rhythm should be attempted. If atrial fibrillation is refractory, rate control and anticoagulation are essential.

Devices and Interventions

Placement of an implantable cardioverter-defibrillator (ICD) should be considered for patients at high risk for sudden death (see Table 19). The absence of any risk factors for sudden death has a negative predictive value of greater than 90%.

Surgical myectomy or alcohol septal ablation should be considered in patients with outflow obstruction and septal wall thickness of at least 18 mm who have New York Heart Association functional class III or IV heart failure and are refractory to medical therapy. Long-term comparative outcome studies are not available, and there is concern that myocardial necrosis using the percutaneous approach may not be as beneficial for prevention of sudden death as surgical removal of tissue. However, in elderly or high-risk surgical patients, the percutaneous approach may be better tolerated.

KEY POINTS

- Major risk factors for sudden cardiac death in patients with hypertrophic cardiomyopathy are previous cardiac arrest, sustained ventricular tachycardia, and family history of sudden death.
- Strenuous exercise and competitive sports should be avoided in all patients with hypertrophic cardiomyopathy.

Cardiac Tumors

Pathophysiology

Primary cardiac tumors are rare: a tumor affecting the heart is 20 times more likely to represent metastatic disease or direct extension from a noncardiac cause. Myxoma represents 50% of all benign primary cardiac tumors. On echocardiography, a myxoma typically presents as a globular left atrial mass attached to the intra-atrial septum (**Figure 11**). The myxoma may prolapse through the mitral valve in diastole, resulting in Doppler ultrasound and physical examination findings of obstructed ventricular filling similar to mitral stenosis. Other common benign cardiac tumors include lipomatous hypertrophy of the interatrial septum and papillary fibroelastomas, which typically appear as small masses attached to a valve, mimicking vegetations. Sarcomas are the most common type of malignant primary cardiac tumor; others include angiosarcoma, rhabdomyosarcoma, and osteosarcoma.

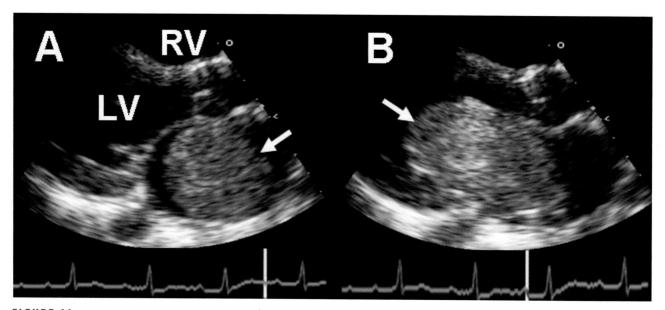

FIGURE 11.
Echocardiographic Appearance of Myxoma.
Parasternal long-axis echocardiographic views in systole (Panel A) and diastole (Panel B) of the left (LV) and right (RV) ventricles. Panel A shows a globular mass (*arrow*) in the left atrium characteristic of myxoma. In Panel B, during diastole, the mass protrudes through the mitral valve, obstructing flow (*arrow*).

Any noncardiac tumor can affect the heart, but lung and breast carcinoma are most common because of their overall prevalence. Noncardiac tumors most often affect the heart via hematogenous spread, but direct extension from breast or lung cancer also occurs. Pericardial involvement is common, and the initial clinical manifestations often are caused by pericardial effusion and tamponade physiology. Tumors that grow within and along blood vessels reach the heart by venous extension; for example, renal, hepatocellular, and adrenal carcinomas may extend into the right side of the heart via the inferior vena cava. Lung carcinoma may extend to the left atrium via the pulmonic veins.

Clinical Presentation and Evaluation

Symptoms from cardiac tumors include dyspnea, fatigue, chest pain, and constitutional symptoms. Cardiac tumors may present with embolic events, syncope, and sudden death. Pericardial tumors may cause cardiac tamponade or constriction. Endocardial tumors may cause valve dysfunction, systemic emboli, or cavity obliteration. Myocardial tumors may trigger arrhythmias or cause conduction abnormalities.

Transthoracic echocardiography is the initial imaging procedure of choice, but transesophageal echocardiography, CT, or CMR imaging often is needed for better delineation. A specific diagnosis requires histologic examination of tissue obtained by biopsy or at surgery.

Management

Benign cardiac tumors are often amenable to resection. Annual echocardiography following resection is warranted to assess for recurrences, which occur in about 5% of patients overall. Left atrial myxoma should be surgically removed even when the patient is asymptomatic to avoid systemic embolic events. In patients with prior systemic emboli, surgical removal should be considered if no other more likely cause can be identified, particularly with left-sided lesions. The prognosis of malignant primary or metastatic tumors is often poor.

KEY POINTS

- Left atrial myxoma should be surgically removed even when the patient is asymptomatic to avoid systemic embolic events.

- Myxomas may be recurrent, and periodic long-term surveillance is appropriate.

Bibliography

Elliott PM, Gimeno JR, Thaman R, et al. Historical trends in reported survival rates in patients with hypertrophic cardiomyopathy. Heart. 2006;92(6):785-791. [PMID: 16216855]

Falk, RH. Diagnosis and management of the cardiac amyloidoses. Circulation. 2005; 112(13):2047-2060. [PMID: 16186440]

Maron BJ, Estes NA 3rd, Maron MS, Almquist AK, Link MS, Udelson JE. Primary prevention of sudden death as a novel treatment strategy in hypertrophic cardiomyopathy. Circulation. 2003;107(23):2872-2875. [PMID: 12814983]

Nishimura RA, Holmes DR Jr. Clinical practice. Hypertrophic obstructive cardiomyopathy [erratum in N Engl J Med. 2004;351(10):1038.]. N Engl J Med. 2004;350(13):1320-1327. [PMID: 15044643]

Pieroni M, Chimenti C, De Cobelli F, et al. Fabry's disease cardiomyopathy: echocardiographic detection of endomyocardial glycosphingolipid compartmentalization. J Am Coll Cardiol. 2006;47(8):1663-1671. [PMID: 16631007]

Smedema JP, Snoep G, van Kroonenburgh MP, et al. Evaluation of the accuracy of gadolinium-enhanced cardiovascular magnetic resonance in the diagnosis of cardiac sarcoidosis. J Am Coll Cardiol. 2005; 45(10):1683-1690. [PMID: 15893188]

Weidemann F, Strotmann JM, Breunig F, et al. Misleading terms in Anderson-Fabry disease. Eur J Clin Invest. 2008;38(3):191-196. [PMID: 18257782]

Zipes DP, Camm AJ, Borggrefe M, et al. ACC/AHA/ESC 2006 Guidelines for Management of Patients With Ventricular Arrhythmias and the Prevention of Sudden Cardiac Death: a report of the American College of Cardiology/American Heart Association Task Force and the European Society of Cardiology Committee for Practice Guidelines. Circulation. 2006;114(10):e385-484. [PMID: 16935995]

Arrhythmias

Approach to the Patient with Bradycardia

Clinical Presentation and Evaluation

Bradycardia is defined as a heart rate of less than 60/min, although slower sinus rates are often very well tolerated. Asymptomatic resting bradycardias, particularly in the young and in athletes, are not pathologic and do not require treatment. Pathologic bradycardias are caused by disorders of impulse generation (impaired automaticity) or impulse conduction (heart block). Idiopathic causes include fibrosis and calcification of the sinus node and conduction system. The few reversible causes include Lyme disease, hypothyroidism, hyperkalemia, medications, and ischemia. Symptoms of bradycardia may range from fatigue and exercise intolerance to dizziness and syncope. A 24-hour ambulatory electrocardiogram (ECG) or event monitor should be used to correlate symptoms with heart rate. Evaluation of bradycardia includes assessment of heart rhythm, symptoms (constant versus intermittent), medications, and associated medical conditions (hypothyroidism, electrolyte abnormalities, coronary artery disease, and cardiomyopathy). Symptomatic bradycardia is treated by alleviation of the underlying cause or insertion of a permanent pacemaker. If bradycardia is caused by a medication, an alternative agent should be considered unless the benefit of the drug outweighs the risk of pacemaker placement. In patients with a pacemaker or other implanted cardiac device, MRI is contraindicated owing to possible device malfunction when exposed to strong magnetic waves.

Sick Sinus Syndrome

The terms *sick sinus syndrome* and *sinus node dysfunction* encompass various disorders of the sinus node, including reduced automaticity of the sinoatrial node, exit block, and sinus arrest. The syndrome primarily affects the elderly, and is associated with paroxysmal atrial fibrillation or flutter in approximately 50% of patients and with distal conduction disease in up to 11% of patients, presumably due to progression of the underlying degenerative process. A frequently encountered subtype is *tachycardia-bradycardia syndrome*, characterized by periods of slow sinus rhythm alternating with periods of atrial fibrillation with rapid ventricular response. Bradycardia can be worsened by rate control medications, and therefore management of the syndrome usually requires an implanted pacemaker.

Atrioventricular Block

Atrioventricular (AV) block is usually caused by fibrosis and degeneration of the conduction system but also has important associations with ischemic heart disease and medications. Symptoms are related to cerebral hypoperfusion from an inadequate heart rate. AV block can occur at the level of the AV node or in the distal conduction system and is categorized by degree and site of conduction block.

In first-degree AV block, all atrial impulses are conducted to the ventricle but there is delay, usually within the AV node, that results in a prolonged PR interval on ECG (>200 msec).

Second-degree AV block comprises two subtypes: Mobitz I and Mobitz II. Mobitz I, or Wenckebach block, consists of progressive prolongation of conduction from the atria to the ventricles, usually within the AV node, resulting in progressive prolongation of the PR interval until loss of conduction to the ventricle occurs (**Figure 12**). Mobitz I block is rarely symptomatic and does not require treatment.

Mobitz II AV block is characterized by a constant PR interval with intermittent failure of conduction from the atria to the ventricles (**Figure 13**). The pattern of dropped beats can vary from occasional to as frequently as 3:1 or 2:1. The terms *high-grade AV block* and *advanced second-degree AV block* are used to describe the occurrence of two or more consecutive nonconducted P waves with some conducted beats.

Complete heart block (third-degree heart block) (**Figure 14**) is characterized by a complete lack of conduction from the atria to the ventricles; the ventricular rate must, therefore, be slower than the atrial rate. (A complete lack of conduction with the ventricular rate faster than the atrial rate is termed *AV dissociation* and does not necessarily imply complete heart block.) A junctional escape rate is generally between 40 and 60 beats/min and demonstrates a relatively narrow QRS complex, whereas a ventricular escape rate is slower, less reliable, and demonstrates a wide QRS complex. Escape rhythms are quite regular; an irregular rhythm is likely due to intermittent AV conduction. If the cause is reversible (AV blocking drugs that can be safely withheld, ischemia with plans for revascularization, or antibiotic therapy for Lyme disease) the patient can be monitored for improvement in conduction. A pacemaker is indicated for symptomatic bradycardia due to advanced second- or third-degree heart block.

KEY POINT

- A pacemaker is indicated for symptomatic bradycardia due to advanced second- or third-degree heart block.

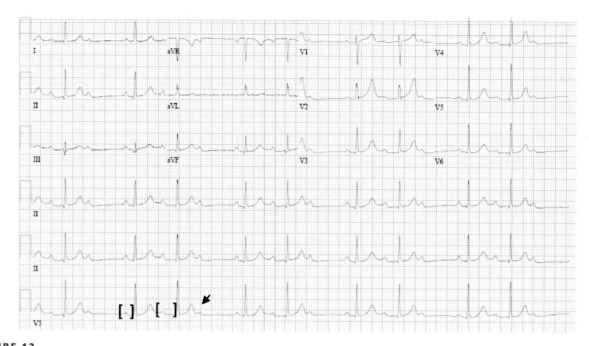

FIGURE 12.
Mobitz I Second-Degree Atrioventricular Block.
Electrocardiogram showing Mobitz I second-degree (Wenckebach) heart block. Note prolongation of PR intervals (*brackets*) followed by nonconducted P waves (*arrow*).

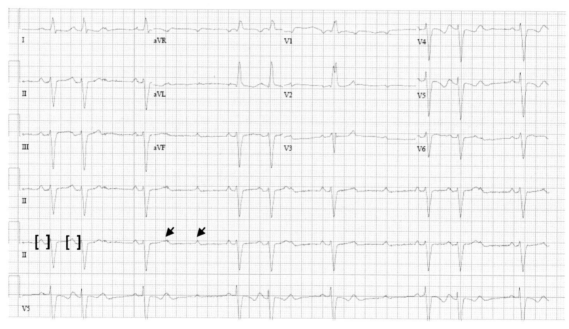

FIGURE 13.
Mobitz II Second-Degree Atrioventricular Block.
Electrocardiogram showing Mobitz II second-degree heart block. Note absence of PR prolongation (*brackets*) and successive nonconducted P waves (*arrows*).

Approach to the Patient with Tachycardia

Evaluation and Initial Management

Evaluation of patients presenting with a tachyarrhythmia starts with a resting ECG; however, symptoms of palpitations often are episodic, and recording the heart rhythm during symptoms with an ambulatory recording device is usually needed. Management of tachyarrhythmias depends on the clinical stability of the patient. Narrow-complex tachycardia is either supraventricular in origin or uses the AV node and distal conduction system as part of its circuit. Narrow-complex tachycardia can be further subdivided into irregular and regular (**Figure 15**). This differentiation helps distinguish atrial

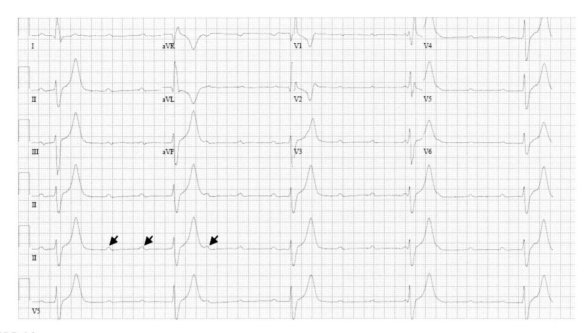

FIGURE 14.
Complete Heart Block.
Electrocardiogram showing complete heart block. Note stable R-R intervals and lack of relation of P waves (*arrows*) to the QRS complex.

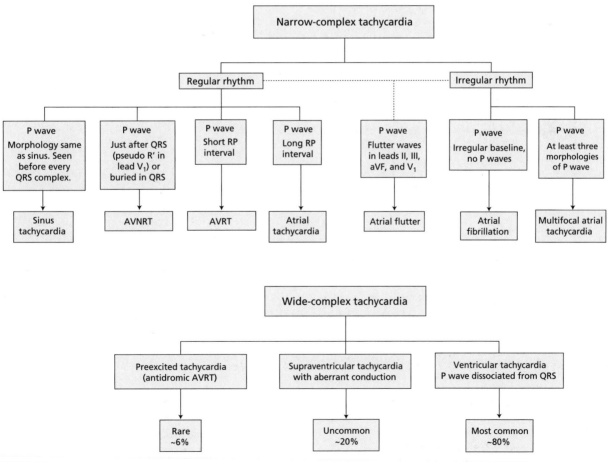

FIGURE 15.
Classification of Narrow- and Wide-Complex Tachycardias.

AVNRT = atrioventricular nodal reentry tachycardia; AVRT = atrioventricular reentry tachycardia.

fibrillation and atrial flutter from other supraventricular arrhythmias. The differential diagnosis of a wide-complex tachycardia (QRS duration >120 msec) is ventricular tachycardia (VT), supraventricular tachycardia with aberrant conduction (bundle branch block), and preexcited tachycardia due to antegrade conduction via an accessory pathway (see Figure 15). VT cannot be ruled out on the basis of hemodynamic stability of the patient, and intravenous calcium channel blockers or adenosine—appropriate for the patient with a supraventricular tachycardia—may precipitate hemodynamic collapse in the patient with VT. If the diagnosis of supraventricular tachycardia with aberrancy or of an accessory pathway–mediated tachycardia cannot be made reliably, the patient should be treated as if the rhythm is VT because statistically, VT is the most likely diagnosis.

Immediate cardioversion is the treatment of choice for patients in extremis and often is the safest choice even in hemodynamically stable patients, particularly in those with wide complex tachycardia. After termination of the arrhythmia, the ECG can provide clues regarding the presence of prior myocardial infarction, left ventricular hypertrophy, or long QT syndrome, and an echocardiogram provides evaluation for structural heart disease and assessment of left ventricular function. Exercise testing can screen for significant coronary artery disease and provoke exercise-associated tachycardias. In newly diagnosed cardiomyopathy, cardiac catheterization is often necessary to evaluate for coronary artery disease as the cause of myocardial dysfunction. Many patients with symptomatic tachycardia benefit from referral to an arrhythmia specialist to determine the utility of further invasive risk stratification or therapy, as ablation procedures are often safer and more effective than antiarrhythmic drug management.

Antiarrhythmic Drugs

Antiarrhythmic drugs are classified based on the major ion channel effect of the drug (**Table 20**). Both class I and class III antiarrhythmic drugs can cause dangerous proarrhythmia, and their use is often limited by side effects and toxicity. When used to treat atrial fibrillation, class IC agents can sometimes "organize" fibrillation to atrial flutter. Since flutter waves are less inhibiting to the AV node, the ventricular response in this situation can be very rapid. For this reason, additional AV nodal blocking agents (β-blockers, nondihydropyridine calcium-channel blockers, digoxin) should always be used in conjunction with class IC agents in atrial fibrillation. Class IC agents are contraindicated in patients with coronary artery disease owing to an increased risk of sudden cardiac death. Class III agents can prolong the QT interval and place the

TABLE 20 Antiarrhythmic Drugs

Vaughan Williams Classification	General Mechanism	Commonly Used Drugs	Clinical Uses
IA	Fast sodium channel blockade; prolongs AP duration	Procainamide	Preexcited AF, SVTs, ventricular arrhythmias
IB	Fast sodium channel blockade; shortens AP duration	Lidocaine	Ventricular arrhythmias, particularly in setting of ischemia
IC	Fast sodium channel blockade; slows conduction	Flecainide	Life-threatening ventricular arrhythmias, SVT, PAF, AFL
		Propafenone	Life-threatening ventricular arrhythmias, PAF, PAFL, PSVT
II	β-Blockade	Atenolol, metoprolol, propranolol	Adrenergically mediated tachycardias, rate control of AF, AFL, SVTs using AV node, ventricular arrhythmias, reduction in SCD after MI
III	Potassium channel blockade	Amiodarone	Useful in a wide spectrum of ventricular and supraventricular arrhythmias
		Sotalol	VT, AF, AFL, SVT
		Dofetilide	SVT, particularly AF, AFL
IV	Calcium channel blockade	Verapamil, diltiazem	Termination of SVTs, rate control of AF, AFL, therapy of SVTs, tachycardias mediated by triggered activity

AF = atrial fibrillation; AFL = atrial flutter; AP = accessory pathway; AV = atrioventricular; MI = myocardial infarction; PAF = paroxysmal atrial fibrillation; PAFL = paroxysmal atrial flutter; PSVT = paroxysmal supraventricular tachycardia; SCD = sudden cardiac death; SVT = supraventricular tachycardia; VT = ventricular tachycardia.

NOTE: For specific indications and precautions, please refer to labeling information of the medications listed.

patient at risk for torsades de pointes VT and sudden cardiac death. Initiation of sotalol and dofetilide, therefore, is usually on an inpatient basis. Despite the various toxic effect of amiodarone and QT prolongation on ECG, the risk of ventricular arrhythmia is significantly less with amiodarone than with the other class III agents.

Digoxin is widely used as an oral AV nodal blocking agent, and is particularly effective in elderly or inactive patients as its mechanism of action depends on increasing vagal activity. Adenosine is an intravenous agent that transiently blocks AV nodal conduction; it is effective at terminating supraventricular tachycardia where the electrical circuit is dependent on the AV node.

KEY POINTS

- A wide-complex tachycardia should be treated as ventricular tachycardia unless the diagnosis of supraventricular tachycardia with aberrancy or of an accessory pathway–mediated tachycardia is certain.

- Adenosine and calcium channel blockers should be avoided in patients with possible ventricular tachycardia, particularly those with myocardial dysfunction.

Atrial Fibrillation

Atrial fibrillation is the most common clinical arrhythmia and is characterized by disorganized atrial activity and an irregular ventricular response to the chaotic input into the AV node. Atrial fibrillation may be categorized as paroxysmal, persistent, or permanent.

Clinical Presentation and Evaluation

Symptoms of atrial fibrillation include palpitations, fatigue, exercise intolerance, dyspnea, chest discomfort, dizziness, and syncope; atrial fibrillation can also be asymptomatic. Patients may present with heart failure or with a stroke. Symptoms can lessen over time, particularly if atrial fibrillation becomes permanent.

Several factors play a role in the development of symptomatic atrial fibrillation, including the ventricular response rate (either too slow or too fast), decreased cardiac output due to loss of atrial contraction, variability in R-R intervals (experienced as an uncomfortable awareness of irregularity), and impaired coronary blood flow. Atrial function during episodes of atrial fibrillation tends to decline over time as a result of electroanatomic remodeling of the atria as well as underlying atrial disease. In patients with long-standing uncontrolled high ventricular rates (>130 beats/min), a tachycardia-related cardiomyopathy can develop.

Hypertension is commonly associated with atrial fibrillation. Associated cardiovascular conditions include coronary artery disease; valvular heart disease; dilated, hypertrophic, and restrictive cardiomyopathies; heart failure; and preexcitation syndromes.

Atrial fibrillation is a common, but generally self-limited, postoperative complication of cardiothoracic surgery. Other common reversible causes include alcohol, thyroid disorders, myocarditis or pericarditis, and pulmonary embolism.

Acute Management

Approximately 50% of episodes of atrial fibrillation spontaneously convert. Patients with adverse or marginal hemodynamic status or acute coronary ischemia due to a rapid ventricular response should be immediately cardioverted. Otherwise stable patients with a rapid ventricular response are usually managed with AV nodal blocking agents. β-Blockers and calcium channel blockers are preferred to digoxin owing to digoxin's lack of efficacy in the presence of normal sympathetic tone. Digoxin can be useful as an adjunct to other rate control agents, particularly in the setting of heart failure and in elderly or sedentary patients. In preexcited atrial fibrillation with a rapidly conducting accessory pathway, AV nodal blocking agents should be avoided because of the risk of increasing conduction through the accessory pathway, thereby provoking ventricular fibrillation. A patient who presents with asymptomatic rate-controlled atrial fibrillation can often be managed as an outpatient. Rapid or bradycardic ventricular response or signs and symptoms of heart failure, ischemia, or other distress should prompt admission.

Acute Anticoagulation

Not all patients with newly diagnosed atrial fibrillation require acute anticoagulation with heparin. Asymptomatic patients with good rate control who require long-term anticoagulation with aspirin or warfarin can have this initiated as an outpatient. If heparin is initiated as an inpatient, it will usually be continued until the patient is therapeutically anticoagulated on warfarin. Limited data are available to support the use of low-molecular-weight heparin.

Cardioversion

Synchronized direct-current cardioversion is an effective method of converting atrial fibrillation to sinus rhythm. Patients who have been in atrial fibrillation for less than 48 hours may be cardioverted without anticoagulation. In patients with atrial fibrillation of longer or unknown duration, cardioversion can be performed after at least 3 weeks of anticoagulation with warfarin (INR 2.0-3.0). Alternatively, the patient can undergo transesophageal echocardiography to rule out thrombus in the left atrial appendage while anticoagulated on intravenous heparin. Following cardioversion, oral anticoagulation is initiated and maintained for at least 4 weeks after the procedure because the risk of subsequent thromboembolism remains high owing to mechanical dysfunction of the left atrium and appendage.

Cardioversion is safe in patients with implanted pacemakers and defibrillators, although care should be taken to position the cardioversion pads away from the generator to reduce the risk of electromagnetic interference.

Long-Term Management

Rate Control Versus Rhythm Control

There are two strategies in the treatment of persistent or paroxysmal atrial fibrillation: controlling the ventricular response rate to atrial fibrillation (rate control) and using antiarrhythmic drugs to maintain sinus rhythm (rhythm control). The use of anticoagulation for stroke prevention is not affected by choice of approach. The Atrial Fibrillation Follow-up Investigation of Rhythm Management (AFFIRM) trial showed no survival advantage to a rhythm control strategy. However, the average age of patients in the trial was 70 years, and patients were relatively asymptomatic and could tolerate randomization to either approach. In younger, symptomatic patients, restoration of sinus rhythm has been shown to decrease left atrial size and improve left atrial contractility. In addition, quality of life may be improved with maintenance of sinus rhythm.

Whether atrial fibrillation is paroxysmal or persistent is important because the ability to maintain sinus rhythm is reduced in patients with persistent episodes. When significant structural heart disease is present, correction of the structural or hemodynamic abnormality may be necessary before atrial fibrillation can be effectively managed. Medications that block AV nodal conduction—normally β-blockers or nondihydropyridine calcium-channel blockers—are preferred for rate control treatment of chronic atrial fibrillation (see Table 20). Reasonable rate control is defined as a ventricular rate of 60-80/min at rest with an increase with exercise to 90-115/min. Bradycardia can be an adverse effect of rate-control agents, particularly in the elderly. Occasionally, pacemaker placement is required for bradycardia resulting from the medication dose needed to provide adequate control of rapid ventricular rates.

Preferred rhythm control medications are class III and class IC agents. Class IC agents should not be given for atrial fibrillation without additional AV nodal blockade. Amiodarone is the most effective antiarrhythmic agent, and in patients with structural heart disease, amiodarone has a low risk of proarrhythmia in comparison with other agents. Even with rhythm control drugs, the recurrence rate of symptomatic atrial fibrillation is 20% to 50% in the long term (>1 year).

Anticoagulation to Reduce Stroke Risk

The annual risk of stroke in atrial fibrillation patients is 1%-18%. The classification of type of atrial fibrillation (paroxysmal, persistent, or permanent) does not affect the decision to anticoagulate, as the amount and duration of atrial fibrillation have not been shown to alter the risk of stroke. The $CHADS_2$ risk score for assessing the risk of stroke associated with atrial fibrillation and the benefit of warfarin has been validated in a large population (**Table 21**).

The choice of aspirin or warfarin for anticoagulation to prevent thromboembolism is dependent on the patient's

TABLE 21 Anticoagulation in Atrial Fibrillation

$CHADS_2$ Score[a]	Stroke Risk	Warfarin
0	Low	No
1	Intermediate	Individualized[b]
2	Intermediate or high[c]	Individualized
3	High	Yes
4	High	Yes
5	High	Yes
6	High	Yes

[a]$CHADS_2$ score is calculated by assigning 1 point each for the presence of chronic heart failure, hypertension, age 75 years or older, and diabetes mellitus; and 2 points for history of stroke or transient ischemic attack.

[b]For patients at intermediate risk, the risks and benefits of anticoagulation are assessed based on individual factors such as comorbidities, risk of hemorrhage, and patient preference.

[c]History of stroke or transient ischemic attack confers high risk regardless of score.

individual risk. Patients with nonvalvular atrial fibrillation at high risk of stroke (for example, with rheumatic mitral stenosis or prior thromboembolism) should be maintained on warfarin with a goal INR of 2.0-3.0. Warfarin (INR 2.0-3.0) is also recommended for those with one or more moderate risk factors (age >75 years, hypertension, diabetes mellitus, heart failure, or ejection fraction <35%). For patients with just one of these risk factors, aspirin is a reasonable choice. Warfarin is not recommended for patients younger than 60 years without other associated risk factors. For patients with atrial fibrillation and mechanical heart valves, the intensity of anticoagulation depends on the type of valve. Warfarin has repeatedly been shown to significantly reduce the risk of stroke associated with atrial fibrillation by about 60%, compared with 20% with aspirin, with a risk of major bleeding of approximately 1% to 2% per year. The restoration and maintenance of sinus rhythm have not been shown to decrease the risk of stroke; therefore, anticoagulation or aspirin based on the $CHADS_2$ score remains appropriate in patients with a history of atrial fibrillation.

Nonpharmacologic Therapies

Atrioventricular Junction Ablation and Pacing

In patients with an uncontrollable ventricular response in whom other strategies have failed, or to treat or prevent the development of a tachycardia-related cardiomyopathy, atrioventricular junction ablation and pacemaker placement can be performed. Because the patient is rendered pacemaker-dependent, this procedure is usually restricted to elderly patients in whom other options have been exhausted.

Radiofrequency Ablation

In curative radiofrequency ablation procedures for atrial fibrillation, a catheter is used to apply radiofrequency energy to selected areas of the left atrium, rendering the ablated tissue unable to conduct electrical current. The success rate of the procedure can be greater than 80%, although the specific techniques and methods continue to evolve. Candidates for atrial fibrillation ablation generally consist of patients who cannot tolerate a rate control strategy who have failed to benefit from at least one rhythm control drug. Significant valvular disease or hypertrophic cardiomyopathy and advanced age are relative contraindications.

Surgical Maze Procedures

Surgical "maze" procedures to cure atrial fibrillation have been quite successful; however, they have been limited by the necessity for cardiopulmonary bypass and are usually performed in concert with other cardiac surgical procedures. Reported success rates range from **70% to 95%**, and the development of less invasive techniques (minimally invasive or thoracoscopic approaches) is an active area of research.

KEY POINTS

- Anticoagulation with warfarin is recommended for patients with atrial fibrillation and one or more risk factors for thromboembolism.

- Patients with atrial fibrillation and a history of stroke or transient ischemic attack should receive warfarin.

- For patients with asymptomatic atrial fibrillation, a rate control management strategy is acceptable.

- Patients with atrial fibrillation who are symptomatic despite rate control and those whose rates cannot be controlled may require a rhythm control strategy.

Atrial Flutter

Atrial flutter is often associated with atrial fibrillation, but the underlying arrhythmic mechanism and many aspects of clinical management differ. Approximately 90% of cases are considered typical or common atrial flutter, consisting of a well-described macro-reentrant electrical circuit that traverses around the tricuspid valve. This circuit passes through the cavotricuspid isthmus, a narrow rim of tissue between the tricuspid valve and the inferior vena cava. The atrial circuit usually travels at about 240-340 cycles/min in the counterclockwise direction around the valve (as seen from a traditional left anterior oblique fluoroscopic view), which accounts for the characteristic negative sawtooth deflections in ECG leads II, III, and aVF, with a positive deflection in V_1 (**Figure 16**). The circuit can also travel in the opposite direction, inscribing the ECG in a reverse manner.

Clinical Presentation and Evaluation

Medical conditions that are more often associated with atrial flutter rather than fibrillation include congenital heart disease, pulmonary disease, hypertension, diabetes, obesity, thyroid disorders, sick sinus syndrome, and major cardiothoracic surgery. Compared to atrial fibrillation, atrial flutter is characterized by fewer and more regular electrical impulses reaching the AV node; the ventricular response to atrial flutter, therefore, is often very fast—2:1 conduction results in a ventricular rate of 150/min.

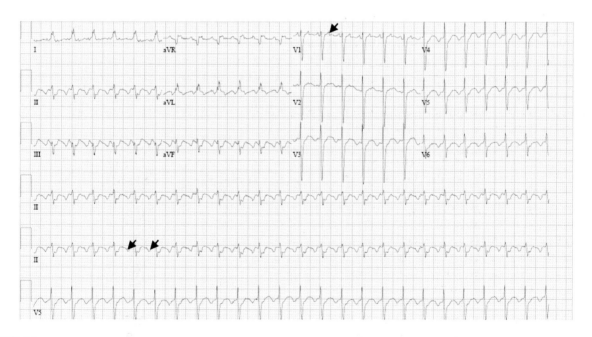

FIGURE 16.
Atrial Flutter.
Electrocardiogram showing typical atrial flutter with 2:1 conduction to the ventricles. Flutter waves (*arrows*), with cycle length of approximately 300/min, are most easily seen in the inferior leads (II, III, aVF) and lead V_1.

Acute Management

Early cardioversion often is needed because of the rapid ventricular response to atrial flutter. Cardioversion is highly effective at terminating atrial flutter; however, pharmacologic approaches can be tried first in hemodynamically stable patients. For pharmacologic conversion to sinus rhythm, class I agents are less effective in atrial flutter than in atrial fibrillation; class III agents are often more efficacious in atrial flutter. Rate control agents include β-blockers and nondihydropyridine calcium-channel blockers (class II and class IV agents). Digoxin is not particularly useful as a first-line agent in atrial flutter but can be an effective adjunct. Acute anticoagulation guidelines for patients with atrial flutter are the same as those for atrial fibrillation.

Chronic Management

Percutaneous radiofrequency ablation is first-line therapy for recurrent atrial flutter; it has a success rate of greater than 90%, a recurrence rate less than 10%, and a 1% to 2% risk of major complications (vascular damage, heart block, stroke, tamponade, death). The recurrence rate for atrial flutter that has not been ablated is 60% (>6 months). The occurrence of other arrhythmias after radiofrequency ablation is relatively common (usually atrial fibrillation or atypical atrial flutter— an atrial-based electrical circuit that does not revolve around the tricuspid valve). Therefore, for patients with risk factors for stroke, anticoagulation may still be required after ablation. Current guidelines recommend using the atrial fibrillation risk assessment to determine the benefits of anticoagulation.

KEY POINT

- Radiofrequency ablation is a successful and low-risk option for treatment of typical atrial flutter.

Supraventricular Tachycardias

Epidemiology and Electrophysiology

The term *supraventricular tachycardia* generally comprises AV nodal reentrant tachycardia (AVNRT), which has a reentrant circuit within the AV node; AV reentrant tachycardia (AVRT), which uses an accessory bypass tract; and atrial tachycardia. This group is often referred to as paroxysmal supraventricular tachycardias. Other rare narrow-complex tachycardias include inappropriate sinus tachycardia, sinus node reentrant tachycardia, and junctional tachycardia.

AVNRT accounts for approximately 60% of cases, AVRT for 30%, and atrial tachycardia for 10%. Reentry using two pathways from atrium to ventricle is the underlying mechanism of both AVNRT and AVRT. In *typical* AVNRT, anterograde conduction occurs via the *slow pathway*, and retrograde conduction occurs via the *fast pathway*. On the surface electrocardiogram, the P wave is seen either just after the QRS complex (short RP) or buried within it (no RP). In *atypical* AVNRT, the circuit is reversed. Because the slow pathway conducts more slowly, the P wave is seen on the surface electrocardiogram much later, just preceding the next QRS complex (long RP).

Accessory pathways or bypass tracts, present in AVRT, typically connect atrial with ventricular myocardium, bypassing the AV node and resulting in electrical activation of the ventricle earlier than expected (preexcitation). Accessory pathways that conduct anterograde (from atrium to ventricle) are characterized as *manifest,* and ventricular preexcitation can be seen on ECG as a delta wave (a slurred upstroke just before the QRS). Accessory pathways that can only conduct retrograde are termed *concealed* and cannot be identified on ECG. Preexcitation of the ventricle can be intermittent, owing to the conduction properties of the accessory pathway or to preferential conduction down the AV node. Accessory pathways usually demonstrate rapid conduction even at high rates of input similar to His-Purkinje tissue or myocardium. In contrast, the AV node is characterized by "decremental" conduction (progressive delay in conduction with increasing rate of input).

Atrial tachycardia (**Figure 17**) usually results from enhanced automaticity of a group of atrial cells. Triggered activity (spontaneously generated heart beats due to afterdepolarizations that reach the threshold potential) or reentry (particularly in patients with congenital heart disease or prior cardiac surgery) are less common mechanisms.

Clinical Presentation and Evaluation

Most patients with a supraventricular tachycardia have acute-onset episodic palpitations that may be associated with chest or neck pounding, dyspnea, lightheadedness, anxiety, and, rarely, syncope. Supraventricular tachycardias are commonly characterized by abrupt onset and termination and often respond well to vagal maneuvers, such as a guided Valsalva maneuver, squatting, carotid sinus massage, or cold water facial immersion.

In addition to a resting ECG, the arrhythmias should be recorded using an event monitor (or a loop recorder, if the patient experiences syncope). Evaluation for exacerbating factors (anemia, hyperthyroidism) is appropriate. An echocardiogram should be considered if there are symptoms or signs of structural heart disease.

In patients with symptoms and manifest preexcitation on ECG (Wolff-Parkinson-White syndrome), referral to an electrophysiologist for percutaneous ablation of the accessory pathway is considered first-line therapy because of the very small, yet persistent, risk of sudden death in this population. Early referral should also be considered for patients with syncope, dyspnea, or heart failure.

Acute Management

Initial management for a supraventricular tachycardia depends on the patient's hemodynamic stability. Many patients respond well to vagal maneuvers. Adenosine bolus injection is

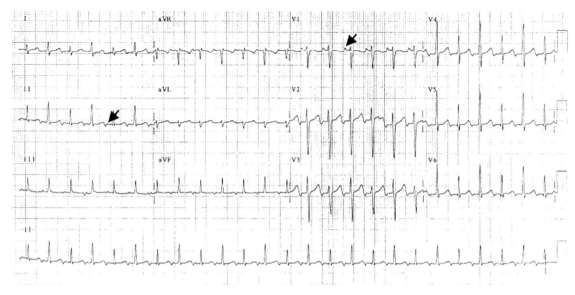

FIGURE 17.
Atrial Tachycardia.
Electrocardiogram showing atrial tachycardia. P waves are most clearly seen in lead V_1 and at the end of the T wave in other leads (*arrows*).

highly effective at terminating tachycardias that use the AV node as part of the circuit as well as providing diagnostic information in unclear cases (such as revealing flutter waves during AV block or revealing an underlying atrial tachycardia). A continuous rhythm strip should be run during the time of injection. It can be helpful to inform patients that the half-life of the drug is seconds and warn that they may experience uncomfortable or distressing sensations during the procedure. Adenosine is contraindicated in patients with severe bronchospastic disease. Intravenous calcium channel blockers are also recommended for termination of a tachycardia. Intravenous β-blockers or amiodarone may be used as second-line therapy. Although it is rarely necessary, cardioversion is effective at terminating reentry supraventricular tachycardias. Cardioversion and adenosine are often ineffective for atrial tachycardia because the usual mechanism is enhanced automaticity, and even if briefly terminated, the arrhythmia will resume. However, the underlying mechanism of supraventricular tachycardia is not always definitive on ECG, and synchronized cardioversion is very low risk.

Long-Term Management

Patients with extremely rare episodes of supraventricular tachycardia that can be easily terminated with Valsalva maneuvers may opt for a watchful approach. Obvious triggers of episodes, such as caffeine and dehydration, can often be avoided. Low-dose β-blockers or calcium channel blockers can abbreviate or eliminate episodes, although these agents are relatively contraindicated in patients with preexcitation. Antiarrhythmic drugs are a management option, although they are less frequently used as first-line therapy than previously because of the low risk and high success rate of ablation

therapy. Catheter ablation is a safe and effective treatment, with success rates of 95% to 99% in AVNRT and AVRT and low rates of complications (1%-2%). The success rate of catheter ablation for atrial tachycardia is somewhat lower than for other supraventricular tachycardias, but the risk of complications is also quite low.

Wolff-Parkinson-White Syndrome

The Wolff-Parkinson-White (WPW) syndrome is characterized by ventricular preexcitation and symptomatic tachycardia (**Figure 18**). In these patients, AVRT is the most common arrhythmia. Other preexcited tachycardias are seen in patients with WPW syndrome in which the accessory pathway is not a critical part of the supraventricular tachycardia circuit but acts as a bystander. Owing to the rapid conduction properties of some accessory pathways, atrial fibrillation can be a life-threatening arrhythmia in these patients due to rapidly conducting atrial fibrillation degenerating to ventricular fibrillation. In addition, patients with WPW syndrome appear to have an increased risk of atrial fibrillation; this risk is reduced with radiofrequency ablation of the accessory pathway. Patients with WPW syndrome have an increased risk of sudden cardiac death, but it is very rarely the first symptomatic manifestation of the syndrome.

Treatment of a narrow-complex tachycardia is standard in patients with WPW syndrome, but care should be taken in preexcited, usually wide-complex, tachycardia. AV-nodal blocking agents should be used with caution in patients with WPW syndrome because of the risk of atrial fibrillation and rapid conduction down the bypass tract. AV-nodal blocking agents are absolutely contraindicated in patients with WPW syndrome and preexcited atrial fibrillation. In

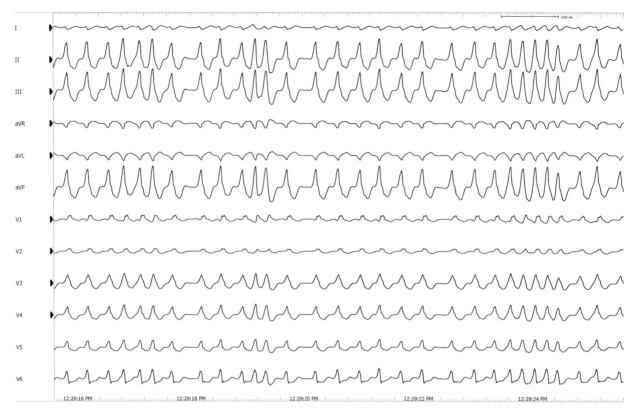

FIGURE 18.
Preexcited Atrial Fibrillation.
Electrocardiogram showing atrial fibrillation in a patient with an accessory atrioventricular pathway. In patients with Wolff-Parkinson-White syndrome and atrial fibrillation, the rapid atrial impulses travel to the ventricle through both the normal conduction system and the accessory pathway. Because of the chaotic electrical activity in the atria, the degree of conduction via both pathways is quite variable. Therefore, the electrocardiogram shows variable degrees of preexcitation (manifested by variable QRS complex widths) and great irregularity.

this circumstance, antiarrhythmic medications such as procainamide should be used to treat the arrhythmia. For long-term treatment, drug management is rarely used in patients with WPW syndrome owing to the high success rates of radiofrequency ablation and the persistent risk of sudden cardiac death when ablation is not performed.

The role of electrophysiology study and ablation in asymptomatic patients with manifest preexcitation is controversial because the vast majority of these patients have an excellent prognosis. Invasive studies are sometimes performed in patients with high-risk occupations (such as airplane pilots).

KEY POINTS

- Radiofrequency ablation is first-line therapy for Wolff-Parkinson-White syndrome.
- Atrioventricular nodal blockade is contraindicated in patients with preexcited atrial fibrillation.

Premature Ventricular Complexes

Premature ventricular complexes (PVCs) often are not associated with symptoms, although they can cause palpitations or

a sensation that the heart has stopped, owing to the post-PVC compensatory pause. PVCs at rest in the setting of a structurally normal heart appear to be associated with little to no increased risk of cardiovascular events, particularly in patients younger than 30 years. However, some studies have shown an increased mortality risk with exercise- and recovery-induced PVCs. This risk increase is small and constitutes a marker of cardiovascular disease, not an indication to treat the arrhythmia. Repetitive or complex ectopy in the setting of heart disease is associated with increased mortality risk, although the risk is due to the underlying pathophysiologic substrate, and suppression of ambient ventricular arrhythmias does not reduce mortality.

If symptoms can be clearly correlated with PVCs, treatment may be appropriate, although many patients respond well to reassurance. First-line therapy is almost always a β-blocker or calcium channel blocker. Class IC and III agents also can be useful. Radiofrequency ablation may be appropriate for patients with severe symptoms that are refractory to drug therapy.

Nonsustained Ventricular Tachycardia

Nonsustained ventricular tachycardia (VT) is defined as three or more sequential ventricular complexes, with a total duration of less than 30 seconds. The prevalence of nonsustained VT increases with age, left ventricular dysfunction, and the presence of cardiomyopathies. The prevalence of nonsustained VT in patients with chronic heart failure ranges from 30% to 80%. Nonsustained VT in patients with structurally normal hearts is not associated with an increased risk of sudden death.

Nonsustained VT in the setting of an acute myocardial infarction (within 48 hours) does not confer additional risk. However, nonsustained VT occurring in the year following myocardial infarction is associated with increased mortality. Management includes treatment of reversible ischemia, but if ejection fraction is normal, no other therapy for asymptomatic VT is indicated. If the ejection fraction is 35% or less, most patients are candidates for an implantable cardioverter-defibrillator (ICD). Electrophysiology study can be used for further risk stratification in patients with moderately reduced ventricular function (ejection fraction 35%-55%), and ICD placement is indicated for prevention of sudden death if the electrophysiology study shows inducible sustained VT.

Therapy for symptomatic nonsustained VT is similar to treatment for PVCs. β-blockers are the mainstay, although calcium channel blockers also may be used in patients with structurally normal hearts. The most frequently used class III antiarrhythmic agents are amiodarone and sotalol; class IC agents such as flecainide and propafenone are limited to use in patients without coronary artery disease.

Patients in whom drug therapy for nonsustained VT fails can be referred for radiofrequency ablation. Suppression of nonsustained VT by medical therapy in patients with a high risk of sudden death has not shown a mortality benefit.

Sustained Ventricular Tachycardia

VT is considered sustained if the rate is greater than 100/min with an episode lasting longer than 30 seconds (or less than 30 seconds if cardioversion is required). Most commonly, the mechanism of VT is reentry, which occurs around an area of conduction block usually caused by prior myocardial infarction. Other, less frequent causes are triggered activity and enhanced automaticity.

The prognosis of a patient with monomorphic (all complexes showing the same morphology) VT is dependent on the presence or absence of structural heart disease. In contrast, polymorphic VT is most often related to an underlying genetic defect predisposing to often fatal cardiac arrhythmias. Sustained, symptomatic VT in ischemic or nonischemic cardiomyopathy is an adverse prognostic indicator with a high risk of recurrence.

Ventricular Tachycardia with Structural Heart Disease

Sustained VT occurs most commonly in patients with prior myocardial infarction, and it is the scar formed by the infarction that provides the anatomic substrate for reentry. Areas of fibrosis interspersed with viable myocardial tissue are present in the border zone of dense scar tissue and impart the required conduction delay critical to the establishment of reentry circuits. Symptoms depend on the underlying state of the patient, and some patients can be asymptomatic, particularly if the VT rate is slow.

In general, medical therapy does not improve survival in patients with VT and structural heart disease; thus, most such patients are candidates for ICD placement. Large clinical trials have demonstrated that ICD therapy improves survival rates in patients with hemodynamically unstable VT after cardiac arrest who have ischemic or nonischemic cardiomyopathy and ejection fractions below 35%. Electrophysiology study can be useful to establish the diagnosis of VT if there is uncertainty or for radiofrequency ablation if a patient has recurrent shocks from the ICD.

Idiopathic Ventricular Tachycardia

Idiopathic VT occurs most commonly as right ventricular outflow tract tachycardia. The condition is usually benign, although there is some overlap between right ventricular outflow tract tachycardia and arrhythmogenic right ventricular cardiomyopathy. As part of initial evaluation, many of these patients undergo cardiac MRI to assess for fibrofatty infiltrate of the right ventricle (the hallmark of arrhythmogenic right ventricular cardiomyopathy) in addition to standard evaluations.

Idiopathic right ventricular outflow tract tachycardia has a characteristic ECG morphology with a left bundle branch block and tall, monophasic R waves in the inferior leads. The origin is usually high in the right ventricular outflow tract under the pulmonic valve. Typically, this arrhythmia is very catecholamine-sensitive and is triggered by exercise or stress.

If symptoms are mild and infrequent, no therapy is necessary. If treatment is necessary, the arrhythmia can often be suppressed by calcium channel blockers or β-blockers. Class I or class III antiarrhythmic drugs also can be used. Radiofrequency ablation has a success rate of greater than 90% with a low risk of complications.

Sudden Cardiac Death

Epidemiology and Risk Factors

Sudden cardiac death (SCD) is usually defined as collapse occurring within 1 hour of symptom development. The majority of SCD events occur out of the hospital, and 50% of events are the first expression of undiagnosed coronary artery disease. The mechanism is usually a ventricular tachyarrhythmia.

Ventricular fibrillation is the most commonly recorded rhythm, although this can represent a degeneration of prior monomorphic or polymorphic VT. Asystole is a significantly less frequent cause of SCD.

Risk factors for SCD include diabetes, hypertension, hypercholesterolemia, family history of coronary artery disease, smoking, obesity, physical inactivity, heart failure, left ventricular hypertrophy, and heavy alcohol use. Triggers of SCD include electrolyte disturbances, drugs (cocaine, QT-prolonging drugs, antiarrhythmic drugs), acute exercise, and emotional stress. However, most SCD victims do not have identifiable risk factors (**Figure 19**).

Genetics

A predisposition to SCD has been described for certain mutations in familial dilated cardiomyopathy, arrhythmogenic right ventricular cardiomyopathy, and hypertrophic cardiomyopathy; mutations that cause primary electrical disorders (ion "channelopathies"); and polymorphisms in several genes that

confer increased risk of SCD on a population basis, without affecting cardiac structure.

The long QT syndrome is characterized by prolonged ventricular repolarization and a predisposition to the development of torsades de pointes, polymorphic VT, and SCD. Patients can be diagnosed after presenting with syncope, or a prolonged QTc interval can be an incidental finding on ECG. Risk of arrhythmic events is predicted by the presence of a QTc interval greater than 500 msec, female sex, and genotype. β-blockers are the mainstay of therapy. ICD implantation is usually performed in patients at high risk of SCD (recurrent events on β-blockers, strong family history of SCD).

The Brugada syndrome is distinguished by a characteristic ECG pattern of J-point elevation in leads V_1 through V_3 and right bundle branch block (**Figure 20**). The pattern can be intermittent, making diagnosis difficult. Patients with a history of syncope and a spontaneous Brugada pattern on ECG are significantly more likely to have cardiac arrest than patients with the Brugada pattern and no syncope. SCD in

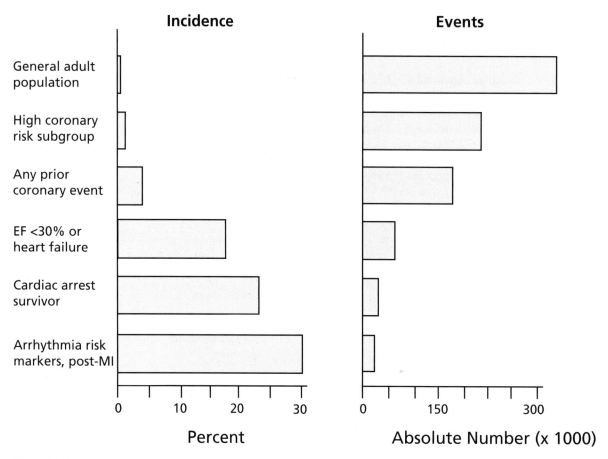

FIGURE 19.
Epidemiology of Sudden Cardiac Death.
Relation between incidence and total number of sudden cardiac deaths annually in the general population and in increasingly higher risk subgroups.

EF = ejection fraction; MI = myocardial infarction.

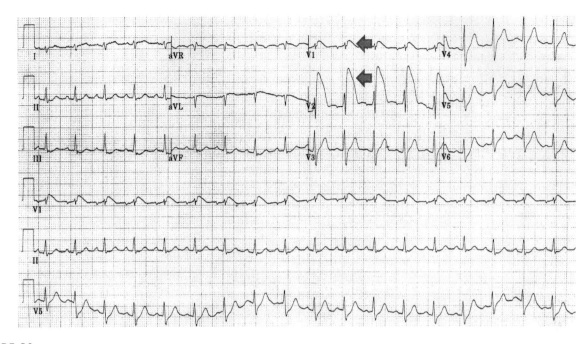

FIGURE 20.
Brugada Syndrome.
Electrocardiogram showing type I Brugada sign with coved-type ST-segment elevation (*arrows*) and a right bundle branch block pattern in the right precordial leads.
Image courtesy of Patrick T. Ellinor, MD, PhD, Massachusetts General Hospital.

the Brugada syndrome is caused by polymorphic VT or ventricular fibrillation, often occurring during sleep. ICD implantation is indicated for symptomatic patients.

Other described inherited arrhythmic disorders include short QT syndrome (QT interval <300 msec), which carries a high risk of SCD; and catecholaminergic polymorphic VT, caused by cardiac ryanodine receptor mutations and characterized by VT that develops during physical activity or emotional stress.

Most cardiomyopathies, both dilated and infiltrative, substantially increase the risk of SCD. Even within subtypes of a disease, certain gene mutations may confer additional risk of arrhythmia. Patients with arrhythmogenic right ventricular cardiomyopathy tend to be affected more by arrhythmias than by heart failure. SCD can be the first manifestation of arrhythmogenic right ventricular cardiomyopathy, and although it usually occurs in patients with right ventricular abnormalities visible on echocardiogram, it also can occur in persons with only microscopic abnormalities on autopsy.

Acute Management

Survival in cardiac arrest is proportional to intervention time and falls rapidly without intervention. Ventricular arrhythmias are treated with cardioversion or defibrillation, although some studies have indicated improved survival after a brief period of cardiopulmonary resuscitation if there is a delay in responding of more than 1 or 2 minutes. The most recent guidelines recommend a one-shock strategy rather than three successive shocks to allow quick resumption of chest

compressions. Epinephrine or vasopressin is recommended for hemodynamic support. Amiodarone has largely replaced other antiarrhythmic agents for resistant VTs, although lidocaine can be useful in coronary ischemia. The induction of mild to moderate hypothermia after resuscitation has demonstrated improved neurologic outcome.

Pulseless electrical activity and asystole differ markedly in underlying pathophysiology from ventricular tachyarrhythmias, and identification of either of these conditions should lead to consideration of potentially reversible causes, including pulmonary embolism, myocardial infarction, tamponade, tension pneumothorax, acidosis, drug overdose, hyperkalemia, hypothermia, and hypoxia. In addition to epinephrine, atropine is often used in these patients to increase heart rate.

Long-Term Management and Secondary Prevention

Most cardiac arrest survivors and patients with malignant ventricular arrhythmias have a 20% to 50% risk of recurrence, and no trials of antiarrhythmic drugs have shown a benefit in outcome from their use in these patients. In contrast, randomized clinical trials have demonstrated a marked benefit of ICD implantation. The landmark Antiarrhythmic Versus Implantable Defibrillator (AVID) trial showed a 27% to 39% reduction in mortality in patients randomized to ICD placement compared with antiarrhythmic drugs (primarily amiodarone).

Inappropriate ICD shocks are common and may be caused by mechanical lead dysfunction, supraventricular tachycardias, sinus tachycardia, and electromagnetic interference. In the absence of symptoms, an isolated shock does not require emergent evaluation. However, patients experiencing cardiac symptoms or multiple shocks should be referred to the emergency department. In most cases, the ICD can be temporarily disabled by magnet application pending further assessment. The response of an ICD to magnet application differs from the response of a pacemaker. Magnet application to a pacemaker causes temporary reversion to "magnet mode"—asynchronous pacing at a preset rate (usually 80-100 beats/min). Magnet application to an ICD only disables tachycardia therapy—it does not affect the pacemaker function of the ICD. ICD shocks are usually painful and frightening, and anxiolytics can be helpful in the treatment of both appropriate and inappropriate shocks.

KEY POINTS

- Ventricular fibrillation is the most common mechanism of sudden cardiac death.

- Implantable cardioverter-defibrillator placement reduces the risk of sudden cardiac death and overall mortality in patients with impaired ejection fraction and cardiomyopathy.

- Implantable cardioverter-defibrillator placement reduces the risk of recurrent sudden cardiac death in cardiac arrest survivors.

Bibliography

Bardy GH, Lee KL, Mark DB, et al; Sudden Cardiac Death in Heart Failure Trial (SCD-HeFT) Investigators. Amiodarone or an implantable cardioverter-defibrillator for congestive heart failure [erratum in N Engl J Med. 2005;352(20):2146.]. N Engl J Med. 2005;352(3):225-237. [PMID: 15659722]

Blomström-Lundqvist C, Scheinman MM, Aliot EM, et al. ACC/AHA/ESC guidelines for the management of patients with supraventricular arrhythmias—executive summary: a report of the American College of Cardiology/ American Heart Association Task Force on Practice Guidelines and the European Society of Cardiology Committee for Practice Guidelines (Writing Committee to Develop Guidelines for the Management of Patients With Supraventricular Arrhythmias). Circulation. 2003;108(15):1871-1909. [PMID: 14557344]

Epstein AE, DiMarco JP, Ellenbogen KA, et al. ACC/AHA/HRS 2008 Guidelines for Device-Based Therapy of Cardiac Rhythm Abnormalities: a report of the American College of Cardiology/ American Heart Association Task Force on Practice Guidelines (Writing Committee to Revise the ACC/AHA/NASPE 2002 Guideline Update for Implantation of Cardiac Pacemakers and Antiarrhythmia Devices): developed in collaboration with the American Association for Thoracic Surgery and Society of Thoracic Surgeons. Circulation. 2008;117(21):e350-408. [PMID: 18483207]

Fuster V, Rydén LE, Cannom DS, et al. ACC/AHA/ESC 2006 Guidelines for the Management of Patients with Atrial Fibrillation: a report of the American College of Cardiology/American Heart Association Task Force on Practice Guidelines and the European Society of Cardiology Committee for Practice Guidelines (Writing Committee to Revise the 2001 Guidelines for the Management of Patients With Atrial Fibrillation): developed in collaboration with the European Heart Rhythm Association and the Heart Rhythm Society. Circulation. 2006;114(7):e257-354. [PMID: 16908781]

Gregoratos G, Abrams J, Epstein AE, et al. ACC/AHA/NASPE 2002 guideline update for implantation of cardiac pacemakers and antiarrhythmia devices: summary article: a report of the American College of Cardiology/American Heart Association Task Force on Practice Guidelines (ACC/ AHA/NASPE Committee to Update the 1998 Pacemaker Guidelines). Circulation. 2002;106(16):2145-2161. [PMID: 12379588]

Moss AJ, Zareba W, Hall WJ, et al; Multicenter Automatic Defibrillator Implantation Trial II Investigators. Prophylactic implantation of a defibrillator in patients with myocardial infarction and reduced ejection fraction. N Engl J Med. 2002;346(12):877-883. [PMID: 11907286]

Oral H, Pappone C, Chugh A, et al. Circumferential pulmonary-vein ablation for chronic atrial fibrillation. N Engl J Med. 2006; 354(9):934-941. [PMID: 16510747]

Wyse DG, Waldo AL, DiMarco JP, et al; Atrial Fibrillation Follow-up Investigation of Rhythm Management (AFFIRM) Investigators. A comparison of rate control and rhythm control in patients with atrial fibrillation. N Engl J Med. 2002;347(23):1825-1833. [PMID: 12466506]

Zipes DP, Camm AJ, Borggrefe M, et al. ACC/AHA/ESC 2006 Guidelines for Management of Patients With Ventricular Arrhythmias and the Prevention of Sudden Cardiac Death: a report of the American College of Cardiology/American Heart Association Task Force and the European Society of Cardiology Committee for Practice Guidelines (writing committee to develop Guidelines for Management of Patients With Ventricular Arrhythmias and the Prevention of Sudden Cardiac Death): developed in collaboration with the European Heart Rhythm Association and the Heart Rhythm Society. Circulation. 2006;114(10):e385-484. [PMID: 16935995]

Pericardial Disease

Acute and Recurrent Pericarditis

Clinical Presentation

Acute pericarditis, or inflammation of the pericardium, has numerous causes (**Table 22**). Chest pain from acute pericarditis is sharp and pleuritic, worsened by assuming a supine position, and may last for days. These characteristics aid in distinguishing it from chest pain of an acute myocardial infarction or unstable angina (**Table 23**). Although the chest pain of acute pericarditis is most frequently retrosternal, it is often left precordial in location and may radiate to the left trapezius ridge.

Acute pericarditis recurs in 10% to 30% of patients. Recurrent pericarditis can be debilitating and may recur for 2 to 5 years, rarely for 15 years or more. Risk factors for recurrence are failure to respond to aspirin therapy or NSAIDs and prior treatment with corticosteroids.

Acute pericarditis may occur within 1 or 2 days of an acute myocardial infarction and is less common in patients who have been treated with a thrombolytic agent than in those who have not received such drugs. Post–myocardial infarction syndrome, or Dressler syndrome, develops several weeks to months after a myocardial infarction and accounts for fewer cases of pericarditis.

TABLE 22 Causes of Acute Pericarditis and Pericardial Effusion

Cause	Notes
Idiopathic	40% of all causes when only conventional diagnostic testing employed; specialized testing can lower frequency of apparently idiopathic cases to less than 5%
Viral infection	20% of all causes; diagnostic testing (cultures and titers) generally not recommended; obtain HIV studies in individuals with risk factors
Bacterial infection	About 7% of all causes; suspect in patients with bacteremia, endocarditis, and contiguous infection; pericardiocentesis and culture mandatory
Fungal infection	Most commonly in immunocompromised patients with evidence of disseminated disease; pericardiocentesis and culture mandatory
Tuberculosis	Although infrequent in developed countries, missing the diagnosis of tuberculous pericarditis has serious consequences and makes its consideration appropriate in all cases; tuberculin skin test recommended for patients at risk
Uremia	6% of causes; obtain creatinine and blood urea nitrogen to confirm
Autoimmune disorders	Most autoimmune diseases are potential causes; during the course of systemic lupus erythematosus, 20% to 40% of patients will have pericarditis
Acute myocardial infarction	Less frequent in reperfusion era; pericardial friction rub is transient and typically occurs for ≤3 days after infarction; course usually benign
Post–myocardial infarction	Patients typically have severe malaise; tamponade and constrictive pericarditis are rare complications
Postpericardiotomy	Occurs >1 week after cardiac surgery; typical course is self-limited but often prolonged; tamponade may occur
Neoplasm	7% of causes; common malignancies include lung, breast, lymphoma, and leukemia; factors suggesting neoplasia: history of malignancy, large pericardial effusion, inadequate response to NSAIDs
Medications	Culprit drugs include hydralazine, procainamide, warfarin, heparin, methysergide, doxorubicin, penicillins
Chest irradiation	Radiation pericarditis occurs in 20% of patients if entire pericardium is in the field, but in <3% if heart is shielded; acute pericarditis may occur immediately or months after radiation; pericarditis occurring during radiation usually does not preclude completion of radiation treatment; constrictive pericarditis may occur up to 15 years after radiation but is not predicted by development of pericarditis during treatment
Blunt or penetrating chest trauma	Uncomplicated traumatic pericarditis usually resolves; most significant complications are hemopericardium and cardiac tamponade, which require surgery
Aortic dissection with leakage into pericardial cavity	Leads to cardiac tamponade; life-threatening, requiring immediate surgery; percutaneous pericardiocentesis may exacerbate condition

Evaluation

Diagnosis of acute pericarditis is made by the presence of at least two of the three classic features: (1) pleuritic chest pain; (2) friction rub; and (3) diffuse concordant ST-segment elevation on electrocardiography (ECG), often with depression of the PR segment. A pericardial friction rub is virtually pathognomonic of pericarditis. The classic pericardial friction rub has three components related to cardiac motion and occurs during atrial systole, ventricular contraction, and rapid ventricular filling. The sound of the rub can be squeaky, scratchy, high-pitched, or swooshing. The rub may be auscultated across the precordium, but is best heard at the lower left sternal border. Its detection is enhanced by listening during inspiration or full expiration, with the patient sitting and leaning forward. Importantly, a pericardial friction rub is evanescent and changes in quality, and frequent examinations may be required for its detection.

Typical ECG changes in acute pericarditis are diffuse concave upward ST-segment elevation (except in leads V_1 and aVR) and PR-segment depression in all limb and precordial leads except aVR (**Figure 21**). These findings, along with other ECG features, help in the differentiation of patients with acute pericarditis versus acute myocardial infarction. The chest radiograph may show enlargement of the cardiac silhouette from an associated pericardial effusion, but is usually of little diagnostic usefulness. Chest radiography is useful in excluding other potential conditions that may present similarly to acute pericarditis, such as pneumothorax and pneumonia.

Blood test results are nonspecific, with leukocytosis and an elevated erythrocyte sedimentation rate reflecting the inflammatory condition. Tumor marker analysis, polymerase chain reaction, and immunohistochemistry tests on pericardial fluid or tissue have lowered the frequency of apparently

TABLE 23 Differentiation of Pericardial Chest Pain from Myocardial Ischemic Chest Pain

Characteristic	Pericardial Pain	Myocardial Ischemic Pain
Quality	Sharp, pleuritic	Pressure, heaviness, tightness, constricting
Location	Left precordial or retrosternal	Retrosternal
Radiation pattern	Left trapezius ridge	Left shoulder, left arm
Duration	Hours or days	1-15 minutes (angina)
		>20 minutes (unstable angina)
		Hours (myocardial infarction)
Relation to exercise	Unrelated	Related (stable angina)
		Unrelated (unstable angina or myocardial infarction)
Relation to position	Relieved by leaning forward	Unrelated
	Aggravated by assuming a recumbent position	
ECG findings	Initial ECG changes that accompany onset of chest pain: ST-segment elevation that is upwardly concave and diffuse (occurs in all leads except aVR and V_1)	ST-segment elevation is downwardly concave and localized; or ST-segment depression
	T waves invert after ST-segment elevation resolves and not associated with loss of R-wave voltage or Q waves (occurs several days after onset of chest pain)	T waves invert while ST-segment elevation is present. May be associated with loss of R-wave voltage or appearance of Q waves
	PR-segment depression present in 80% (occurs in all limb and precordial leads except aVR); reciprocal PR-segment elevation may occur in aVR	PR-segment depression rarely present
	Q waves absent	Q waves may be present
Echocardiographic findings	No left ventricular regional wall motion abnormality	Left ventricular regional wall motion abnormality in distribution of coronary artery

idiopathic cases; however, these tests are not widely available, and their use is not warranted in most patients.

Only about 60% of patients with pericarditis have a pericardial effusion; echocardiography should be performed promptly on patients with pericarditis who have hypotension, pulsus paradoxus greater than 10 mm Hg, or signs of heart failure to evaluate for pericardial effusion and tamponade physiology.

Management

In patients with acute pericarditis, hospitalization is prompted by an associated myocardial infarction, pyogenic infection, or tamponade. Outpatient management is appropriate if other potentially serious causes of chest pain are excluded, hemodynamic status is normal, and a moderate or large pericardial effusion is excluded by echocardiography.

In the absence of a specific cause for acute pericarditis, anti-inflammatory therapy is the mainstay of treatment. High-dose aspirin or high-dose NSAIDs should be started and tapered after several weeks (**Table 24**). Aspirin is preferred over

NSAIDs if acute myocardial infarction is the cause of acute pericarditis. NSAIDs may promote ventricular rupture by impairing myocardial scar formation. Patients who take high-dose aspirin or NSAIDs on a long-term basis should be monitored for adverse renal and gastrointestinal effects. Those at high risk for gastrointestinal bleeding from NSAIDs may be candidates for prophylactic therapy. Maintenance treatment can be stopped after 3 to 4 weeks.

Colchicine in combination with aspirin is an alternative regimen in the treatment of acute pericarditis. In comparison with aspirin alone, this combination therapy has been shown to be more effective in reducing recurrences of pericarditis. Colchicine may also be considered as an alternative agent in the treatment of acute pericarditis when aspirin or an NSAID is contraindicated. Maintenance therapy is 3 months.

If pain is not relieved within 24 hours of use of aspirin or an NSAID, the dosage may be increased or an alternative NSAID used. If pain is not relieved by an alternative NSAID, alternative causes of chest pain should be considered. Patients with acute pericarditis being treated with aspirin or an NSAID

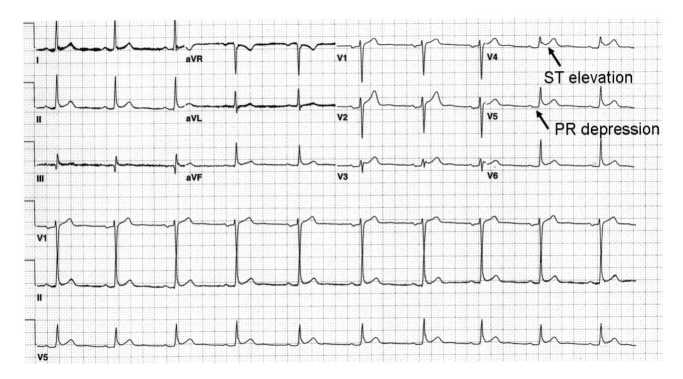

FIGURE 21.
Acute Pericarditis with ST-Segment Elevation.
12-lead electrocardiogram shows upwardly concave ST-segment elevation and PR-segment depression.

	Conventional First-Line Agents		Alternative First-Line Agent[a]	Third-Line Agent (for Refractory Cases)
Treatment Phase	**Aspirin**	**NSAID**	**Colchicine**	**Corticosteroid[b]**
Initiation	650 mg every 4-6 h	Ibuprofen 400-800 mg every 6-8 h	Body weight <70 kg: 0.6 mg every 12 h (use for 1 day only if combined with aspirin or NSAID) Body weight ≥70 kg: 0.6 mg every 8 h (use for 1 day only if combined with aspirin or NSAID)	Prednisone 60 mg/d until improved
Taper	↓ 650 to 975 mg weekly until off	After 2 weeks begin taper to maintenance dose	NA	↓ 5 mg every 3 days until 20 mg/d dose reached
Maintenance	NA	Variable (200-300 mg TID)	Body weight <70 kg: 0.6 mg/d Body weight ≥70 kg: 0.6 mg BID	Taper slowly after reaching 20 mg/d dose
Duration	3-4 weeks	3-4 weeks	3 months	Months

TABLE 24 Pharmacologic Treatment of Acute Pericarditis

BID = twice daily; NA = not applicable; TID = three times daily.

[a]When aspirin and NSAID contraindicated or used as adjunctive therapy to conventional first-line agent when therapeutic response to conventional therapy is suboptimal.

[b]Contraindicated in setting of acute myocardial infarction. Preferred in systemic inflammatory diseases or uremia.

Recommendations based on Maisch B, Seferović PM, Ristić AD, et al. Guidelines on the diagnosis and management of pericardial diseases executive summary; The Task force on the diagnosis and management of pericardial diseases of the European Society of Cardiology. Eur Heart J. 2004;25(7):587-610. [PMID: 15120056]; and Spodick DH. Acute pericarditis: current concepts and practice. JAMA. 2003;289(9):1150-1153. [PMID: 12622586]; and Imazio M, Bobbio M, Cecchi E, et al. Colchicine in addition to conventional therapy for acute pericarditis: results of the COlchicine for acute PEricarditis (COPE) trial. Circulation. 2005;112(13):2012-2016. [PMID: 16186437] who have persistent chest pain, persistent fever, new or enlarging pericardial effusion, or worsening general health should also be given colchicine.

Corticosteroids are used in acute pericarditis due to systemic inflammatory diseases or uremia. Corticosteroids also should be considered in patients who are refractory to or have contraindications to aspirin, NSAIDs, and colchicine. However, corticosteroids may promote the development of recurrent pericarditis and should not be used in patients with acute pericarditis due to bacterial infection or tuberculosis. They should also be avoided in patients with post-infarction pericarditis because of the risk of ventricular aneurysm formation.

Anticoagulation with heparin or warfarin should be avoided in most patients with acute pericarditis because of the risk of hemopericardium, but prophylactic heparin may be considered in patients at high risk for deep venous thrombosis if alternative nonpharmacologic measures are not possible. In patients who develop acute pericarditis from an acute myocardial infarction, anticoagulation should be continued if indicated for the acute coronary syndrome but discontinued if pericardial effusion develops or increases. Colchicine is the treatment of choice for recurrent acute pericarditis and can prevent recurrences (**Table 25**), thus avoiding the use of corticosteroids. Pericardiectomy does not prevent recurrence and is not recommended for acute or recurrent pericarditis without constriction.

KEY POINTS

- Diagnosis of acute pericarditis is made by the presence of at least two of the three classic features: pleuritic chest pain, friction rub, and diffuse concordant ST-segment elevation on ECG, often with depression of the PR segment.

- Many patients with acute pericarditis do not have an effusion; therefore, absence of an effusion on echocardiography does not rule out the diagnosis.

- Corticosteroids should be considered only in patients with acute pericarditis who are refractory to or have contraindications to the use of aspirin, NSAIDs, and colchicine.

- Colchicine is the treatment of choice for recurrent pericarditis.

Pericardial Effusion Without Cardiac Compression

Clinical Presentation and Evaluation

Unless accompanied by pericarditis, most patients with a pericardial effusion are asymptomatic if intrapericardial pressure is not increased. Physical examination is nonspecific with muffled heart sounds and dullness percussible beyond the apex with a large effusion.

Abnormalities on ECG may include reduced QRS voltage and, in the presence of large effusions, electrical alternans. Echocardiography is the mainstay for diagnosis and assessment of hemodynamic significance of a pericardial effusion (**Figure 22**). Chest radiography is not sensitive for detection of pericardial effusions. Both CT and MRI provide a wider tomographic view than echocardiography and so are helpful for defining masses or lymphadenopathy associated with an effusion and evaluation of loculated effusions.

Extensive laboratory testing will yield a diagnosis, but reasonable studies include complete blood count, serum electrolytes, blood urea nitrogen and creatinine, thyroid-stimulating hormone, antinuclear antibodies, and tuberculin skin test. Pericardiocentesis may be indicated for diagnosis of bacterial, tubercular, or systemic inflammatory disease causes of pericarditis. Pericardial fluid should be sent for culture, cytology, and determination of adenosine deaminase activity (for possible tuberculous pericarditis). Surgical pericardial biopsy is important in the diagnosis of malignancy or systemic disease because of its greater sensitivity as compared with pericardiocentesis.

Management

An idiopathic pericardial effusion in stable patients requires no specific therapy, but serial echocardiography is advisable. Echocardiography is more sensitive than monitoring of clinical findings for detecting the development of a hemodynamically significant pericardial effusion. In addition, echocardiography is useful in assessing for progression or regression of the effusion. Pericardiocentesis is advisable if an effusion persists for longer than 3 months. In patients with idiopathic effusions, pericardiocentesis is often curative. Anticoagulants should be avoided because of the risk of hemopericardium.

KEY POINTS

- Pericardiocentesis may be indicated for diagnosis of suspected bacterial, tubercular, or systemic inflammatory disease causes of pericardial effusion.

- Pericardiocentesis is advisable if a pericardial effusion persists for longer than 3 months.

Cardiac Tamponade

Clinical Presentation and Evaluation

Clinical features of cardiac tamponade include dyspnea, tachycardia, jugular venous distention, hemodynamic instability, and hypotension. Tamponade results from increased intrapericardial pressure from the accumulation of pericardial fluid. Cardiac tamponade typically presents acutely, but it may present subacutely (for example, after acute viral pericarditis). Conditions that may present similarly to acute cardiac tamponade include massive pulmonary embolism and myocardial infarction.

TABLE 25 Pharmacologic Treatment of Recurrent Pericarditis

Treatment Phase	Colchicine	NSAID (Added to Colchicine)	Third-Line Agents (for Refractory Cases)
Initiation	Body weight <70 kg: 0.6 mg every 12 h Body weight ≥70 kg: 0.6 mg every 8 h	Ibuprofen 800 mg every 6 h	Prednisone 1 to 1.5 mg/kg daily for 1 month
Taper	NA	After 2 weeks begin 600 mg QID At 4 weeks begin 400 mg QID	Taper over 3 months; for recurrent symptoms during taper, return to prior dose for 2-3 weeks and thereafter taper
Maintenance	Body weight <70 kg: 0.6 mg/d Body weight ≥70 kg: 0.6 mg twice daily	400 mg QID	Add aspirin, NSAID, or azathioprine near end of taper and continue this agent for additional 3 months
Duration	6 months	3 months	≥4 months

NA = Not applicable; QID = four times daily.

Recommendations based on Maisch B, Seferović PM, Ristić AD, et al. Guidelines on the diagnosis and management of pericardial diseases executive summary; The Task force on the diagnosis and management of pericardial diseases of the European Society of Cardiology. Eur Heart J. 2004;25(7):587-610. [PMID: 15120056]; and Imazio M, Bobbio M, Cecchi E, et al. Colchicine as first-choice therapy for recurrent pericarditis: results of the CORE (COlchicine for REcurrent pericarditis) trial. Arch Intern Med. 2005;165(17):1987-1991. [PMID: 16186468]; and Artom G, Koren-Morag N, Spodick DH, et al. Pretreatment with corticosteroids attenuates the efficacy of colchicine in preventing recurrent pericarditis: a multi-centre all-case analysis. Eur Heart J. 2005;26(7):723-727. [PMID: 15755753]

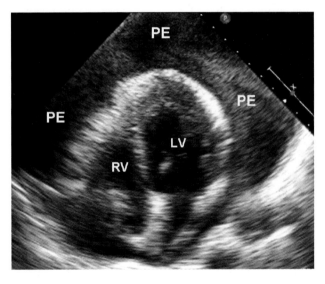

FIGURE 22.
Pericardial Effusion.
Two-dimensional echocardiographic image of a large circumferential pericardial effusion (PE) surrounding the left (LV) and right (RV) ventricles.

In tamponade, pericardial effusion is usually circumferential but may be loculated. The rapidity of fluid accumulation is a greater factor in the development of tamponade than the absolute volume of the effusion. A pulsus paradoxus (systolic pressure variation with respiration >10 mm Hg) supports the diagnosis. Even when tamponade is present, pulsus paradoxus may be absent if there is coexisting significant aortic regurgitation, atrial septal defect, left ventricular hypertrophy, pulmonary hypertension, or right ventricular hypertrophy.

Echocardiography is the procedure of choice for diagnosing tamponade. It confirms elevated intrapericardial pressure as manifested by invagination or diastolic "collapse" of right-sided heart chambers, increased respiratory variation in peak mitral and tricuspid inflow velocities, and inferior vena cava dilatation and plethora (that is, the inferior vena cava remains distended throughout the respiratory cycle). The absence of a pericardial effusion on echocardiography virtually excludes tamponade.

Management

In subacute tamponade, hemodynamic compromise may be mild and conservative therapy can be instituted, with serial noninvasive hemodynamic monitoring (blood pressure, heart rate, pulsus paradoxus) and echocardiography, volume resuscitation, and treatment of the causative illness.

When overt hemodynamic compromise is evident, acute management includes maintenance of systemic blood pressure with aggressive volume resuscitation and vasopressors. Pericardial fluid should be drained by pericardiocentesis or surgery. Complications from pericardiocentesis are minimized when guided by echocardiography, which identifies the site and direction of safe needle entry into the pericardial space. Inotropic agents such as dobutamine may be needed in select patients if ventricular function was impaired prior to the development of tamponade. Intra-aortic balloon counterpulsation should be employed for refractory hypotension, particularly if there is coexisting myocarditis and ventricular dysfunction.

Mechanical ventilation with high positive end-expiratory pressure reduces venous return, exacerbating hemodynamic compromise in patients with tamponade, and should therefore be avoided. Oversedation can reduce the compensatory sympathetic drive and result in sudden hemodynamic collapse. In tamponade caused by aortic dissection, pericardiocentesis can further exacerbate hemodynamic instability, and surgical pericardial drainage, therefore, is appropriate.

Cardiac tamponade should be considered as a possible cause of pulseless electrical activity. If indicated, pericardiocentesis should be promptly performed.

Constrictive Pericarditis

Clinical Presentation and Evaluation

Patients with constrictive pericarditis present with dyspnea, fatigue, jugular venous distention, peripheral edema, hepatomegaly, and ascites. Notably, pulmonary congestion is absent. A pericardial knock may be present. Jugular veins may engorge with inspiration (Kussmaul sign). Atrial fibrillation occurs in more than 20% of patients with constrictive pericarditis, likely due to long-standing elevated atrial pressures and atrial enlargement.

In the United States, constrictive pericarditis commonly occurs following cardiac surgery and as a result of viral infection or acute pericarditis. Other causes include mediastinal irradiation and rheumatoid arthritis or connective tissue disease. Effusive constrictive pericarditis is a disease characterized by components of tamponade from pericardial fluid and constriction from a rigid pericardium. This disease may become apparent after pericardiocentesis in patients initially diagnosed with isolated tamponade. It is important to distinguish constrictive pericarditis from restrictive cardiomyopathy (**Table 26**).

Echocardiography shows an excessively high peak transmitral or peak tricuspid early filling velocity and a rapid rate of decline in the early filling velocities after achieving the peak velocity. In constrictive pericarditis, the normally modest influence of respirations on increasing and decreasing ventricular filling is enhanced and demonstrable by Doppler echocardiography (**Figure 23**). In addition, the ventricles compete during diastole owing to the pericardial restraint, as manifested by shifting of the ventricular septum to and fro during diastole as a manifestation of the right and left ventricle competing for a confined space during diastolic expansion. Importantly, these findings are not seen in restrictive cardiomyopathy.

MRI and CT are useful for confirming pericardial thickening. Calcification of the pericardium on chest radiograph or

TABLE 26 Differentiation of Constrictive Pericarditis from Restrictive Cardiomyopathy

Finding	Constrictive Pericarditis	Restrictive Cardiomyopathy
Electrocardiography		
Presence of left or right bundle branch block	Not supportive	Supportive
Presence of left or right ventricular hypertrophy	Not supportive	Supportive
Chest Radiography		
Pericardial calcification	May be present	Absent
Echocardiography		
Presence of left ventricular hypertrophy	Absent	Present
Accentuated drop in peak left ventricular filling during inspiration	Present	Absent
Reduced tissue Doppler velocities	Absent	Present
To-and-fro diastolic motion of ventricular septum	Present	Absent
MRI/CT		
Increased pericardial thickness	Present in 80%	Absent
Hemodynamic Right and Left Heart Catheterization		
Elevated and equalized diastolic left and right ventricular pressures (within 5 mm Hg)	Present	Absent
Left and right ventricular systolic pressure changes with respiratory cycle	Discordant	Concordant

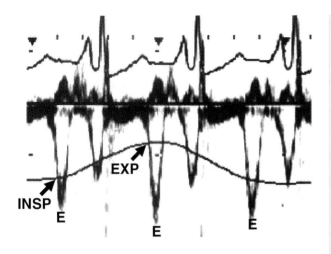

FIGURE 23.
Constrictive Pericarditis on Doppler Echocardiography.
Pulsed Doppler echocardiography of mitral valve inflow shows accentuated rise and fall in early mitral valve peak velocities (E) during onset expiration (EXP) and inspiration (INSP) from constrictive pericarditis, respectively.

Reproduced from Rajagopalan N, Garcia MJ, Rodriguez L, et al. Comparison of new Doppler echocardiographic methods to differentiate constrictive pericardial heart disease and restrictive cardiomyopathy. Am J Cardiol. 2001;87:86-94. [PMID: 11137840] Copyright 2001, with permission from Elsevier.

CT strongly supports the diagnosis. Chest radiograph as well as ECG findings are typically nonspecific. Cardiac catheterization may be needed for diagnosis. In constrictive pericarditis, left and right ventricular pressure recordings show a dip-and-plateau waveform, also called a "square root sign"—a rapid and steep decrease followed by an increase in early diastolic pressure (dip) followed by relatively unchanged mid and late diastolic pressures (plateau).

Management

Diuretics may help relieve dyspnea and peripheral edema in patients with constrictive pericarditis. However, these patients depend on higher than normal filling pressures to maintain stroke volume, and overly aggressive diuresis may reduce cardiac output, causing orthostatic hypotension and dizziness. Heart rate control is necessary if atrial fibrillation is present. However, a compensatory increase in heart rate is to be expected, and overly aggressive rate slowing could be harmful.

Although constrictive pericarditis is typically chronic, it may resolve spontaneously or after anti-inflammatory therapy. Transient causes of constrictive pericarditis include pericardiotomy, viral infection, connective tissue disease, trauma, and malignancy. Treatment for these causes may include NSAIDs, chemotherapy, or antibiotics. Thus, in stable patients a 2- to 3-month trial of conservative management is warranted before surgical pericardiectomy.

Pericardiectomy is effective for constrictive pericarditis. However, it is unnecessary in patients with mild peripheral edema, mild jugular venous distention, or who are in New York Heart Association (NYHA) functional class I with medical therapy. In patients with cachexia, cirrhosis, markedly reduced cardiac output, or NYHA class IV symptoms, the surgical mortality rate is high (6%-19%) and the benefit negligible. Thus, pericardiectomy is advisable in patients with chronic constrictive pericarditis who have NYHA functional class II or III symptoms. In some patients, resolution of symptoms after pericardiectomy may take months. In addition, ejection fraction may decrease after surgery, resulting in symptoms that necessitate the use of diuretics, digoxin, and/or vasodilators.

KEY POINTS

- Constrictive pericarditis presents with dyspnea, fatigue, jugular venous distention, peripheral edema, hepatomegaly, and ascites; pulmonary congestion is absent.

- In stable patients with a transient cause of constrictive pericarditis, a 2- to 3-month trial of conservative management is warranted before surgical pericardiectomy.

Bibliography

Hoit BD. Management of effusive and constrictive pericardial heart disease. Circulation. 2002;105(25):2939-2942. [PMID: 12081983]

Imazio M, Bobbio M, Cecchi E, et al. Colchicine as first-choice therapy for recurrent pericarditis: results of the CORE (COlchicine for Recurrent pericarditis) trial. Arch Intern Med. 2005;165(17):1987-1991. [PMID: 16186468]

Imazio M, Bobbio M, Cecchi E, et al. Colchicine in addition to conventional therapy for acute pericarditis: results of the COlchicine for acute Pericarditis (COPE) trial. Circulation. 2005;112(13):2012-2016. [PMID: 16186437]

Ling LH, Oh JK, Schaff HV, et al. Constrictive pericarditis in the modern era: evolving clinical spectrum and impact on outcome after pericardiectomy. Circulation. 1999;100(13):1380-1386. [PMID: 10500037]

Maisch B, Ristic´ AD. The classification of pericardial disease in the age of modern medicine. Curr Cardiol Rep. 2002;4(1):13-21. [PMID: 11743917]

Maisch B, Seferovic´ PM, Ristic´ AD, et al. Guidelines on the diagnosis and management of pericardial diseases executive summary; The Task Force on the Diagnosis and Management of Pericardial Diseases on the European Society of Cardiology. Eur Heart J. 2004;25(7):587-610. [PMID: 15120056]

Mercé J, Sagristà-Sauleda J, Permanyer-Miralda G, Soler-Soler J. Should pericardial drainage be performed routinely in patients who have a large pericardial effusion without tamponade? Am J Med. 1998;105(2):106-109. [PMID: 9727816]

Troughton RW, Asher CR, Klein AL. Pericarditis. Lancet. 2004; 363 (9410):717-727. [PMID: 15001332]

Valvular Heart Disease

Diagnosis and Evaluation of Valvular Heart Disease

History and Physical Examination

Acute, severe valve disease nearly always presents with heart failure. However, symptom onset may be insidious in chronic or slowly progressive valve lesions, and patients may unconsciously curtail activities to compensate.

The first indications of an abnormality may be a heart murmur heard on physical examination. Murmur descriptions should include intensity, duration, radiation, and timing in the cardiac cycle (**Table 27**). Additional physical examination features that help to identify the source of a murmur include apical impulse palpation, distal pulses, timing of S_1 and S_2, ejection clicks and other extra heart sounds, and response to Valsalva and other maneuvers. Midsystolic murmurs of low intensity (grade 1/6 or 2/6) are usually benign and are attributable to minor aortic valve abnormalities or physiologic increases in blood flow, such as in anemia, sepsis, or pregnancy.

Diagnostic Evaluation

Transthoracic echocardiography is indicated in symptomatic patients, in those with a systolic murmur grade 3/6 intensity or greater, and in those with any continuous murmur (a murmur that begins after S_1 and extends beyond S_2) or diastolic murmur (**Figure 24**). Echocardiography allows diagnosis of lesion etiology and severity, identification of coexistent lesions, diagnosis of pulmonary hypertension, and assessment of ventricular size and function (**Table 28**). For stenotic lesions, Doppler-derived transvalvular velocities allow calculation of valve area and pressure gradients across the valve and are the strongest predictor of clinical outcome. For regurgitant lesions, assessment includes color jet size, the width of the narrowest segment of the regurgitant jet (*vena contracta*), and jet signal strength. Quantitative measurements of the size of the regurgitant orifice and volume of regurgitant flow are increasingly reported and are strongly associated with prognosis and clinical outcome. However, these measurements are technically demanding to acquire. Despite this, the 2006 American College of Cardiology/American Heart Association (ACC/AHA) valvular heart disease guidelines now emphasize quantitative measures in reporting regurgitation severity. Transesophageal echocardiography is recommended in some patients with valve disease, including severe mitral regurgitation, prosthetic valves, and endocarditis.

When symptoms or findings from the physical examination are discrepant from echocardiographic findings, elevated B-type natriuretic peptide levels may indicate early hemodynamic significance of the lesion. Exercise testing with echocardiography assesses lesion significance by measuring exercise-induced changes in pulmonary pressures. Exercise tolerance and duration are predictors of progression to need for intervention.

Dobutamine stress echocardiography can be used in patients with aortic stenosis and systolic dysfunction to assess whether a small calculated aortic valve area is the result of true stenosis or whether the poorly functioning left ventricle cannot generate sufficient systolic pressure to fully open only mildly stenotic valve leaflets. If the calculated valve area increases with dobutamine-augmented cardiac output, then the "obstruction" was due to the inability of the left ventricle to open the valve well (*pseudostenosis*). If the valve area does not increase, the aortic stenosis is present.

Cardiac catheterization is no longer recommended for primary evaluation of valvular disease except for preoperative assessment for coronary artery disease in patients with atherosclerotic risk factors to determine whether concurrent bypass grafting is needed at the time of surgery.

KEY POINTS

- Transthoracic echocardiography for the evaluation of valvular heart disease is indicated in symptomatic patients, in those with a systolic murmur grade 3/6 intensity or greater, and in those with any continuous or diastolic murmur.
- Compared with transthoracic echocardiography, transesophageal echocardiography provides improved imaging quality, particularly for the mitral valve and left atrial appendage, for prosthetic valves, and for evaluation of endocarditis.

General Principles of Management of Valvular Heart Disease

Timing of intervention for valvular heart disease is predicated on the presence of cardiopulmonary symptoms attributable to the lesion or evidence of adverse hemodynamic consequences Cardiopulmonary symptoms in patients with mild or moderate lesions should prompt evaluation for other superimposed or primary disease processes.

Serial clinical evaluation and echocardiography are indicated in asymptomatic patients to monitor for symptoms and hemodynamic effects on the left ventricle and pulmonary pressures, dependent on the type of valve lesion and the severity of valve dysfunction (**Table 29**). When more rapid lesion progression is suspected, shorter evaluation intervals are indicated. In the absence of exertional syncope or known life-threatening exertional arrhythmia, patients with valvular heart disease can usually participate in competitive sports. Most asymptomatic patients with significant disease who need noncardiac surgery can be managed conservatively with a cardiac anesthesiologist and careful intraoperative attention to fluid balance.

Measures to decrease preload, control volume overload, and manage arrhythmia do not supplant surgical intervention in symptomatic patients or in those with evidence of hemodynamic compromise. Asymptomatic patients with severe disease who are having other cardiac surgery, such as coronary artery bypass grafting, should also undergo surgical correction.

TABLE 27 Cardiac Murmurs and Associated Findings

Cause of Murmur	Characteristic	Location	Radiation	Associated Findings
Systolic Murmurs				
Innocent flow murmur	Soft, midsystolic	Base	None	Normal splitting of S_2
Aortic stenosis	Crescendo-decrescendo, midsystolic	Base	Carotids	Single S_2, pulsus parvus, S_4, palpable apical impulse
Bicuspid aortic valve	Crescendo-decrescendo, midsystolic	Base	Carotids	Valve opening click in young adults, diastolic murmur if concurrent aortic regurgitation
Pulmonic stenosis	Crescendo-decrescendo, midsystolic	Base	None	Valve opening click, right-sided S_4
Hypertrophic obstructive cardiomyopathy	Crescendo, mid- or late systolic	Base	Carotids	Bifid carotid impulse; murmur decreases with passive leg elevation or hand grip, increases with Valsalva
Mitral regurgitation	Holo- or late systolic	Apex	Axilla or back	Hyperdynamic apical impulse; apical displacement if left ventricle is enlarged; murmur increases with isometric exercise; best heard in left lateral decubitus position
Mitral valve prolapse with mitral regurgitation	Late systolic	Apex	Axilla	With Valsalva, murmur decreases and midsystolic click moves closer to S_1; other findings similar to mitral regurgitation of any cause
Papillary muscle dysfunction or rupture	Transient, during myocardial ischemia	Apex	Axilla	Acute coronary syndrome, heart failure
Atrial septal defect	Usually only a pulmonic flow murmur is present	LLSB	None	Fixed splitting of S_2; RV heave, tricuspid rumble
Ventricular septal defect	Holosystolic	LLSB	None	Palpable thrill; murmur increases with isometric exercise, decreases with amyl nitrate
Tricuspid regurgitation	Holosystolic	LLSB	LRSB	Prominent *v* waves in neck, hepatic pulsation; murmur increases with inspiration; in severe TR, abdominal ascites, pedal edema; with pulmonary hypertension, loud pulmonic component of S_2
Diastolic Murmurs				
Aortic regurgitation	Decrescendo	LLSB	None	Enlarged apical impulse, widened pulse pressure, bounding carotid pulses; murmur best heard in upright position, leaning forward, end-expiration
Pulmonic regurgitation	Mid-diastolic	LLSB	None	Loud S_2 if pulmonary hypertension is present
Mitral stenosis	Low-pitched rumble	Apex	None	Murmur best heard in left lateral decubitus position; opening snap; palpable P_2; irregular pulse if atrial fibrillation is present
Tricuspid stenosis	Low-pitched rumble	LLSB	RUQ	Right ventricular heave
Continuous Murmurs				
Patent ductus arteriosus	Machinery-like	Base	Back	May have widened pulse pressure
Mammary souffle	Soft, humming	Between breast and sternum	None	Usually heard over the breast during pregnancy or lactation
Coarctation of the aorta	Accentuation midsystole, but continuous	Over back	Back	Higher blood pressure in arms versus legs

LLSB = lower left sternal border; LRSB = lower right sternal border; RUQ = right upper quadrant of the abdomen; RV = right ventricular; TR = tricuspid regurgitation.

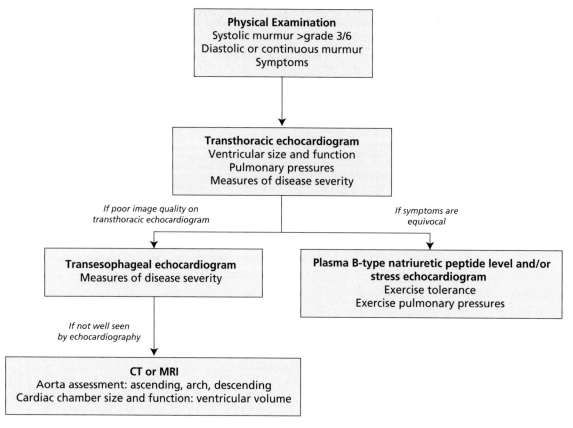

FIGURE 24.
Diagnostic Pathway for Valvular Heart Disease.

TABLE 28 Normal Cardiac Measurements	
Parameter	**Normal Value**
Ejection fraction	>55%
Left ventricular end-diastolic dimension	<60 mm
Left ventricular end-systolic dimension	<40 mm
Left atrial dimension	<40 mm
Pulmonary artery systolic pressure	<30 mm Hg
Ascending aorta diameter	<3.5 cm

Aortic Stenosis

Pathophysiology

Progressive calcification of a normal trileaflet or congenitally bicuspid aortic valve is the most common cause of aortic stenosis in the United States. Less common causes include rheumatic disease and noncalcified congenital valve disease. Progressive obstruction of left ventricular outflow increases afterload and intracavitary systolic pressure. The initial compensatory mechanism is myocardial hypertrophy with impaired diastolic filling and preservation of systolic function. In the later stages, increased myocardial wall stress may cause impaired systolic function and ventricular dilation.

Calcific stenosis is an active disease process, akin to atherosclerosis, with disruption of the basement membrane, inflammatory cell infiltration, progressive calcification, and lipid deposition. There is a long latency period; calcific stenosis of a trileaflet aortic valve usually presents clinically in the sixth or seventh decade of life.

Risk factors associated with aortic stenosis include diabetes mellitus, male sex, smoking, hypertension, older age, and hyperlipidemia. Several small clinical trials have investigated the use of lipid-lowering therapy or angiotensin-converting enzyme (ACE) inhibitors to retard or halt this disease process. However, larger prospective, randomized trials have shown no effect on valve disease progression or cardiovascular death.

Aortic valve sclerosis, or valve thickening without outflow obstruction, is present in more than 25% of persons older than 65 years. Patients are often diagnosed when an asymptomatic murmur is auscultated or following an incidental echocardiographic finding. If leaflet thickening causes malcoaptation of the leaflets, regurgitation may be present, but it is usually mild. The progression from aortic sclerosis to stenosis is slow, and fewer than 20% of patients develop valve obstruction over the next 10 years. Once mild stenosis is present, however, there is an average annual

TABLE 29 Serial Evaluation of Asymptomatic Patients with Left-Sided Valvular Conditions

Factors Considered	Lesion Severity	Frequency
Aortic Stenosis		
Stenosis severity; rate of progression	Mild (V_{max} <3 m/s, AVA >1.5 cm^2)	Clinical eval yearly
		Echo every 3-5 y
	Moderate (V_{max} 3-4 m/s, AVA 1.0-1.5 cm^2)	Clinical eval yearly
		Echo every 1-2 y
	Severe (V_{max} >4 m/s, AVA <1.0 cm^2)	Clinical eval yearly
		Echo yearly
Mitral Stenosis		
Stenosis severity; rate of progression	Mild (MVA >1.5 cm2, MPG <5 mm Hg, PASP <30 mm Hg)	Clinical eval yearly
		Echo every 3-5 y
	Moderate (MVA 1.0-1.5 cm^2, MPG 5-10 mm Hg, PASP 30-50 mm Hg)	Clinical eval yearly
		Echo every 1-2 y
	Severe (MVA <1.0 cm^2, MPG >10 mm Hg, PASP >50 mm Hg)	Clinical eval yearly
		Echo yearly
Aortic Regurgitation		
Regurgitation severity; rate of progression; EF; LV chamber size; ascending aorta dilation	Mild (VC <0.3 cm, ROA <0.10 cm^2, RV <30 mL/beat); normal EF	Clinical eval yearly
		Echo every 2-3 y
	Severe (VC >0.6 cm, ROA ≥0.3 cm^2, RV ≥60 mL/beat, RF >50%)	
	EF >50%; LV size normal	Clinical eval every 6-12 mo
		Echo yearly
	EF >50%; LV size increased	Clinical eval every 6 mo
		Echo every 6 to 12 mo
Mitral Regurgitation		
Regurgitation severity; rate of progression; EF; LV chamber size; pulmonary pressure	Mild (VC <0.3 cm, ROA <0.10 cm^2, RV <30 mL/beat); normal EF mL/beat); EF normal; LV size normal	Clinical eval yearly
		Echo only if symptomatic
	Severe (VC ≥0.7 cm, ROA ≥0.4 cm^2, RV ≥60 mL/beat, RF >50%)	Clinical eval every 6-12 mo
		Echo every 6-12 mo

AVA= aortic valve area; echo = echocardiography; EF = ejection fraction; eval = evaluation; LV = left ventricle; MPG = mean pressure gradient; MVA = mitral valve area; PASP = pulmonary artery systolic pressure, RF = regurgitant fraction; ROA = regurgitant orifice area; RV = regurgitant volume; VC = vena contracta width; V_{max} = maximum aortic jet velocity.

Recommendations based on American College of Cardiology/American Heart Association Task Force on Practice Guidelines; Society of Cardiovascular Anesthesiologists; Society for Cardiovascular Angiography and Interventions; Society of Thoracic Surgeons, Bonow RO, Carabello BA, Kanu C, et al. ACC/AHA 2006 guidelines for the management of patients with valvular heart disease: a report of the American College of Cardiology/American Heart Association Task Force on Practice Guidelines (writing committee to revise the 1998 Guidelines for the Management of Patients With Valvular Heart Disease): developed in collaboration with the Society of Cardiovascular Anesthesiologists: endorsed by the Society for Cardiovascular Angiography and Interventions and the Society of Thoracic Surgeons. Circulation. 2006;114(5):e84-231. [PMID: 16880336]

increase of 7 mm Hg in mean transvalvular pressure gradient and an annual decrease of 0.1 cm^2 in valve area. Clinical factors associated with more rapid progression include severity of valve calcification, renal disease, and older age. Although significant outflow obstruction is not present with aortic sclerosis, there is a 50% increased risk of myocardial infarction or death due to cardiovascular disease over 5 years, likely due to the association between aortic sclerosis and total atherosclerotic burden.

Bicuspid Aortic Valve

About 50% of adults undergoing surgery for calcific aortic stenosis have a congenital bicuspid valve. Because a bicuspid valve is subject to higher mechanical and shear stress than a tricuspid valve, the disease process is accelerated, and clinical presentation tends to be earlier—in the fourth or fifth decades of life. A bicuspid aortic valve also is associated with aortic dilation and an increased risk of aortic dissection. Therefore, serial imaging of the aorta is indicated if aortic dilation is diagnosed. If the ascending aorta is not seen well by transthoracic echocardiography, serial CT or cardiac MRI of the aorta may be used. Aortic root replacement is indicated if diameter exceeds 5.0 cm but should be considered earlier if progression is rapid, there is a family history of dissection, or if there is a known underlying connective tissue disease. Most patients with bicuspid valves eventually develop significant abnormalities requiring surgery.

Clinical Presentation

Classic manifestations of aortic stenosis are angina, syncope, and heart failure. In early stages, aortic stenosis may present subtly, with dyspnea or a decrease in exercise tolerance. Atrial fibrillation can be associated with severe clinical deterioration. Angina occurs in more than 50% of patients with severe stenosis, due in part to maldistribution of coronary flow in the hypertrophied myocardium. Patients with aortic stenosis have increased sensitivity to ischemic injury and subsequent higher mortality. Frank syncope associated with aortic stenosis is rare, with prospective studies documenting sudden cardiac death rates below 1% annually.

Auscultatory features of aortic stenosis include a mid- to late-peaking systolic murmur that radiates to the carotid arteries, an S_4, a single S_2 due to loss of the aortic closure component, and delayed timing and decreased amplitude in the carotid pulses (pulsus parvus et tardus) (see Table 27).

Management

Once severe aortic stenosis is diagnosed in asymptomatic patients, yearly echocardiography aids in monitoring pulmonary pressure, ventricular hypertrophy, and worsening valve hemodynamics.

In the absence of valve replacement, the overall 1-year mortality rate in symptomatic patients with severe aortic stenosis is poor, approaching 50%. Definitive markers to predict timing and symptom onset are lacking, but most asymptomatic patients with transaortic velocities greater than 4 m/s eventually develop symptoms. Symptom provocation during exercise testing and an elevation in B-type natriuretic peptide levels may be early predictors for symptom onset.

Aortic valve replacement is the treatment of choice for symptomatic disease (**Table 30**). Patients with preoperative systolic dysfunction may recover some function after valve replacement with relief of afterload on the heart. Urgent valve replacement is indicated in patients who present in acute heart failure. Although studies suggest the relative safety and benefit of intravenous nitroprusside to transiently improve cardiac function as a bridge to valve replacement, this and other afterloading agents do not supplant valve replacement in symptomatic patients. Aortic valve replacement is associated with a perioperative mortality rate of 3% to 4%. Complications include thromboembolism, bleeding, prosthetic valve dysfunction, and endocarditis. Prophylactic valve replacement in asymptomatic patients is considered if other cardiac surgery is planned in patients with greater than moderate aortic

stenosis, those with systolic dysfunction, in women contemplating pregnancy, and in patients who live far from health care facilities.

Early studies with percutaneous valve replacement show promising results, but the data are still preliminary. Percutaneous balloon aortic valvotomy is generally not performed for calcific aortic stenosis because serious complications occur in more than 10% of patients, and restenosis or recurrent symptoms occur within 1 year in most patients.

KEY POINTS

- Auscultatory features of aortic stenosis include a mid- to late-peaking systolic murmur that radiates to carotid arteries, a single S_2, and a decrease and delay in the carotid pulses.
- Valve replacement for aortic stenosis is indicated once symptom onset occurs.
- Bicuspid aortic valves are associated with aortic stenosis, regurgitation, and aortic dilation.

Mitral Stenosis

Pathophysiology

Mitral stenosis is almost always caused by rheumatic valve disease, and more than 80% of patients are women. Recurrent rheumatic fever leads to progressive inflammatory injury and valvular dysfunction. Depending on the extent and location of injury, patients can develop stenotic valvular lesions, regurgitant lesions, or both. In the United States, clinical presentation tends to be in the fifth decade of life, or 20 to 30 years after the initial episode of rheumatic fever, but severe disease presents at much younger ages (adolescent to young adult) in immigrants from areas where rheumatic fever is endemic.

Clinical Presentation

Patients with moderate mitral stenosis (mean valvular pressure gradients 5-10 mm Hg) may be asymptomatic at rest, but develop dyspnea with increased cardiac demand, such as exercise, anemia, or pregnancy. Once symptoms develop, another decade can pass before symptoms are disabling. Progressive obstruction of mitral inflow leads to increases in left atrial pressure and dilation. Atrial fibrillation occurs in more than 30% of all symptomatic patients and is associated with worsening symptoms and poorer long term-outcome. Measures to restore sinus rhythm are usually unsuccessful or unsustained.

The auscultatory findings for rheumatic mitral stenosis include an opening snap with a low pitched mid-diastolic murmur that accentuates presystole (see Table 27). S_1 may be intensified owing to higher left atrial pressures. The echocardiographic appearance is one of commissural fusion, leaflet thickening, calcification, and restricted leaflet motion. The mitral valve may appear "domed" in diastole owing to the inability to fully open. Involvement of the chordae and subvalvular apparatus is common. In severe mitral stenosis,

TABLE 30 Timing of Intervention for Severe Left-Sided Valvular Conditions

Aortic Stenosis	Mitral Stenosis	Chronic Aortic Regurgitation	Chronic Mitral Regurgitation
INTERVENTION	*INTERVENTION*	*INTERVENTION*	*INTERVENTION*
Aortic valve replacement	Percutaneous valvotomy if anatomy amenable *and* if less than moderate mitral regurgitation *and* no left atrial appendage clot by TEE[a]; otherwise, mitral valve replacement	Aortic valve replacement with aortic root replacement if needed	Mitral valve repair if anatomy amenable; otherwise, mitral valve replacement
IF	*IF*	*IF*	*IF*
Patient symptomatic	Patient symptomatic	Patient symptomatic	Patient symptomatic
OR	*OR*	*OR*	*OR*
Ejection fraction <50%		Ejection fraction <50%	Ejection fraction <60%
OR		*OR*	*OR*
		End-systolic dimension >55 mm *or* end-diastolic dimension > 70 mm	End-systolic dimension >40 mm
		OR	*OR*
Patient needs other cardiothoracic surgery (e.g., CABG)	Abnormal hemodynamic response to exercise (PAP increases by 25 mm Hg)	Abnormal hemodynamic response to exercise (PAP increases by 25 mm Hg)	(Consider if) pulmonary hypertension or atrial fibrillation
OTHERWISE	*OTHERWISE*	*OTHERWISE*	*OTHERWISE*
Serial evaluation (see Table 29)	Serial evaluation (see Table 29)	Serial evaluation (see Table 29)	Serial evaluation (see Table 29)

CABG = coronary artery bypass surgery; PAP = pulmonary arterial pressure; TEE = transesophageal echocardiography.

[a]All patients considered for percutaneous valvotomy should undergo TEE to assess for left atrial appendage clot and mitral regurgitation severity whether or not the patient is in sinus rhythm or atrial fibrillation.

Recommendations based on American College of Cardiology/American Heart Association Task Force on Practice Guidelines; Society of Cardiovascular Anesthesiologists; Society for Cardiovascular Angiography and Interventions; Society of Thoracic Surgeons; Bonow RO, Carabello BA, Kanu C, et al. ACC/AHA 2006 guidelines for the management of patients with valvular heart disease: a report of the American College of Cardiology/American Heart Association Task Force on Practice Guidelines (writing committee to revise the 1998 Guidelines for the Management of Patients With Valvular Heart Disease): developed in collaboration with the Society of Cardiovascular Anesthesiologists: endorsed by the Society for Cardiovascular Angiography and Interventions and the Society of Thoracic Surgeons [erratum in Circulation. 2007;115(15):e409.]. Circulation. 2006;114(5):e84-231. [PMID: 16880336]

transmitral pressure gradients are greater than 10 mm Hg, the left atrium is enlarged, and pulmonary arterial pressures are usually above 60 mm Hg.

Management

Conservative medical management is a reasonable approach for patients with asymptomatic mild mitral stenosis. Rate control for atrial fibrillation with atrioventricular nodal blocking agents may improve diastolic filling time and decrease symptoms. Anticoagulation with warfarin is recommended in patients with atrial fibrillation or embolic stroke; prophylactic use of anticoagulation in other mitral stenosis patients has not shown benefit. Prognosis is excellent in asymptomatic and minimally symptomatic patients (>80% survival rate at 10 years), but once patients develop significant symptoms, the 10-year survival rate drops to below 15% without intervention. Death from rheumatic mitral stenosis results from progressive pulmonary congestion, systemic embolism, and infection.

In symptomatic patients, percutaneous valvotomy is indicated in symptomatic patients with a valve area of less than 1.0 cm² or pulmonary pressures above 50 mm Hg (see Table 30).

Percutaneous valvotomy also is recommended in asymptomatic patients with moderate or severe obstruction if valve anatomy is favorable. Valve characteristics that favor a successful valvotomy include pliable mitral valve leaflets, minimal commissural fusion, and minimal valvular/subvalvular calcification as evaluated by echocardiography. Pulmonary hypertension is not a contraindication, as this typically improves immediately following the procedure and continues to improve over the ensuing year. Major complications include severe mitral regurgitation, systemic embolization, and tamponade; the mortality rate is approximately 1%, with improved success rates at more experienced centers. Percutaneous valvotomy should not be attempted if the anatomy is unfavorable or if preprocedure transesophageal echocardiography demonstrates moderate or severe mitral regurgitation or the presence of a left atrial appendage thrombus. Symptom recurrence following valvotomy is more commonly due to mitral regurgitation than to recurrent stenosis.

In patients whose anatomy is not amenable to valvotomy or who have significant mitral regurgitation, valve replacement is recommended. In patients referred for mitral valve replacement surgery who have atrial fibrillation, concurrent left atrial radiofrequency ablation and left atrial appendage ligation should be considered to reduce postoperative atrial fibrillation rates.

- Mitral stenosis is almost always caused by rheumatic valve disease.
- Patients with mild mitral stenosis may be asymptomatic at rest but develop dyspnea with increased cardiac demand.
- Percutaneous valvotomy is the intervention of choice for moderate to severe mitral stenosis with favorable anatomy.

Acute Valvular Regurgitation

Acute, severe left-sided (aortic or mitral) valvular regurgitation causes sudden left ventricular volume overload. The initial cardiac response is increased heart rate to maintain forward cardiac output. Cardiac chamber size is generally preserved, with normal or hyperdynamic systolic function to accommodate the increased volume. When forward cardiac output cannot be maintained, heart failure, pulmonary edema, respiratory failure, and/or hemodynamic shock ensue. Patients are always symptomatic.

Acute valvular regurgitation is a medical emergency, regardless of the cause. Afterload reduction and inotropic medications may initially help stabilize the patient by increasing forward flow but do not usually supplant urgent surgical intervention.

Acute Aortic Regurgitation

The most common causes of acute aortic regurgitation are aortic dissection with retrograde propagation to the aortic valve and valve destruction from endocarditis. In acute aortic regurgitation, forward cardiac output is decreased and patients present with tachycardia and hemodynamic shock. During cardiac auscultation, the S_2 may be soft owing to early closure of the mitral valve, and an S_3 is often present. A low-pitched early diastolic murmur may be heard over the right sternal border. However, this may be difficult to discern if the patient is tachycardic or if the intensity of the murmur is lessened with sudden elevation in left ventricular diastolic pressure decreasing the relative pressure gradient across the aortic valve. Characteristic features of chronic aortic regurgitation (bounding peripheral pulses, widened pulse pressure) are less prominent because of a decrease in overall mean arterial pressure and inadequate time for compensatory changes in cardiac chamber size and function to augment forward stroke volume.

If acute aortic regurgitation is suspected, transthoracic echocardiography is diagnostic. Once diagnosed, surgical valve repair or replacement should be performed expeditiously. If an aortic dissection is suspected, additional imaging with transesophageal echocardiography, CT, or MRI aids in determining whether concurrent aortic root replacement is needed. Intra-aortic balloon pump placement is contraindicated, as diastolic inflation exacerbates aortic regurgitation.

Acute Mitral Regurgitation

Acute mitral regurgitation most commonly results from myxomatous mitral valve disease and chordal rupture; endocarditis with leaflet perforation, destruction, or malcoaptation; or papillary muscle dysfunction or rupture following myocardial infarction. Acute mitral regurgitation should be suspected in patients with myocardial infarction and acute respiratory failure. Heightened suspicion is critical, as these patients are often misdiagnosed with pneumonia or acute respiratory distress syndrome. Patients often do not present until several days after their infarct, once ischemic tissue becomes necrotic and rupture occurs.

Clinical presentation for acute mitral regurgitation includes tachycardia, heart failure, and hemodynamic shock. On physical examination, peripheral pulses are weak and pulmonary edema is evident. An S_3 is often present. With significant pulmonary hypertension, the pulmonic component of S_2 may be prominent. A parasternal systolic murmur is usually heard but may be diminished in hypotensive or tachycardic patients.

Transthoracic echocardiography is diagnostic for severe mitral regurgitation and can aid in diagnosing etiology by identifying papillary muscle rupture, flail mitral valve leaflets, large vegetations, or valve perforation. Left ventricular systolic function may appear normal or hyperdynamic, as left ventricular ejection volume is directed anterograde through the aortic valve and concurrently into the low-pressured left atrium.

Acute mitral regurgitation is a medical emergency. Although inotropic drugs, afterload-reducing drugs, and intra-aortic balloon pump support can provide temporary hemodynamic improvement in unstable patients, urgent surgical intervention is usually indicated.

- Clinical presentation in acute valvular regurgitation includes tachycardia, heart failure, pulmonary edema, and hemodynamic shock.
- Acute mitral regurgitation should be suspected in patients with myocardial infarction and acute respiratory failure.
- Afterload-reducing and inotropic medications may initially stabilize patients with acute valvular regurgitation but do not supplant urgent surgical intervention.

Chronic Valvular Regurgitation

Patients with mild or moderate left-sided valve regurgitation are usually asymptomatic and most do not progress to severe disease. In patients with severe regurgitation, compensatory changes in cardiac chamber size and function occur over time, allowing for maintenance of forward flow despite increased regurgitant stroke volume. Most patients eventually develop cardiopulmonary symptoms or a decline in exercise tolerance. Other, less common symptoms include arrhythmia and angina. Surgical intervention is indicated in all symptomatic patients with severe regurgitation (New York Heart Association functional class II-IV).

Although most patients with significant regurgitation are symptomatic prior to ventricular enlargement or dysfunction, some remain asymptomatic. Enlarged ventricular chamber size and the extent and duration of systolic dysfunction are important predictors of subsequent adverse events. Therefore, periodic clinical evaluation is indicated to evaluate ventricular size and function and aid in optimal timing of surgery. Serial evaluation is usually performed with echocardiography, but radionuclide angiography or MRI may be used to assess left ventricular volume and function if echocardiography is equivocal or nondiagnostic. Frequency of evaluation depends on the severity of valve dysfunction, the rapidity of lesion progression, and the symptom status of the patient (see Table 29).

Chronic Aortic Regurgitation

Chronic aortic regurgitation can result from annular dilation or primary leaflet dysfunction. Causes of primary leaflet dysfunction include bicuspid aortic valve, endocarditis, and leaflet prolapse. Aortic root enlargement due to various causes, such as Marfan syndrome, bicuspid aortic valve, and hypertension, can stretch the valve annulus, causing poor coaptation of the valve leaflets and regurgitation. The left ventricle dilates in response to the increased regurgitant volume, which allows maintenance of cardiac output. In this compensatory phase, patients may remain asymptomatic for a long time period. However, with eventual ventricular chamber enlargement or dysfunction due to the increased hemodynamic load, patients usually develop dyspnea, decreased exercise tolerance, and heart failure.

Physical examination in patients with chronic severe aortic regurgitation shows a widened pulse pressure with bounding peripheral and carotid pulses. With ventricular enlargement, the point of maximal impulse may be diffuse and displaced laterally. Auscultatory findings include an early- to holodiastolic murmur along the left upper sternal border which is high pitched and may be better heard when the patient is at end-expiration, leaning forward.

Valve replacement is indicated for symptomatic patients with severe aortic regurgitation, as the mortality rate in untreated patients exceeds 10% per year. In addition, long-term outcome is worse when regurgitant volume has had an adverse hemodynamic effect on ventricular size or function. Surgery is also indicated in some asymptomatic patients because approximately 15% of patients with significant regurgitation develop left ventricular dysfunction without

symptoms (see Table 30). Concurrent aortic root replacement should be considered if the ascending aorta diameter exceeds 5 cm, or 4.5 cm in those with a bicuspid valve.

In asymptomatic patients with chronic aortic regurgitation and normal left ventricular function, serial clinical evaluation to monitor for lesion progression is indicated. In these patients, oral afterload reduction with nifedipine or angiotensin-converting enzyme inhibitors to slow the rate of ventricular dilation by reducing regurgitant volume and improving forward stroke volume is controversial. Although a study of nearly 1000 patients found no change in symptom development or time to aortic valve replacement over 7 years with nifedipine or enalapril, several previous studies suggested that these agents helped delay the time to surgery. These medications are a reasonable choice for initial antihypertensive therapy in patients with aortic regurgitation, but surgical intervention should not be withheld if surgical criteria are met.

Chronic Mitral Regurgitation

Primary causes of chronic mitral regurgitation include mitral valve prolapse and endocarditis. Functional, or secondary, regurgitation of otherwise anatomically normal mitral valve leaflets can occur with leaflet tethering or dilation of the mitral valve annulus and is usually a consequence of ischemic myocardial dysfunction or dilated cardiomyopathy. In chronic mitral regurgitation, ventricular systolic function is initially hyperdynamic. However, progressive regurgitant volume and increased hemodynamic cardiac load can lead to ventricular chamber enlargement or dysfunction. Most patients with severe mitral regurgitation develop cardiopulmonary symptoms before onset of systolic dysfunction.

Physical examination findings of chronic mitral regurgitation in patients with hyperdynamic systolic function include a prominent apical impulse with normal pulse pressure. The murmur is usually holosystolic, heard best at the apex, and radiates laterally or posteriorly. In patients with mitral valve prolapse, the murmur may occur or be concentrated later in systole, once leaflet buckling leads to regurgitation. Physical examination findings in patients with left ventricular enlargement and systolic dysfunction include a laterally displaced apical impulse, an S_3, and evidence of pulmonary hypertension (prominent pulmonary component of S_2, increased jugular venous pressure, pulmonary congestion, and pedal edema). Echocardiography is integral to visualizing leaflet anatomy, assessing ventricular geometry, estimating pulmonary pressures, and predicting likelihood of valve repairability.

Treatment strategies for chronic mitral regurgitation are dependent on the underlying cause of mitral valve dysfunction. When mitral regurgitation occurs in volume-overloaded states (secondary regurgitation), both pre- and afterload reduction benefit the poorly functioning ventricle by reducing ventricular size, mitral annular diameter, and functional regurgitation. Studies on the use of resynchronization therapy (biventricular pacing) for dilated cardiomyopathy have shown improvement in left ventricular geometry and a decrease in regurgitation.

In patients with primary valve dysfunction and severe regurgitation, mitral valve replacement or repair is the treatment of choice. Mitral valve repair (annuloplasty) is preferred over valve replacement when possible because ventricular function is better preserved and long-term anticoagulation may be avoided. Although surgery is most commonly performed for primary mitral regurgitation, some symptomatic improvement in patients with secondary regurgitation refractory to medical therapy has been reported.

Surgery is indicated in symptomatic patients (NYHA class II-IV). In asymptomatic patients, surgery is recommended once there is evidence of adverse hemodynamic effects on the ventricle. Compared with previous guidelines, these criteria now recommend intervention at a smaller ventricular size (end-systolic diameter criterion has changed from >45 mm to >40 mm); this change is based on improved long-term outcomes with earlier surgical intervention and increased clinical experience with mitral valve repair techniques over time. Some experienced centers advocate even earlier mitral valve repair, including for patients with normal ventricular size and function when regurgitation is severe and the likelihood of a successful repair exceeds 90%.

Mitral Valve Prolapse

The prevalence of mitral valve prolapse in the United States is 2% to 3%, with approximately equal sex distribution. The mechanism of mitral valve prolapse is systolic buckling of the mitral valve leaflets into the left atrium. Mitral regurgitation occurs if there is faulty leaflet coaptation. Acute mitral regurgitation can also occur with chordal rupture.

Auscultatory findings are a midsystolic click followed by a late apical systolic murmur. Physical maneuvers that transiently change cardiac loading conditions can alter timing and character of the murmur. Echocardiography reveals thickened and redundant leaflets with systolic bulging or motion into the left atrium, usually with associated mitral regurgitation. Chordae may also be involved, with thickening and redundancy contributing to poor leaflet coaptation.

Serious complications of mitral valve prolapse can occur, including mitral regurgitation, endocarditis, and arrhythmia. Progressive mitral regurgitation is associated with heart failure, chordal rupture, arrhythmia, and sudden cardiac death. The benefit of pharmacologic therapy, such as afterload reduction or diuretics, is not well proven, and mitral regurgitation tends to worsen over time regardless of therapy. Therefore, early referral to a cardiologist to monitor for disease progression is indicated.

Mitral valve prolapse *syndrome* is a constellation of nonspecific symptoms that cannot be attributed to valvular dysfunction. The syndrome is benign and thought to be secondary to autonomic dysfunction. Commonly described symptoms include palpitations, atypical chest pain, dyspnea, fatigue, orthostatic symptoms, and neuropsychiatric complaints. Conservative management of clinical symptoms is indicated.

KEY POINTS

- Surgical intervention is indicated in symptomatic patients with severe left-sided valvular regurgitation.
- Timing of surgery in asymptomatic patients with chronic valvular regurgitation is primarily determined by left ventricular end-systolic dimension and ejection fraction.

Tricuspid Valve Disease

Primary tricuspid valve disease, usually related to a congenital disorder, is rare. Acquired tricuspid valve dysfunction nearly always manifests as regurgitation. Tricuspid regurgitation most often is due to left-sided heart disease causing pulmonary hypertension, which leads to right ventricular enlargement and annular dilation. Primary pulmonary hypertension and elevated pulmonary pressures due to chronic lung disease also cause tricuspid regurgitation, with the term *cor pulmonale* describing right-sided heart failure owing to pulmonary hypertension in the absence of left-sided heart disease. Other causes of tricuspid regurgitation include endocarditis, injury following pacer lead placement, carcinoid disease, mediastinal irradiation, and trauma. Carcinoid disease causes direct toxicity to the tricuspid valve, seen as leaflet thickening and retraction. The combination of sympathomimetic appetite suppressants fenfluramine and dexfenfluramine has been associated with valvular regurgitation and pulmonary hypertension. A similar valvulopathy has been seen with pergolide, ergotamine, and methysergide. In mild or moderate tricuspid regurgitation, most patients are asymptomatic. In severe tricuspid regurgitation, increased central venous pressures can lead to dyspnea with ascites, hepatic dysfunction, and pedal edema. Echocardiography should be performed in patients with either symptoms or a murmur and prior exposure to any of these drugs.

Severe tricuspid regurgitation from any cause is difficult to treat. Diuretics may aid in managing volume status in patients with significant pedal edema or ascites. Surgical tricuspid valve repair or replacement is usually attempted only if other cardiac surgery is planned. Bioprosthetic valves tend to be preferred over mechanical valves because of the lower risk of thromboembolism.

KEY POINTS

- Significant pulmonary hypertension can cause regurgitation of a normal tricuspid valve.
- Severe tricuspid regurgitation is difficult to treat, and surgery is generally performed only if other cardiac surgery is planned.

Endocarditis

Diagnosis

Endocarditis should be suspected if an abnormal murmur is heard on examination, particularly in patients with a compelling history or concurrent fever. Incidence is higher in patients with underlying valve abnormalities and prosthetic valves. Most cases of native valve endocarditis are caused by streptococcal and staphylococcal species. Less common pathogens causing culture-negative or slow-growing endocarditis include *HACEK* organisms (*Haemophilus*, *Actinobacillus*, *Cardiobacterium*, *Eikenella*, and *Kingella*), fungi, and mycobacteria. However, the most common reason for culture-negative or slow-growing cultures in endocarditis is antibiotic treatment prior to culture.

Diagnostic criteria for endocarditis include bacteriologic evidence, clinical findings, and echocardiographic evidence of endocardial involvement such as valvular dysfunction, vegetation, or paravalvular abscess (**Table 31**). Transthoracic echocardiography has a sensitivity of 50% to 80% for detecting vegetations. Transesophageal echocardiography increases sensitivity and specificity to approximately 95% and better delineates native valvular anatomy. Transesophageal echocardiography is the test of choice to identify a paravalvular abscess.

Persons with known native valve disease, long-term indwelling intravascular access catheters, or permanent devices (prosthetic valves, pacemakers, defibrillators) who present with fever should have blood cultures obtained prior to starting antibiotics. If bacteremia is diagnosed in a patient with a device, early notification of the specialty care provider (for example, an electrophysiologist) is indicated in case the device will need to be removed.

Management

Antibiotic therapy is guided by the causative organism (see MKSAP 15 Infectious Disease). Emergent valve repair or replacement surgery is indicated in patients with hemodynamic instability and should not be delayed until after the acute infection has resolved. However, surgery may be reconsidered if there are severe complications with remote prospect of recovery, such as severe embolic cerebral damage. Up to 50% of endocarditis patients eventually require surgery. Factors favoring earlier surgical intervention include valve destruction, paravalvular abscess, heart block, resistant infections, fungal endocarditis, larger vegetations, and recurrent septic embolic disease. Valve repair is preferred over replacement to reduce the risk of prosthetic infection. All complications of endocarditis occur with higher frequency and are more difficult to treat with prosthetic valves.

Prophylaxis

Previous guidelines recommended prophylaxis to various patients with cardiac abnormalities undergoing certain dental, gastrointestinal, or genitourinary procedures. Guidelines were published in 2007 that reflect a dramatic shift in prophylaxis recommendations (**Table 32**). Endocarditis is now thought more likely to result from frequent exposure to random bacteremia rather than standard dental, gastrointestinal, or genitourinary procedures, and therefore prophylaxis is no longer recommended for most native valve disease. Also, it is not clear that prophylaxis is effective for prevention of endocarditis, and prophylaxis exposes patients to the risks of antibiotic therapy. Prophylaxis regimen options are provided in MKSAP 15 Infectious Disease.

TABLE 31 Clinical Criteria for the Diagnosis of Endocarditis	
Definite Endocarditis	
2 major criteria *or*	
1 major and 3 minor criteria *or*	
5 minor criteria	
Major Criteria	**Minor Criteria**
Persistently positive blood cultures of organisms typical for endocarditis[a]	Predisposing condition or injection drug use
New valvular regurgitation	Fever
Positive echocardiogram	Embolic vascular phenomena
	Immunologic phenomena (eg, glomerulonephritis, rheumatoid factor)
	Positive blood cultures not meeting major criteria

[a]Or a single positive culture for *Coxiella burnetii* or IgG antibody titer >1:800.

Information from Li JS, Sexton DJ, Mick N, et al. Proposed modifications to the Duke criteria for the diagnosis of infective endocarditis. Clin Infect Dis. 2000;30(4):633-638. [PMID: 10770721]

TABLE 32 Patients Requiring Bacterial Endocarditis Prophylaxis for Dental Procedures

Patients with:
Prosthetic heart valves or valve repair with prosthetic material
Prior endocarditis
Congenital heart disease
Unrepaired cyanotic congenital heart disease
Palliative shunts and conduits
Prosthetic valve
Repair with prosthetic material or device for the first 6 months after intervention
Valve disease in heart transplant recipients

Recommendations based on Wilson W, Taubert KA, Gewitz M, et al; American Heart Association Rheumatic Fever, Endocarditis, and Kawasaki Disease Committee; American Heart Association Council on Cardiovascular Disease in the Young; American Heart Association Council on Clinical Cardiology; American Heart Association Council on Cardiovascular Surgery and Anesthesia; Quality of Care and Outcomes Research Interdisciplinary Working Group. Prevention of infective endocarditis: guidelines from the American Heart Association: a guideline from the American Heart Association Rheumatic Fever, Endocarditis, and Kawasaki Disease Committee, Council on Cardiovascular Disease in the Young, and the Council on Clinical Cardiology, Council on Cardiovascular Surgery and Anesthesia, and the Quality of Care and Outcomes Research Interdisciplinary Working Group [erratum in Circulation. 2007;116(15):e376-e377.]. Circulation 2007;116(15):1736-1754. [PMID: 17446442]

KEY POINTS

- Endocarditis should be suspected in patients with a new or abnormal murmur, particularly in patients with fever or a compelling history.

- Blood cultures should be obtained in febrile patients with implanted devices, such as prosthetic valves or pacemakers, and those with known native valve disease before instituting antibiotic therapy for presumed noncardiac infections.

- Endocarditis prophylaxis is no longer indicated in most patients with native valve disease, including those with mitral valve prolapse or a bicuspid aortic valve.

- Emergent surgery is indicated in endocarditis patients with hemodynamic instability and should not be delayed while the acute infection is treated.

Prosthetic Valves

Mechanical prosthetic valves require continuous anticoagulation to reduce valve thrombosis. Advances in valve design have resulted in improved hemodynamic flow profiles and reduced blood stasis over prosthetic valve occluders. As a result, recommended INR values are lower than previous recommendations. For low-risk patients, those with a mechanical aortic valve with no other risk factors, the INR goal is 2.0 to 3.0. In high-risk patients, those with a mechanical mitral valve or aortic valve plus an additional risk factor (atrial fibrillation, left ventricular dysfunction, previous thromboembolism, or hypercoagulable condition), an INR of 2.5 to 3.5 is recommended. The addition of low-dose aspirin (81 mg/d) to warfarin further decreases risk of thromboembolism and is recommended in all patients with prosthetic heart valves.

Bioprosthetic valves consist of biologic material mounted on struts and a sewing ring. Valve thrombosis is much lower for bioprosthetic valves (<1%), and continuous life-long anticoagulation is not recommended. However, warfarin with an INR goal of 2.0 to 3.0 is recommended for bioprosthetic valves in the mitral position for the first 3 postoperative months to allow complete endothelialization of the new valve.

Bioprosthetic valves are less durable than mechanical valves because of the progressive degenerative calcification of the biologic material. In the first generation of bioprosthetic valves, only about 50% of aortic and 30% of mitral prostheses were still working after 15 years. Although newer valves are more durable and have larger valve areas and improved hemodynamics, they are still prone to progressive calcific degeneration. Paradoxically, leaflet degeneration is increased in patients who are younger at the time of implantation.

Valve choice depends on valve characteristics, patient characteristics, and preference. Mechanical valves tend to be implanted in younger patients, but require lifelong anticoagulation. In patients older than 65 years, bioprosthetic valves are recommended for aortic valve disease because anticoagulation can be avoided and valve degeneration is less likely in this age group. Mechanical valves typically are used in the mitral position because of concurrent atrial fibrillation and durability issues, unless there are contraindications to warfarin anticoagulation or in very elderly patients. For both valve types, prosthetic valve endocarditis is a serious potential complication, responsible for approximately 20% of endocarditis cases. The risk of prosthetic valve endocarditis is higher with mechanical prostheses during the first 3 months following valve replacement; by 5 years, however, the rate of long-term infection is comparable at approximately 6%. Endocarditis prophylaxis is required for all patients with prosthetic valves undergoing certain dental, gastrointestinal, or genitourinary procedures.

All patients with a prosthetic valve should have an echocardiogram performed 2 to 3 months after surgery to establish baseline values. Common complications of prosthetic valves include structural valve deterioration, valve thrombosis, embolism, bleeding, and endocarditis. In the immediate postoperative period, valve dehiscence or dysfunction should be suspected in patients who develop acute heart failure.

Prosthetic valve dysfunction should be suspected in patients with new cardiac symptoms, embolic phenomena, hemolytic anemia, or new murmurs. If valve dysfunction is suspected, transesophageal echocardiography is the diagnostic procedure of choice, but findings may be somewhat limited by acoustic shadowing and reverberations from prosthetic material. Thromboembolic events in patients with prosthetic valves should always be assumed to be due to the valve prosthesis unless there is compelling evidence for another cause. Emergency surgery is recommended for patients with mechanical valves who develop left-sided valve thrombosis with heart failure, valve dysfunction, or a large clot burden. With a large clot burden, fibrinolytic therapy is associated with a 15% risk of major cerebral emboli and is unlikely to be effective. However, fibrinolytic therapy may be considered in hemodynamically stable patients with a small clot burden or with right-sided valve thrombosis.

KEY POINTS

- Mechanical valves are durable but require lifelong warfarin anticoagulation.
- Biologic valves do not require lifelong anticoagulation, but are prone to progressive calcific degeneration.
- Surgery is indicated for mechanical valve thrombosis unless the patient is hemodynamically stable and the clot burden is small.

Bibliography

Bonow RO, Carabello BA, Kanu C, et al. ACC/AHA 2006 guidelines for the management of patients with valvular heart disease: a report of the American College of Cardiology/American Heart Association Task Force on Practice Guidelines (writing committee to revise the 1998 Guidelines for the Management of Patients With Valvular Heart Disease): developed in collaboration with the Society of Cardiovascular Anesthesiologists: endorsed by the Society for Cardiovascular Angiography and Interventions and the Society of Thoracic Surgeons. Circulation [erratum in Circulation. 2007; 115(15):e409.]. 2006;114(5):e84-231. [PMID: 16880336]

Douglas PS, Khandheria B, Stainback RF, et al. ACCF/ASE/ACEP/ASNC/SCAI/SCCT/SCMR 2007 appropriateness criteria for transthoracic and transesophageal echocardiography: a report of the American College of Cardiology Foundation Quality Strategic Directions Committee Appropriateness Criteria Working Group, American Society of Echocardiography, American College of Emergency Physicians, American Society of Nuclear Cardiology, Society for Cardiovascular Angiography and Interventions, Society of Cardiovascular Computed Tomography, and the Society for Cardiovascular Magnetic Resonance endorsed by the American College of Chest Physicians and the Society of Critical Care Medicine. J Am Coll Cardiol. 2007;50(2):187-204. [PMID: 17616306]

Evangelista A, Tornos P, Sambola A, Permanyer-Miralda G, Soler-Soler J. Long-term vasodilator therapy in patients with severe aortic regurgitation. N Engl J Med. 2005;353(13):1342-1349. [PMID: 16192479]

Goldbarg S, Elmariah S, Miller MA, Fuster V. Insights into degenerative aortic valve disease. J Am Coll Cardiol. 2007;50(13):1205-1213. [PMID: 17888836]

Hayek E, Gring CN, Griffin BP. Mitral valve prolapse. Lancet. 2005;365(9458):507-518. [PMID: 15705461]

Li JS, Sexton DJ, Mick N, et al. Proposed modifications to the Duke criteria for the diagnosis of infective endocarditis. Clin Infect Dis. 2000; 30(4):633-638. [PMID: 10770721]

Rosenhek R, Rader F, Klaar U, et al. Outcome of watchful waiting in asymptomatic severe mitral regurgitation. Circulation. 2006;113 (18):2238-2244. [PMID: 16651470]

Rossebø AB, Pedersen TR, Boman K, et al; SEAS Investigators. Intensive lipid lowering with simvastatin and ezetimibe in aortic stenosis. N Engl J Med. 2008;359(13):1343-1356. [PMID: 18765433]

Supino PG, Borer JS, Schuleri K, et al. Prognostic value of exercise tolerance testing in asymptomatic chronic nonischemic mitral regurgitation. Am J Cardiol. 2007;100(8):1274-1281. [PMID: 17920370]

Wilson W, Taubert KA, Gewitz M, et al. Prevention of infective endocarditis: guidelines from the American Heart Association: a guideline from the American Heart Association Rheumatic Fever, Endocarditis, and Kawasaki Disease Committee, Council on Cardiovascular Disease in the Young, and the Council on Clinical Cardiology, Council on Cardiovascular Surgery and Anesthesia, and the Quality of Care and Outcomes Research Interdisciplinary Working Group [erratum in Circulation. 2007;116(15):e376-7.]. Circulation. 2007;116(15): 1736-1754. [PMID: 17446442]

Adult Congenital Heart Disease

Epidemiology

It is estimated that more than 85% of infants born with congenital heart disease in North America now reach adulthood, and there are now more adults living with congenital heart disease than children. Adults with a history of congenital cardiac surgery and those with newly diagnosed congenital heart disease require regular specialized cardiovascular care and informed follow-up.

Newly Diagnosed Congenital Heart Disease in Adults

Atrial Septal Defect

Pathophysiology and Genetics

Atrial septal defect, a communication between the atria that persists after birth, may not be diagnosed until adulthood. Atrial septal defects are classified according to their location in the atrial septum (**Figure 25**). An ostium secundum atrial septal defect, located in the midportion of the atrial septum, is the most common type of atrial septal defect, accounting for 75% of cases and usually occurring as an isolated congenital cardiac abnormality. The volume load imposed by the left-to-right shunt through the defect causes right-sided chamber dilatation. An ostium primum atrial septal defect is located in the lowest portion of the atrial septum. These defects are

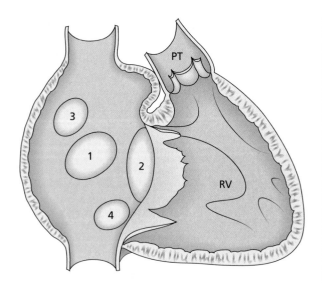

FIGURE 25.
Atrial Septal Defects.
Positions of various atrial septal defects viewed from the right side of the heart.

PT = pulmonary trunk; RV = right ventricle; 1 = ostium secundum; 2 = ostium primum; 3 = sinus venosus; 4 = inferior vena cava.

Redrawn from original supplied courtesy of Dr. William D. Edwards, Department of Laboratory Medicine and Pathology, Mayo Clinic, Rochester, MN.

usually associated with a cleft in the anterior mitral or tricuspid valve leaflets (leading to valve regurgitation) and with a ventricular septal defect or aneurysm of the membranous ventricular septum. A sinus venosus atrial septal defect is located at the uppermost portion of the atrial septum and is usually associated with one or more anomalous right-sided pulmonary veins connecting to the right atrium or superior vena cava. Inferior vena caval and unroofed coronary sinus atrial septal defects are both very rare.

The risk of a woman with a sporadic atrial septal defect transmitting a defect to her offspring is estimated at 8% to 10%. Genetic syndromes with skeletal abnormalities associated with atrial septal defect include various heart-hand syndromes, of which Holt-Oram syndrome is best known. Both ostium secundum and ostium primum atrial septal defects are associated with Down syndrome. Familial occurrence of ostium secundum atrial septal defects is recognized, and a defect has been localized to chromosome 5 in some kindreds. Familial atrial septal defect with a conduction defect is an autosomal dominant trait. Because of the possibility of familial occurrence, a family history should be taken in patients with atrial septal defect, and echocardiographic screening of relatives may be indicated.

Clinical Presentation

Adults with unrepaired atrial septal defects may be asymptomatic or may present with symptoms related to excess pulmonary blood flow, including fatigue, dyspnea, palpitations, or right-sided heart failure. Atrial arrhythmias, including

atrial fibrillation or flutter and sick sinus syndrome, are a common presentation and are caused by long-standing right heart volume and pressure overload. Paradoxical embolism, from peripheral venous or pelvic vein thromboses, unfiltered intravenous infusions, or indwelling venous catheters or pacemakers, is a risk for patients with any atrial septal defect regardless of size. Pulmonary artery hypertension may develop in up to 5% to 10% of persons with atrial septal defect and predominantly affects females.

The characteristic physical examination findings in atrial septal defect are fixed splitting of the S_2 and a right ventricular heave. A pulmonary midsystolic flow murmur and a tricuspid diastolic flow rumble caused by increased flow through the right-sided valves from a large left-to-right shunt may be heard. The jugular venous pressure may be normal, or a and v waves may be equal. Typically, there is absence of sinus arrhythmia (the normal cyclic increase in heart rate with inspiration and decrease with expiration) because sinus arrhythmia depends on separation of the systemic and pulmonary venous return to the heart as well as on normal autonomic control mechanisms.

Diagnostic Evaluation

Transthoracic echocardiography is the diagnostic test of choice for atrial septal defects and allows assessment of the defect location and size as well as associated cardiac manifestations such as right heart size, function, and pulmonary pressures. Transesophageal echocardiography is recommended to confirm the diagnosis when transthoracic imaging is suboptimal or when associated abnormalities are suspected; it is often required to confirm the diagnosis in sinus venosus atrial septal defect. Cardiac magnetic resonance (CMR) imaging provides direct visualization of the atrial septal defect and pulmonary veins but is rarely required when echocardiography is diagnostic. It should be considered primarily in the evaluation of a patient with a suspected anomalous pulmonary venous connection as an alternative to transesophageal echocardiography. In addition, CMR imaging allows quantification of right ventricular volume and function as well as shunt size.

In ostium secundum atrial septal defect, the electrocardiogram demonstrates right axis deviation and incomplete right bundle branch block. The electrocardiogram in ostium primum atrial septal defect characteristically demonstrates first-degree atrioventricular block, left axis deviation, and right bundle branch block. Left atrial enlargement may result from mitral valve regurgitation from the cleft.

The chest radiograph is noteworthy for right atrial and right ventricular enlargement, a prominent pulmonary artery, and increased pulmonary markings in both lung fields. Left atrial enlargement generally does not occur in ostium secundum atrial septal defect in the absence of atrial fibrillation. Diagnostic cardiac catheterization is rarely required unless there are concerns about pulmonary artery hypertension or coronary artery disease that may influence intervention.

Treatment

Treatment of an atrial septal defect depends on size, location, and hemodynamic impact of the defect; available treatments; comorbidities; and patient status and preferences. Small atrial septal defects (<5 mm) with no evidence of right ventricular volume overload may not require closure unless associated with paradoxical embolism. Atrial septal defects with evidence of right ventricular volume overload on echocardiography usually only cause symptoms after the second or third decade of life. Closure is indicated to reduce or prevent long-term complications such as atrial arrhythmias, exercise intolerance, paradoxical embolism, right-sided heart failure, and irreversible pulmonary hypertension. Even in adults, closure of large defects improves survival and relieves symptoms. The rate of late atrial fibrillation after atrial septal defect closure increases with age at the time of intervention; more than half of patients who are older than 40 years when closure is performed develop late atrial arrhythmias.

Ostium secundum atrial septal defect with associated significant right-to-left shunt and no pulmonary hypertension is usually treated by percutaneous device closure. Follow-up data for this treatment are still limited, but a multicenter study with a 12-month follow-up showed that percutaneous device closure is safe, with similar adverse event rates and shorter hospital stays compared with surgical closure. Ostium primum, sinus venosus, and caval types of atrial septal defects require surgical closure by experienced cardiac surgeons.

Aspirin is recommended for 6 months after device closure of an atrial septal defect. Endocarditis prophylaxis is recommended for 6 months after device or prosthetic surgical closure of an atrial septal defect.

KEY POINTS

- Atrial septal defect should be considered in all patients presenting with new-onset atrial arrhythmias.
- Paradoxical embolism is a risk for all patients with an atrial septal defect regardless of the size of the defect.
- The characteristic physical examination findings in atrial septal defect are fixed splitting of the S_2 and the absence of sinus arrhythmia.
- An atrial septal defect should be closed if there is evidence of volume overload of right-sided cardiac chambers or symptoms related to the defect.

Patent Foramen Ovale

Before birth, the foramen ovale allows transfer of oxygenated placental blood to the fetal systemic circulation. This communication usually closes after birth, but in 25% to 30% of the population, a potential pathway remains patent (**Figure 26**). Patent foramen ovale may be incidentally found by echocardiography or suspected in a young patient with cryptogenic stroke.

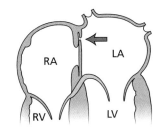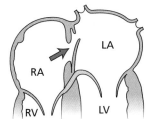

FIGURE 26.
Patent Foramen Ovale.
The *arrow* on the right panel demonstrates the mechanism of right-to-left shunt through the patent foramen ovale.

LA = left atrium; LV = left ventricle; RA = right atrium; RV = right ventricle.

Redrawn from original supplied courtesy of Dr. William D. Edwards, Department of Laboratory Medicine and Pathology, Mayo Clinic, Rochester, MN.

Transesophageal echocardiography is the test of choice to detect a patent foramen ovale. Agitated saline is injected into a peripheral intravenous catheter to demonstrate the right-to-left intracardiac shunt, which is often enhanced by the Valsalva maneuver.

Most patients with a patent foramen ovale are asymptomatic. However, there is an increased prevalence of patent foramen ovale in patients with cryptogenic stroke, which may be related to a paradoxical embolism through the patent foramen ovale. Cryptogenic stroke is more frequent in patients with a patent foramen ovale associated with an atrial septal aneurysm than with patent foramen ovale alone. Current guidelines note that insufficient data exist to make a recommendation regarding closure for secondary stroke prevention after a first stroke. Closure may be considered, however, for patients with recurrent cryptogenic stroke despite medical therapy.

Patent foramen ovale may be related to cyanosis in the setting of tricuspid valve regurgitation, right-sided heart failure, pulmonary artery hypertension, decompression sickness in divers, and orthodeoxia-platypnea (postural dyspnea and cyanosis). Closure may be suggested in such cases.

Patent Foramen Ovale and Migraine

Several observational studies demonstrate an association between patent foramen ovale and migraine headaches; however, evidence to support a causal link is insufficient. Although the results of uncontrolled observational studies suggest that patent foramen ovale closure may have a beneficial effect on migraine frequency, a large randomized trial failed to support this conclusion. Therefore, patent foramen ovale closure should not be performed for the prophylaxis of migraine.

KEY POINTS

- Most patients with a patent foramen ovale are asymptomatic.
- Patent foramen ovale closure may be considered for patients with recurrent cryptogenic stroke despite medical therapy.

Ventricular Septal Defect

Pathophysiology

Ventricular septal defects may be subdivided into four anatomic types according to their location on the ventricular septum (**Figure 27**). *Perimembranous* ventricular septal defects are the most common, accounting for approximately 80% of defects in adults. They are located in the membranous portion of the ventricular septum adjacent to the aortic valve and the septal leaflet of the tricuspid valve. The leaflet may adhere to the defect, forming a pouch or "aneurysm" of the ventricular septum. This pouch limits left-to-right shunting and can result in partial or complete closure of the defect. *Subpulmonary* or *outlet* ventricular septal defects account for approximately 6% of defects in non-Asian populations, but up to 33% in Asian patients. Spontaneous closure of this type of ventricular septal defect is uncommon. *Muscular* ventricular septal defects can occur in any part of the ventricular septum and can be multiple. Spontaneous closure is common, and although these defects account for up to 20% of ventricular septal defects in infants, the incidence is much lower in adults. *Inlet* ventricular septal defects occur in the superior posterior portion of the ventricular septum, adjacent to the tricuspid valve. These defects are rare in adults, but do occur in patients with Down syndrome and as part of the atrioventricular septal defect complex.

Clinical Presentation

Patients with small ventricular septal defects have small left-to-right shunts and present with systolic murmurs. These patients have no left ventricular volume overload and no pulmonary artery hypertension. The small ventricular septal defect causes a loud holosystolic murmur that is sometimes palpable and obliterates the S_2. The murmur is most commonly located at the left lower sternal border.

Patients with moderate-sized ventricular septal defects and small to moderate left-to-right shunts will develop left ventricular volume overload and pulmonary artery hypertension. They may remain asymptomatic for many years or develop symptoms of mild heart failure. A moderate-sized ventricular septal defect with volume overload causes a displaced left ventricular impulse and a systolic murmur. The duration and quality of the systolic murmur depend on the pressure gradient between the left and right ventricle. When the ventricular septal defect is small and the right ventricular pressure is low, the murmur is holosystolic. As the patient develops pulmonary artery hypertension, the murmur becomes an early peaking, short systolic murmur. A mitral diastolic rumble occurs in patients with a moderate or large shunt and is related to increased flow across the mitral valve.

Large ventricular septal defects are usually detected in childhood because of a murmur or the presence of heart failure. Without closure early in life, large ventricular septal defects cause pulmonary artery hypertension with irreversible pulmonary vascular disease and eventual reversal of the shunt from a left-to-right shunt to a right-to-left shunt (Eisenmenger syndrome).

Diagnostic Evaluation

In most patients with a small ventricular septal defect, the electrocardiogram is normal. In patients with significant pulmonary artery hypertension, right ventricular hypertrophy will be evident on the electrocardiogram.

Chest radiograph in patients with a small ventricular septal defect is typically normal. The presence of a significant left-to-right shunt will create the appearance of left atrial and left ventricular enlargement. In patients with severe pulmonary artery hypertension, the chest radiograph demonstrates a prominent pulmonary artery segment and diminished peripheral pulmonary vascular markings.

Transthoracic echocardiography is the primary diagnostic technique in patients with a known or suspected ventricular septal defect. Echocardiography allows identification of the number and location of defects; assessment of chamber sizes, ventricular function, presence or absence of aortic valve prolapse or regurgitation, and presence or absence of tricuspid regurgitation; and estimation of pulmonary pressures. MRI may be useful to confirm the anatomy of unusual ventricular septal defects, such as inlet or apical defects not well seen by echocardiography. Cardiac catheterization is performed in select patients to delineate hemodynamics and the degree of pulmonary hypertension; this is particularly

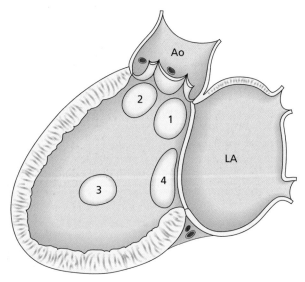

FIGURE 27.
Ventricular Septal Defects.
Positions of various ventricular septal defects viewed from the left side of the heart.

Ao = aorta; LA = left atrium; 1 = perimembranous; 2 = subpulmonary; 3 = muscular; 4 = inlet.

Redrawn from original supplied courtesy of Dr. William D. Edwards, Department of Laboratory Medicine and Pathology, Mayo Clinic, Rochester, MN.

important to help determine the advisability of operation in a patient with a moderate ventricular septal defect.

Treatment

Children and adults with isolated small ventricular septal defects rarely require closure. Closure of the defect is recommended in adults with progressive aortic or tricuspid valve regurgitation, progressive left ventricular volume overload, and, occasionally, recurrent endocarditis. Percutaneous device closure is possible in select ventricular septal defects.

KEY POINTS

- Most ventricular septal defects in adults are small membranous defects that cause a loud murmur with little flow and do not require closure.

- Ventricular septal defect closure is recommended in adults with progressive aortic or tricuspid valve regurgitation, progressive left ventricular volume overload, and, occasionally, recurrent endocarditis.

Coarctation of the Aorta

Clinical Presentation

Aortic coarctation is a narrowing of the aorta that is usually located just beyond the left subclavian artery. It is usually diagnosed in childhood by the association of a systolic murmur with systemic hypertension and reduced femoral pulse amplitude. More than 50% of patients with aortic coarctation also have a bicuspid aortic valve. Aortic coarctation may be associated with Turner syndrome, a chromosomal abnormality (45,X) characterized by a female with short stature, a broad chest, wide-spaced nipples, webbed neck, and cardiac defects.

Hypertension in the upper extremities with reduced blood pressure in the lower extremities is present, resulting in a radial-to-femoral artery delay in pulse appearance. A systolic murmur is common. When coarctation is severe, the murmur may be continuous and a murmur from collateral intercostal vessels may also be audible and palpable. An ejection click and aortic systolic murmur suggest the presence of a bicuspid aortic valve. An S_4 is common. In the presence of dilated collateral vessels, femoral pulses and the measured systolic gradients may not correlate with the degree of coarctation.

Diagnostic Evaluation

The electrocardiogram in aortic coarctation demonstrates left ventricular hypertrophy. When aortic coarctation is severe, the intercostal arteries (usually of ribs 4-8) dilate to accommodate blood flow, bypassing the area of obstruction. This may cause the characteristic radiographic sign of "rib notching." Another radiographic finding is an indentation at the coarctation site resulting in the "figure 3 sign," caused by dilatation of the aorta above and below the area of coarctation (**Figure 28**).

A prominent curvilinear shadow along the mid-right sternal border may be present from a dilated ascending aorta.

Echocardiography is often the initial diagnostic test and confirms the presence of coarctation and associated features such as a bicuspid aortic valve. CMR imaging and CT clearly delineate the location and severity of coarctation, the presence of collateral vessels, and the status of the ascending aorta. These techniques are the preferred means of imaging the aorta in coarctation. Diagnostic cardiac catheterization is mainly justified when associated coronary artery disease is suspected and a catheter-based intervention is to be performed.

Treatment

In persons with aortic coarctation who do not have surgery, survival averages 35 years of age with 75% mortality by 46 years of age. Systemic hypertension, accelerated coronary artery disease, stroke, aortic dissection, and heart failure are common complications in patients who do not have surgery or who have surgery as adults.

Coarctation intervention is usually recommended when the systolic gradient across the coarctation is above 30 mm Hg. Surgical treatment is the treatment of choice for primary coarctation. Percutaneous intervention with balloon and

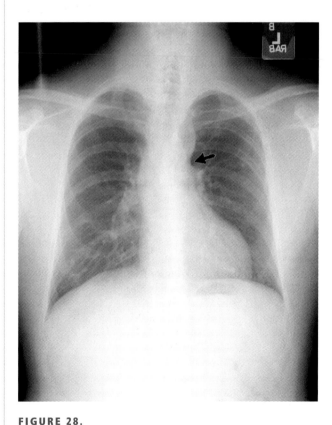

FIGURE 28.
Figure 3 Sign.
Chest radiograph of a patient with aortic coarctation exhibiting the "figure 3 sign," caused by dilatation of the aorta above and below the area of coarctation (*arrow*).

stent dilatation is increasingly performed for both native coarctation and recoarctation.

Patent Ductus Arteriosus

Clinical Presentation

The arterial duct connects the aorta and pulmonary artery in fetal life. Persistence of the ductus arteriosus after birth is associated with maternal rubella and prematurity.

A tiny patent ductus arteriosus may be inaudible and does not require intervention. A small patent ductus arteriosus in the adult produces an arteriovenous fistula with a continuous murmur that envelopes the S_2 and is characteristically heard beneath the left clavicle. Patients with a moderate-sized patent ductus arteriosus may present with symptoms of heart failure, a continuous "machinery-type" murmur best heard at the left infraclavicular area, and bounding pulses with a wide pulse pressure.

Adults may present with pulmonary artery hypertension due to a previously unrecognized patent ductus arteriosus. A clinical clue to the diagnosis is cyanosis and clubbing affecting the feet more than the hands, which result from desaturated blood reaching the lower body.

Diagnostic Evaluation

The electrocardiogram may be normal if the patent ductus arteriosus is small. If there is a moderate left-to-right shunt, the electrocardiogram may show left atrial enlargement and left ventricular hypertrophy. Biventricular hypertrophy may be present if there is associated pulmonary artery hypertension.

With a moderate-sized patent ductus arteriosus, the chest radiograph may show cardiomegaly, increased pulmonary vascular markings, prominent proximal pulmonary arteries indicating elevated pulmonary artery pressure, and an enlarged left atrium and left ventricle. Calcification may be noted in the region of the ductus.

Color Doppler echocardiography is usually diagnostic of a patent ductus arteriosus. However, in patients with significant pulmonary artery hypertension, it may be difficult to see the patent ductus by echocardiography. Cardiac catheterization and angiography may be indicated in these patients to evaluate the degree of shunting, the pulmonary vascular resistance,

and the reactivity of the vascular bed. In addition, angiography can determine the size and shape of the ductus.

Treatment

If the size and shape of the patent ductus arteriosus are suitable, it can be closed percutaneously. Transcatheter closure of a small patent ductus arteriosus should be considered in patients with a past episode of endarteritis. In the absence of symptoms or complications, observation is recommended.

For a moderate-sized patent ductus arteriosus with left heart enlargement and no pulmonary artery hypertension, percutaneous device closure is recommended to avoid progressive heart failure. Patent ductus arteriosus closure should be avoided in patients with irreversible pulmonary artery hypertension, which is confirmed by cardiac catheterization.

Pulmonary Stenosis

Clinical Presentation

Valvular pulmonary stenosis is usually an isolated congenital abnormality and causes obstruction to the right ventricular outflow. It may be associated with Noonan syndrome, an autosomal dominant disorder characterized by short stature, intellectual impairment, unique facial features, neck webbing, and congenital heart disease. Severe valvular obstruction may be tolerated for many years before development of symptoms.

In severe pulmonary stenosis, the jugular venous pressure demonstrates a prominent *a* wave. A right ventricular lift is common. An ejection click is common, and increased proximity of the click to S_1 suggests increasing severity of the stenosis. Eventually, the click is lost as the valve loses pliability. A systolic murmur is present, with the pulmonic component of the S_2 delayed. With severe valvular pulmonary stenosis, the pulmonic component of the S_2 disappears, and a right ventricular S_4 may be present.

Diagnostic Evaluation

In severe pulmonary stenosis, right ventricular hypertrophy, right axis deviation, and right atrial enlargement are noted on the electrocardiogram. The heart size on chest radiograph is usually normal, and dilatation of the main pulmonary artery is common. Calcification of the valve is seen infrequently.

Echocardiography with Doppler evaluation confirms the diagnosis and determines the severity of pulmonary stenosis and the degree of right ventricular hypertrophy. Intervention is recommended when the peak systolic gradient is greater than 50 mm Hg, when right ventricular hypertrophy is present, or when the patient is symptomatic.

Treatment

The treatment of choice for pulmonary stenosis is pulmonary balloon valvuloplasty. In the past, surgical pulmonary valvotomy was performed. Despite near-normal life expectancy, patients with pulmonary stenosis and previous surgical valvotomy or balloon intervention have an increased risk of cardiovascular events. Long-standing pulmonary regurgitation eventually causes enlargement of the cardiac chambers on the right side, dilation of the tricuspid annulus with progressive tricuspid regurgitation, and both atrial and ventricular arrhythmias. Pulmonary valve replacement after pulmonary valvotomy is often required during follow-up, emphasizing the need for lifelong cardiac surveillance.

KEY POINTS

- The treatment of choice for valvular pulmonary stenosis is pulmonary balloon valvuloplasty.

- Lifelong cardiac surveillance is needed in patients who have undergone pulmonary valvotomy or replacement.

Previously Operated Congenital Heart Disease

Postoperative or Postintervention Atrial Septal Defect

Patients with surgically or device-treated atrial septal defect should have periodic cardiovascular reevaluation. The most common cause of morbidity in these patients is atrial fibrillation, the rate of which directly increases with age at intervention. Rare complications that have been reported after device closure of an atrial septal defect include device dislocation, arrhythmias, pericardial effusion, aortic erosion, and sudden death.

Postoperative Ventricular Septal Defect

Although most patients with previous surgical ventricular septal defect closure have an uncomplicated course, periodic cardiovascular evaluation is necessary. Complications following repair include residual or recurrent ventricular septal defect, left ventricular dysfunction, infective endocarditis, pulmonary hypertension, aortic or tricuspid regurgitation, heart block, and atrial or ventricular arrhythmias. The need for reoperation for a residual ventricular septal defect is uncommon. Late reoperation is occasionally required for progressive tricuspid or aortic regurgitation.

Postoperative Aortic Coarctation

Patients with repaired coarctation of the aorta have an increased risk for persistent or recurrent hypertension

(occurring in 50%-75% of patients), coronary artery disease, recoarctation, aortic aneurysm formation or dissection, and endocarditis, even after successful repair. Age at the time of initial repair is the most important predictor of long-term survival. Patients with a bicuspid aortic valve require lifelong follow-up.

Reoperation is often required in patients with a history of coarctation. The most common reasons for reoperation include aortic valve disease, mitral valve disease, recoarctation, ascending or descending aortic aneurysm, and coronary artery disease. Long-standing hypertension causing abnormal left ventricular diastolic function increases the risk of late atrial arrhythmias and associated morbidity. All patients who undergo either interventional catheterization or surgical repair of coarctation should have close follow-up and aggressive management of risk factors for cardiovascular disease.

Tetralogy of Fallot

The anatomic features of tetralogy of Fallot include a large subaortic ventricular septal defect and obstruction to pulmonary outflow at the infundibular or pulmonary valve level. Secondary features include right ventricular hypertrophy and the aorta overriding the ventricular septal defect (**Figure 29**). Tetralogy of Fallot is the most common form of cyanotic congenital heart disease, and unoperated adults are rarely seen.

Chest radiographic features of tetralogy of Fallot include right ventricular enlargement, small pulmonary arteries, and reduced pulmonary blood flow; 25% of patients also have a right aortic arch. The electrocardiogram demonstrates right

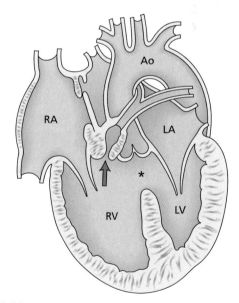

FIGURE 29.
Tetralogy of Fallot.
A subarterial ventricular septal defect (*asterisk*) and pulmonary stenosis (*arrow*) are associated with secondary aortic override and right ventricular hypertrophy.

Ao = aorta; LA = left atrium; LV = left ventricle; RA = right atrium; RV = right ventricle.

Redrawn from original supplied courtesy of Dr. William D. Edwards, Department of Laboratory Medicine and Pathology, Mayo Clinic, Rochester, MN.

ventricular hypertrophy, right axis deviation, and tall peaked P waves. After repair, right bundle branch block is universally present. The diagnosis of tetralogy of Fallot suspected clinically is confirmed by echocardiography. Cardiac catheterization may be required to evaluate the anatomy of the pulmonary and coronary arteries.

Patients with tetralogy of Fallot have an increased risk of fetal loss, and their offspring are more likely to have congenital anomalies than offspring in the general population. Approximately 15% of patients with tetralogy of Fallot have chromosome 22q11.2 microdeletion; screening for the microdeletion should be considered in patients with tetralogy of Fallot, pulmonary artery atresia, or truncus arteriosus (conotruncal abnormalities) prior to pregnancy in order to provide appropriate genetic counseling. In patients with tetralogy of Fallot who have the 22q11.2 deletion, the risk of a child having the microdeletion and congenital heart disease is approximately 50%; the risk in children born to a parent with tetralogy of Fallot without the 22q11.2 microdeletion is 4% to 6%.

Successful surgical repair for tetralogy of Fallot results in the loss of cyanosis and dramatic improvement in functional status. The late survival after repair is excellent, with a 35-year survival of approximately 85%. Residual problems after surgical repair however, do occur, the most common of which is pulmonary valve regurgitation, which results from the transannular patch repair performed for relief of right ventricular outflow tract obstruction. Longstanding pulmonary regurgitation causes right-sided cardiac chamber enlargement, progressive tricuspid regurgitation from annular dilatation, and atrial and ventricular arrhythmias. Residual right ventricular outflow tract obstruction, pulmonary artery stenosis, or ventricular septal defect may also occur after tetralogy of Fallot repair. Additional concerns include right or left ventricular systolic and diastolic dysfunction and sudden death due to ventricular arrhythmias. Continued close follow-up is required after surgical intervention for tetralogy of Fallot, and re-intervention is commonly required.

Adults with Cyanotic Congenital Heart Disease

General Management

Patients with cyanotic congenital heart disease should be evaluated by an adult congenital cardiac specialist annually. Right-to-left intracardiac or extracardiac shunts result in hypoxemia, erythrocytosis, and cyanosis. The increase in erythrocyte mass that accompanies cyanosis is a compensatory response to improve oxygen transport. The resulting physical features include central cyanosis and digital clubbing. Patients with cyanotic congenital heart disease are disposed to hemostatic problems, scoliosis, painful arthropathy or arthritis, gallstones,

pulmonary hemorrhage or thrombus, paradoxical cerebral emboli or cerebral abscess, and renal dysfunction.

Most cyanotic patients have compensated erythrocytosis with stable hemoglobin levels. Rarely, hyperviscosity symptoms occur and are manifested by headaches and reduced concentration. Dehydration should be excluded before considering therapeutic phlebotomy; phlebotomy should be followed by fluid administration and should be performed no more than two to three times per year. Iron deficiency and resultant microcytosis in cyanotic patients are often caused by unnecessary phlebotomy or blood loss, including menstrual bleeding. Microcytes are more rigid than normal erythrocytes, thus microcytosis increases the risk of stroke. The treatment for iron deficiency in a patient with destabilized erythropoiesis is challenging. Oral iron often causes a rapid and dramatic increase in erythrocyte mass. Therefore, administration of 1 tablet daily of ferrous sulfate or ferrous gluconate is recommended, with repeat hemoglobin assessment in 7 to 10 days. Once the hemoglobin level or hematocrit has started to increase, iron therapy should be discontinued.

Cyanosis increases the risk of maternal and fetal complications, including heart failure, preterm delivery, intrauterine growth retardation, and miscarriage. Maternal and fetal mortality are also increased and relate to the degree of cyanosis, ventricular function, and pulmonary pressures. Cyanotic patients with Eisenmenger syndrome should be counseled to avoid pregnancy, which carries up to a 50% risk of maternal mortality.

When hospitalized for medical or surgical problems, cyanotic patients should be seen and followed by a specialist with experience in the management of patients with congenital heart disease. These patients have an increased risk of paradoxical embolism related to air in intravenous lines, and thus air filters are recommended. Early ambulation or pneumatic compression devices are recommended for prevention of venous stasis and thrombophlebitis to reduce the risk of paradoxical embolism. Anticoagulation is generally avoided owing to platelet dysfunction and bleeding tendencies in patients with cyanotic heart disease.

Eisenmenger Syndrome

Eisenmenger syndrome is a cyanotic congenital heart disease characterized by irreversible pulmonary vascular disease due to the presence of a long-standing cardiac shunt with eventual reversal of the shunt. Although the disease is decreasing in frequency, affected patients represent a major proportion of cyanotic adults with congenital heart disease. Conservative medical management is recommended for these patients when minimally symptomatic. Alternative treatment options for symptomatic patients include pulmonary vasodilator therapy and lung transplantation with intracardiac repair or heart-lung transplantation.

Bibliography

Beauchesne LM, Warnes CA, Connolly HM, et al. Prevalence and clinical manifestations of 22q11.2 microdeletion in adults with selected conotruncal anomalies. J Am Coll Cardiol. 2005;45(4):595-598. [PMID: 15708709]

Carminati M, Butera G, Chessa M, et al; Investigators of the European VSD Registry. Transcatheter closure of congenital ventricular septal defects: results of the European Registry. Eur Heart J. 2007; 28(19):2361-2368. [PMID: 17684082]

Drenthen W, Pieper PG, Roos-Hesselink JW, et al; ZAHARA Investigators. Outcome of pregnancy in women with congenital heart disease: a literature review. J Am Coll Cardiol. 2007;49(24):2303-2311. [PMID: 17572244]

Earing MG, Connolly HM, Dearani JA, Ammash NM, Grogan M, Warnes CA. Long-term follow-up of patients after surgical treatment for isolated pulmonary valve stenosis. Mayo Clin Proc. 2005; 80(7):871-876. [PMID: 16007892]

Galiè N, Beghetti M, Gatzoulis MA, et al; Bosentan Randomized Trial of Endothelin Antagonist Therapy-5 (BREATHE-5) Investigators. Bosentan therapy in patients with Eisenmenger syndrome: a multicenter, double-blind, randomized, placebo-controlled study. Circulation. 2006;114(1):48-54. [PMID: 16801459]

Jones TK, Latson LA, Zahn E, et al. Results of the U.S. multicenter pivotal study of the HELEX septal occluder for percutaneous closure of secundum atrial septal defects. J Am Coll Cardiol. 2007;49(22):2215-2221. [PMID: 17543643]

Messé SR, Silverman IE, Kizer JR, et al. Practice parameter: recurrent stroke with patent foramen ovale and atrial septal aneurysm: report of the Quality Standards Subcommittee of the American Academy of Neurology. Neurology. 2004;62(7):1042-1050. [PMID: 15078999]

Murphy JG, Gersh BJ, McGoon MD, et al. Long-term outcome after surgical repair of isolated atrial septal defect. Follow-up at 27 to 32 years. N Engl J Med. 1990;323(24):1645-1650. [PMID: 2233961]

Sacco RL, Adams R, Albers G, et al. Guidelines for prevention of stroke in patients with ischemic stroke or transient ischemic attack: a statement for healthcare professionals from the American Heart Association/ American Stroke Association Council on Stroke: co-sponsored by the Council on Cardiovascular Radiology and Intervention: the American Academy of Neurology affirms the value of this guideline. Stroke. 2006;37(2):577-617. [PMID: 16432246]

Warnes CA, Williams RG, Bashore TM, et al. ACC/AHA 2008 Guidelines for the Management of Adults with Congenital Heart Disease: a report of the American College of Cardiology/American Heart Association Task Force on Practice Guidelines (writing committee to develop guidelines on the management of adults with congenital heart disease). Circulation. 2008;118(23):e714-833. [PMID: 18997169]

Diseases of the Aorta

Introduction

Most diseases of the aorta arise as the result of atherosclerosis, hypertension, smoking, inflammation, or congenital defects involving the metabolism of connective tissue. These diseases tend to follow an indolent, asymptomatic, progressive course culminating in an acute and, very often, life-threatening clinical presentation. Intervention during the chronic phase of aortic disease prevents the acute syndrome and its associated high morbidity and mortality.

Aortic Atheroma

Atherosclerotic changes within the aorta are common, beginning in the second to third decade of life as fatty streaks of subintimal collections of cholesterol, foamy macrophages, and secretory smooth muscle cells. These changes may progress, with thickening, calcification, or, sometimes, with ulceration, destabilization, and the development of mobile projections or embolization. Aortic atheromas are most commonly identified on transesophageal echocardiography or CT in patients being evaluated for stroke or thromboembolism. Atheromas appear as intimal thickening and calcification. Complex atheromas (ulcerated or mobile) also may be noted.

Aortic atheromas may embolize leading to stroke. The size, location, and morphology of the plaque are determinants of risk. In stroke patients, the risk of recurrent stroke is directly proportional to plaque thickness proximal to the left subclavian artery, with a pronounced increase in risk with plaques 4 mm or greater. Whether plaque mobility or ulceration influences risk is controversial. However, the largest prospective study demonstrated that plaque calcification strongly influences relative risk, with noncalcified atheroma carrying a 10-fold increase in the relative risk of stroke, suggesting that calcification may confer greater plaque stability.

Patients in whom an aortic atheroma has been identified should be considered for treatment with an antiplatelet or antithrombotic regimen. Warfarin may be superior to aspirin in prevention of recurrent events. Additionally, reduction of atherosclerotic risk should be encouraged in these patients, such as lipid-lowering therapy and smoking cessation. Descending aorta atheroma is a marker for increased coronary risk but has not been linked to an increased risk of peripheral embolization.

KEY POINT

- Atheromas 4 mm or greater in thickness in the ascending aorta or arch increase the risk of recurrent stroke.

Abdominal Aortic Aneurysm

Clinical Presentation and Natural History

Abdominal aortic aneurysms affect 5% of elderly men who have smoked. The relative risk is substantially increased for men with a first-degree family member affected by abdominal aortic aneurysm. The risk tends to be lower in women than in men, although less is understood about the natural history of abdominal aortic aneurysm in women. Common symptoms associated with threat of rupture include back pain, vague abdominal pain, or an abdominal mass that is painful to palpation; however, most patients remain asymptomatic for many years. The mortality rate associated with rupture of an abdominal aortic aneurysm approaches 80%. The annual rate of rupture of abdominal aortic aneurysms smaller than 5 cm in transverse diameter is 5% or less per year. For each increase in diameter of 1 cm, the annual event rate increases by approximately 10%.

Most small aneurysms enlarge slowly, but the rate of expansion increases as aneurysms dilate. For example, most aneurysms less than 4 cm in diameter enlarge by less than 0.2 cm per year. A typical rate for an aneurysm greater than 4.5 cm in diameter is 0.35 cm per year.

Screening

The U.S. Preventive Services Task Force recommends one-time screening for abdominal aortic aneurysm with ultrasonography for men ages 65 to 75 years who have ever smoked. The American College of Cardiology/American Heart Association guidelines for the management of peripheral arterial disease also include this along with the recommendation that men 60 years or older who have a first-degree relative with an abdominal aortic aneurysm undergo physical examination and ultrasonography screening.

Management

Medical Treatment

Two large studies have confirmed the safety of semi-annual noninvasive surveillance, along with risk factor intervention, in asymptomatic patients with aneurysms 4.0 cm to 5.5 cm as compared with early surgery. Although β-blockers are often prescribed to slow progression, several randomized trials have failed to show a benefit of β-blockers on aneurysm enlargement. Case-controlled studies suggest that aneurysm rupture is less likely in patients treated with angiotensin-converting enzyme inhibitors, but this may be due to effects on matrix remodeling rather than hemodynamic effects.

Development and expansion of abdominal aortic aneurysms are related to inflammation and elaboration of proteases. In animal models, the use of statins or the immune modulators rapamycin or doxycycline appears to reduce formation and progression of aortic aneurysms. A small prospective human trial has demonstrated reduced rates of enlargement in patients treated with simvastatin. The effect of statins appears to be independent of cholesterol level, suggesting that an anti-inflammatory effect may be responsible.

Smoking is the strongest reversible association with abdominal aortic aneurysms, and smoking cessation is therefore recommended for prevention of aneurysms.

Aneurysm Repair

All patients with symptomatic aneurysms, regardless of size, should receive intervention. In selected asymptomatic patients, repair should be performed in aneurysms 5.5 cm in diameter or larger. In addition, intervention in asymptomatic patients has been recommended for smaller aneurysms when progression is much faster than would be expected (0.5 cm per year). Medical therapy without repair might be considered in patients who are at high surgical risk or in whom other disease limits life expectancy.

Two methods of aneurysm repair may be considered: open surgical and endovascular. The choice depends on anatomic considerations and operative risk. Several randomized trials have compared endovascular and open surgical repair, with one study comparing endovascular repair with medical management in patients not considered candidates for surgery. Endovascular repair has a shorter length of hospital stay and lower 30-day morbidity and mortality than open repair but greater in-hospital costs (primarily due to the cost of the stent graft). Endovascular repair does not, however, improve quality of life beyond 3 months or survival beyond 2 years and, compared with open repair, is associated with a higher rate of complications and need for re-intervention, more long-term monitoring, and higher long-term costs. In patients medically unfit for surgery, endovascular repair costs more and has not been shown to improve survival.

> **KEY POINTS**
>
> - The U.S. Preventive Services Task Force recommends one-time screening for abdominal aortic aneurysm with ultrasonography for men ages 65 to 75 years who have ever smoked.
>
> - Asymptomatic patients with an abdominal aortic aneurysm greater than 4 cm in diameter should undergo semi-annual surveillance with abdominal ultrasonography.
>
> - Elective repair should be performed in most patients when an abdominal aortic aneurysm reaches 5.5 cm in diameter or larger or when aneurysm progression is much faster than would be expected.

Thoracic Aortic Aneurysm

Most thoracic aortic aneurysms are discovered incidentally during chest radiography or CT requested for other reasons. Symptoms may include hoarseness, dysphagia, and back pain, but most patients are asymptomatic at the time of discovery.

As with abdominal aortic aneurysm, the risk of rupture is strongly related to size and rapidity of expansion. The indications for repair are slightly different from those for abdominal aortic aneurysm (**Table 33**).

Patients with thoracic aortic aneurysms that do not meet criteria for repair should undergo serial CT or MRI for surveillance and receive medical therapy, including β-blockers and certain angiotensin receptor blockers.

Operative morbidity and mortality rates are higher for thoracic aortic aneurysm and thoraco-abdominal aneurysm repair compared with abdominal aortic aneurysm, with a 20% risk of stroke or paralysis and a short-term mortality rate of up to 10%. Owing to this relatively high risk, interest in the use of endovascular repair has grown in recent years. At least one device has been approved by the U.S. Food and Drug Administration for the endovascular repair of thoracic aortic aneurysm. Early outcomes from endovascular repair suggest lower peri-procedural complication rates, but long-term analysis of a randomized prospective comparison with surgical repair is still lacking.

Marfan Syndrome

Pathophysiology and Clinical Presentation

The Marfan syndrome is an autosomal dominant heritable disorder most frequently involving mutations in the gene encoding fibrillin-1 and with characteristic phenotypic features (**Table 34**). The fibrillin-1 protein is both a structural component of normal connective tissue and a regulatory protein affecting transforming growth factor β (TGF-β) signaling. Patients with the Marfan syndrome develop a dilated aortic root with loss of the normal angle between the sinuses and ascending aorta. This abnormality usually is present by the adolescent or young adult years and progresses with age. Untreated, it may lead to ascending aortic dissection.

Management

The European Society of Cardiology recommends elective aortic root repair at a diameter of 45 mm (or if expansion is faster than 5 mm per year); the American College of

TABLE 33 Indications for Repair of Thoracic Aortic Aneurysms

Symptoms (hoarseness, dysphagia, back pain)
Severe dilation
Ascending aortic diameter >50-60 mm
Descending aortic diameter >60-70 mm
Descending aortic diameter in patients with high surgical risk: ≥70 mm
Rapid growth rate (≥10 mm per year) in aneurysms <50 mm in diameter
Dissection

TABLE 34 Clinical Features of the Marfan Syndrome

Eye
Superior lens dislocation (ectopia lentis)*
Skeleton
Arm span exceeding height (ratio >1.05)
Erosion of lumbosacral vertebrae due to dural ectasia*
Joint hypermobility
Long digits (arachnodactyly)
Reduced elbow extension (<170 degrees)
Scoliosis
Sternal deformity (carinatum type)
Tall stature
Thumb sign (distal phalanx protrudes beyond border of clenched fist)
Wrist sign (thumb and fifth digit overlap when around the wrist)
Oral Cavity
Crowded dentition
High palate
Mandible malocclusion
Cardiac
Aortic dissection*
Aortic root dilatation*
Mitral valve prolapse
Pulmonary
Spontaneous pneumothorax
Central Nervous System
Dural ectasia*

*Asterisks represent the most specific findings.

Data from De Paepe A, Devereux RB, Dietz HC, Hennekam R, Pyeritz RE. Revised diagnostic criteria for the Marfan syndrome. Am J Med Genet. 1996;62(4):417-426. [PMID: 8723076]

Cardiology/American Heart Association recommends repair at 50 mm (or expansion of 10 mm per year). Given the proximal nature of the abnormality, the aortic root size can be followed noninvasively and serially every 6 to 12 months by echocardiography. This has the added benefit of assessment of aortic regurgitation and associated ventricular size and function.

Pregnant women with the Marfan syndrome are at high risk for dissection, estimated to exceed 10% in women with an aortic root dimension of more than 40 mm. American College of Cardiology/American Heart Association guidelines recommend elective aortic root repair in women considering pregnancy once the aortic root measures 45 mm or greater.

Patients with the Marfan syndrome who do not meet criteria for elective surgery should be counseled to avoid strenuous activity, especially weight lifting or "burst" activity.

β-Blockers have been demonstrated to reduce the rate of aortic root dilation. In animal studies, losartan, but not propanolol, prevented aortic root dilation, independent of hemodynamic effect. Early results in humans also support a beneficial effect of angiotensin receptor blockers. These promising trials may reflect an important role of angiotensin receptor blockade in TGF-β signaling.

KEY POINTS

- Treatment with β-blockers or angiotensin receptor blockers may slow the rate of aortic root dilation in Marfan syndrome.
- In patients with Marfan syndrome, elective surgical repair should be performed when the aortic root is 45 to 50 mm in diameter.
- Pregnancy increases the risk of aortic dissection in patients with Marfan syndrome.

Takayasu Arteritis

Takayasu arteritis is a chronic vasculitis involving the aorta and major tributaries that largely affects young women. The early symptoms are constitutional, with symptoms of vascular involvement becoming more apparent as the disease progresses. Arterial inflammation, similar pathologically to giant cell arteritis, leads to thickening, stenosis, and aneurysmal dilation of the aorta and major branches. Late manifestations include arm or leg claudication and distal ulceration. Carotid or vertebral artery involvement may provoke headache, vertigo, syncope, or visual impairment. Angina may occur with involvement of the ostial portion of the coronary arteries, and renovascular hypertension may result from mid-aortic involvement. The diagnosis and treatment of Takayasu arteritis are reviewed in MKSAP 15 Rheumatology.

Acute Aortic Syndromes

Pathophysiology and Clinical Presentation

Acute aortic syndromes include acute aortic dissection, aortic intramural hematoma, and penetrating atherosclerotic ulcer. Aortic dissection is characterized by an intimal tear and formation of a false lumen within the media of the artery. Aortic intramural hematoma is a crescent of fresh hematoma contained within the media but without an intimal tear or false lumen and without involvement of the aortic valve, pericardium, or major branch vessels. It is thought to represent rupture of the vasa vasorum and is considered by many to be a precursor of dissection. Penetrating atherosclerotic ulcer represents avulsion of a mural atherosclerotic plaque with erosion of the media and pseudoaneurysmal adventitial containment.

Patients with an acute aortic syndrome present with the abrupt onset of severe pain within the thorax. Blood pressure is variable. Pain described as "ripping" or "tearing" occurs in only about 50% of patients, and migrating pain is distinctly unusual. The physical finding of a pulse deficit is uncommon. At least one third of patients have no electrocardiographic abnormality, and at least 40% of patients lack widening of the mediastinum on plain chest radiograph. An acute aortic syndrome must, therefore, be considered in any patient with unexplained new severe thoracic pain regardless of the results of these initial diagnostic tests.

Diagnosis

Diagnosis of a suspected acute aortic event is made by MRI, contrast CT, or transesophageal echocardiography. CT scanning can be performed rapidly and demonstrates the aortic arch, great vessels, and infradiaphragmatic aorta and tributaries well; however, it requires intravenous contrast. MRI may take longer and may require patient transport; in addition, it is contraindicated in patients with pacemakers and implanted defibrillators. Transesophageal echocardiography can be performed at bedside and allows definition of the ascending and descending aorta, evaluation of the pericardium, inspection of aortic valve structure and competence, and evaluation of left ventricular function; however, this modality is limited with regard to definition of the aortic arch, great vessels, and abdominal aorta. The choice, therefore, depends on institutional availability and expertise.

Acute aortic syndromes have been categorized according to the Stanford classification scheme originally developed for the description of dissection: *type A* originates within the ascending aorta or arch; *type B* originates distal to the left subclavian artery.

Treatment

Type A aortic syndromes are surgical emergencies, and medical therapy to control heart rate, blood pressure, and pain should be instituted while awaiting surgery.

Type B aortic syndromes are usually treated medically. Patients with type B aortic syndromes are usually hypertensive at presentation, and therapy should include initiation of intravenous β-blockers followed by a rapidly titratable parenteral antihypertensive agent, such as sodium nitroprusside, fenoldopam, or enalaprilat. The goal of therapy is a heart rate of 60/min to 80/min and the lowest level of mean arterial pressure that allows vital organ perfusion. Therapy also includes analgesia to prevent pain worsening both hypertension and tachycardia. Surgical therapy of type B aortic syndromes may also be indicated but is associated with significant morbidity and mortality (**Table 35**).

The few studies of endovascular grafts for type B repair have reported acute mortality rates ranging from 0% to 20%. There are no long-term results assessing the durability of this therapy.

Type B aortic dissections can undergo aneurysmal transformation, and intramural hematoma may progress to aneurysm or dissection over time. Therefore, surveillance

TABLE 35 Indications for Interventional Therapy in Type B Acute Aortic Syndromes

Occlusion of a major aortic branch with visceral or limb ischemia
Progressive dilation or extension despite appropriate medical therapy
Contained aortic rupture of type B dissection
Penetrating atherosclerotic ulcers >20 mm diameter and >10 mm depth
Penetrating atherosclerotic ulcers associated with hematoma

imaging of medically treated type B aortic syndromes is reasonable at 1, 3, and 6 months from the index event and every 6 to 12 months thereafter if aneurysmal dilatation is present.

Distal penetrating ulcers with broad-based or deep ulceration are most commonly treated with surgery or endovascular repair. Distal shallow and narrow ulcers without evidence of threatened rupture have been treated conservatively; however, outcome data regarding conservative therapy for penetrating atherosclerotic ulcer are not currently available. Penetrating ulcer with associated intramural hematoma has been reported to be a particularly aggressive form of this disease, and urgent surgical or endovascular repair has been suggested.

KEY POINTS

- An acute aortic syndrome should be considered in any patient who presents with the abrupt onset of severe pain within the thorax.

- "Classic" findings of an acute aortic syndrome, including tearing pain, a pulse deficit, and electrocardiographic and radiographic abnormalities, are often absent.

- Type A acute aortic syndromes (originating in the ascending aortic artery) are surgical emergencies.

- Type B acute aortic syndromes (originating distal to the left subclavian artery) are usually treated medically.

Bibliography

Brooke BS, Habashi JP, Judge DP, Patel N, Loeys B, Dietz HC 3rd. Angiotensin II blockade and aortic-root dilation in Marfan's syndrome. N Engl J Med. 2008;358(26):2787-2795. [PMID: 18579813]

EVAR trial participants. Endovascular aneurysm repair and outcome in patients unfit for open repair of abdominal aortic aneurysm (EVAR trial 2): randomised controlled trial. Lancet. 2005;365(9478):2187-2192. [PMID: 15978926]

EVAR trial participants. Endovascular aneurysm repair versus open repair in patients with abdominal aortic aneurysm (EVAR trial 1): randomised controlled trial. Lancet. 2005;365(9478):2179-2186. [PMID: 15978925]

Hirsch AT, Haskal ZJ, Hertzer NR, et al. ACC/AHA 2005 guidelines for the management of patients with peripheral arterial disease (lower extremity, renal, mesenteric, and abdominal aortic): executive summary: a collaborative report from the American Association for Vascular Surgery/Society for Vascular Surgery, Society for Cardiovascular Angiography and Interventions, Society for Vascular Medicine and Biology, Society of Interventional Radiology, and the ACC/AHA Task Force on Practice Guidelines (Writing Committee to Develop Guidelines for the Management of Patients With Peripheral Arterial Disease) endorsed by the American Association of Cardiovascular and Pulmonary Rehabilitation; National Heart, Lung, and Blood Institute; Society for Vascular Nursing; TransAtlantic Inter-Society Consensus; and Vascular Disease Foundation. J Am Coll Cardiol. 2006;47(6):1239-1312. [PMID: 16545667]

Kronzon I, Tunick PA. Aortic atherosclerotic disease and stroke. Circulation. 2006;114(1):63-75. [PMID: 16818829]

Lederle FA, Wilson SE, Johnson GR, et al; Aneurysm Detection and Management Veterans Affairs Cooperative Study Group. Immediate repair compared with surveillance of small abdominal aortic aneurysms. N Engl J Med. 2002;346(19):1437-1444. [PMID: 12000813]

Sundt TM. Intramural hematoma and penetrating atherosclerotic ulcer of the aorta. Ann Thorac Surg. 2007;83(2):S835-S841. [PMID: 17257937]

Thenappan T, Ali Raza J, Movahed A. Aortic atheromas: current concepts and controversies—a review of the literature. Echocardiography. 2008;25(2):198-207. [PMID: 18269565]

Tunick PA, Nayar AC, Goodkin GM, et al; NYU Atheroma Group. Effect of treatment of the incidence of stroke and other emboli in 519 patients with severe thoracic aortic plaque. Am J Cardiol. 2002;90(12):1320-1325. [PMID: 12480041]

The UK Small Aneurysm Trial Participants. Mortality results for randomised controlled trial of early elective surgery or ultrasonographic surveillance for small abdominal aortic aneurysms. Lancet. 1998; 352(9141):1649-1655. [PMID: 9853436]

Peripheral Arterial Disease

Evaluation of Peripheral Arterial Disease

Clinical Presentation and Differential Diagnosis

Peripheral arterial disease (PAD) is most commonly the result of atherosclerosis, and the annual cardiovascular event rate in patients with PAD is 5% to 7%. Current recommendations for who should be evaluated for PAD are shown in **Table 36**. Fewer than 20% of patients present with classic intermittent claudication—muscle cramping with effort relieved by rest. Patients with mild to moderate lower extremity PAD are more likely to report leg fatigue, difficulty walking, and atypical leg pain. When classic claudication is present, the location of the pain provides important clues as to the site of arterial compromise (**Table 37**). Signs of severe PAD include pain while at rest, ulceration, and gangrene.

The differential diagnosis of lower extremity discomfort includes musculoskeletal disorders, neuropathies, and venous thrombosis (**Table 38**). The discomfort of spinal stenosis has been termed *pseudoclaudication*; however, this type of pain is not necessarily related to exertion; is provoked by standing; and is relieved by sitting, lying down, or leaning forward.

TABLE 36 Persons at Risk for Lower Extremity Peripheral Arterial Disease

Age <50 years, with diabetes and one other atherosclerosis risk factor (smoking, dyslipidemia, hypertension, or hyperhomocysteinemia)
Age 50-69 years and history of smoking or diabetes
Age ≥70 years
Leg symptoms with exertion (suggestive of claudication) or ischemic rest pain
Abnormal lower extremity pulse examination
Known atherosclerotic coronary, carotid, or renal artery disease

Adapted from Hirsch AT, Haskal ZJ, Hertzer NR, et al; American Association for Vascular Surgery; Society for Vascular Surgery; Society for Cardiovascular Angiography and Interventions; Society for Vascular Medicine and Biology; Society of Interventional Radiology; ACC/AHA Task Force on Practice Guidelines; American Association of Cardiovascular and Pulmonary Rehabilitation; National Heart, Lung, and Blood Institute; Society for Vascular Nursing; TransAtlantic Inter-Society Consensus; Vascular Disease Foundation. ACC/AHA 2005 guidelines for the management of patients with peripheral arterial disease (lower extremity, renal, mesenteric, and abdominal aortic): executive summary: a collaborative report from the American Association for Vascular Surgery/Society for Vascular Surgery, Society for Cardiovascular Angiography and Interventions, Society for Vascular Medicine and Biology, Society of Interventional Radiology, and the ACC/AHA Task Force on Practice Guidelines (Writing Committee to Develop Guidelines for the Management of Patients With Peripheral Arterial Disease). J Am Coll Cardiol. 2006;47(6):1239-1312. [PMID: 16545667] Copyright 2006 American College of Cardiology Foundation, with permission from Elsevier.

Physical Examination and Diagnostic Studies

Physical examination of patients at risk for PAD should include palpation and auscultation of the carotid and femoral arteries; auscultation of the abdomen for bruits; and palpation of the popliteal, dorsalis pedis, and posterior tibial arteries. Femoral bruits suggest aortoiliac disease. The skin should be examined for ulceration, hair loss, and changes in coloration.

The ankle-brachial index (ABI) is a simple, sensitive, and specific method of initial evaluation. The ABI is a ratio of lower extremity to upper extremity systolic blood pressures (ABI = ankle pressure/brachial pressure). There are a variety of methods for calculating the ABI; the following represents the method espoused by the American Heart Association and the American College of Cardiology. Systolic pressures are measured in the posterior tibial and dorsalis pedis arteries of each foot using a Doppler probe (**Figure 30**); the highest systolic pressure recorded in each ankle is divided by the highest brachial pressure to obtain the ABI for each lower extremity. The interpretation of ABI results is shown in **Table 39**.

When the ABI is greater than 1.30, a toe-brachial index may provide a better assessment of lower extremity perfusion. Great toe pressures are normally lower than ankle or brachial pressures, and a toe-brachial index of less than 0.70 is considered diagnostic of PAD. When high clinical suspicion for PAD persists despite a normal ABI, exercise testing may be useful. A decrease of the ABI by 20% after exercise suggests significant PAD.

Segmental limb pressure recordings can be obtained with a series of plethysmographic cuffs placed at the upper thigh, lower thigh, calf, and ankle to better localize the point of arterial obstruction. Segmental pressure recordings are useful in patients with moderate to severe disease with limiting symptoms despite medical therapy in whom surgical or endovascular intervention is being considered. A 20 mm Hg drop in pressure across adjacent zones signifies underlying disease. When used in combination with pulse volume recordings (noninvasive arterial waveform analysis), this technique has a diagnostic accuracy of greater than 95%.

Further anatomic data can be obtained noninvasively using gadolinium-enhanced magnetic resonance angiography or contrast-enhanced multi-detector CT angiography. MRI is contraindicated in patients with implanted defibrillators, and gadolinium has been associated with nephrogenic systemic fibrosis in patients with severe kidney disease. In addition, patients with kidney disease are at risk of contrast-induced nephropathy from iodinated contrast agents used in CT angiography. Invasive contrast angiography is reserved for patients in whom revascularization is already planned.

Management of Peripheral Arterial Disease

Cardiovascular Risk Factor Modification

Randomized controlled studies have demonstrated a 20% reduction in major cardiovascular events and need for revascularization in patients with PAD when LDL cholesterol level is lowered to approximately 100 mg/dL (2.6 mmol/L) with a statin. Patients at the highest cardiac risk and patients at very high PAD risk benefit from further reduction to 70 mg/dL (1.8 mmol/L). Patients at very high PAD risk include those with multiple major risk factors (particularly diabetes), severe and poorly controlled risk factors, or the metabolic syndrome. Additionally, treatment with a fibric acid derivative is reasonable in patients with PAD, low HDL cholesterol, normal LDL cholesterol, and elevated triglyceride levels.

TABLE 37 Claudication Site and Corresponding Vascular Territory in Peripheral Arterial Disease

Claudication Site	Vascular Territory
Buttock/hip	Aortoiliac
Thigh	Common femoral or aortoiliac
Upper calf	Superficial femoral
Lower calf	Popliteal

TABLE 38 Differential Diagnosis of Peripheral Arterial Disease

Disease	Notes
Osteoarthritis	Pain often locates to the hips and knees; pain with variable activity and certain positions; common in the same age group as those affected by, and may accompany, peripheral arterial disease
Sensory neuropathy	Pain is not usually dependent on activity and is more often position-related; symptoms may include numbness or burning pain; patients often younger than those with PAD; often associated with diabetes mellitus
Musculoskeletal disease	Diffuse muscle pains, often unrelated to activity; typical in patients with fibromyalgia and systemic autoimmune diseases
Venous disease	Limb pain may worsen with activity and standing; limb elevation often relieves the pain; usually associated with edema; patients are younger and may have a history of deep venous thrombosis; leg pruritus, hyperpigmentation, and medial malleolar ulcers may be present
Lumbar radiculopathy	Pain may be burning and localized to the back of the leg; patient usually has a history of back problems or pain occurs in the setting of back injury
Popliteal entrapment syndrome	Pain affects the calves and worsens with vigorous physical activity; a drop in the ABI occurs with dorsiflexion; occurs primarily in young athletes
Chronic compartment syndrome	Pain affects calves and is worse after a long duration of physical activity; ABI is not affected; occurs primarily in young athletes

ABI = ankle-brachial index.

Lowering blood pressure in hypertensive patients with PAD reduces overall cardiovascular risks and mortality. The blood pressure goal is less than 140/90 mm Hg. For patients with diabetes, the goal is less than 130/80 mm Hg. The Heart Outcomes Prevention Evaluation study demonstrated that angiotensin-converting enzyme inhibitors reduced major cardiovascular events in patients with PAD; however, the Appropriate Blood Pressure Control in Diabetes trial suggested that in patients with diabetes and PAD, the intensity of blood pressure treatment may be more important than the class of drug employed.

β-Blockers are appropriate treatment for secondary prevention in patients with prior myocardial infarction and reduce perioperative risk in patients with PAD undergoing noncardiac surgery.

Aspirin therapy can reduce the need for vascular intervention and retard the progression of PAD. Although individual trials of aspirin in patients with PAD have been inconclusive, a large meta-analysis demonstrated a 25% reduction in the risk of stroke, myocardial infarction, or death with antiplatelet therapy in both men and women. The CAPRIE trial demonstrated a significant benefit of clopidogrel over aspirin with regard to these major adverse events. Based on the level of evidence, aspirin remains first-line therapy, with clopidogrel an acceptable alternative. Recently, the CHARISMA trial demonstrated further benefit of combined clopidogrel and aspirin in patients with prior myocardial infarction, ischemic stroke, or PAD. However, sub-group analysis suggests that patients with PAD alone may not share the benefit shown by the entire cohort.

No prospective trial has demonstrated that tight diabetic control (hemoglobin A_{1c} ≤7%) is associated with a reduction

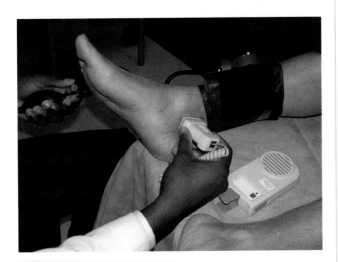

FIGURE 30.
Determining the Ankle-Brachial Index.
A Doppler probe is used to measure the posterior tibial systolic pressure.

TABLE 39 Interpretation of the Ankle-Brachial Index

Ankle-Brachial Index	Interpretation
>1.30	Noncompressible (calcified) vessel (uninterpretable result)
1.00-1.30	Normal
0.91-0.99	Borderline
0.41-0.90	Mild to moderate PAD
0.00-0.40	Severe PAD

PAD = peripheral arterial disease.

in macrovascular complications. Observational data from the UK Prospective Diabetes Study demonstrated that each one percentage point increase in hemoglobin A_{1c} was associated with a 28% increase in the incidence of PAD over a 6-year period.

KEY POINTS

- Aggressive cardiovascular risk factor modification is indicated for all patients with peripheral arterial disease regardless of symptoms or ankle-brachial index score.
- Antiplatelet therapy may reduce progression of peripheral arterial disease and the need for vascular intervention.

Medical Treatment of Symptomatic Patients

Noninvasive treatment of symptomatic PAD should include medical and exercise therapy in addition to risk factor modification. The use of atorvastatin or simvastatin, besides lowering overall cardiovascular risk, increases pain-free walking duration. In a meta-analysis, *Ginkgo biloba* extract also has been shown to improve pain-free walking duration.

Cilostazol, a phosphodiesterase inhibitor, increases pain-free and overall walking distance in PAD patients with lifestyle-limiting claudication in the absence of heart failure; cilostazol, however, is contraindicated in patients with heart failure.

Pentoxifylline, garlic, L-carnitine, and chelation therapy have not been shown to be effective in randomized trials for treatment of symptoms of PAD. Warfarin is also not effective in reducing symptoms or progression of PAD.

A supervised exercise program consisting of repeated walking to the point of near-maximal pain significantly increases pain-free walking time and overall walking distance. Over time, results with exercise training approach those achieved with angioplasty or antiplatelet therapy. Consistency must be stressed because therapeutic gains are quickly lost when exercise is stopped.

KEY POINTS

- Atorvastatin, simvastatin, *Ginkgo biloba* extract, and cilostazol have been shown to increase pain-free walking duration in patients with peripheral arterial disease.
- Properly supervised exercise to the point of near-maximal pain increases pain-free walking duration and distance in patients with peripheral arterial disease.

Endovascular and Surgical Management

Invasive management of PAD is indicated to salvage a threatened limb and improve symptoms in patients with short-distance or lifestyle-limiting claudication refractory to conservative therapy. Several aspects must be considered carefully before offering endovascular or surgical intervention:

- Patients should demonstrate an inadequate response to medical and exercise therapy.
- Patients should demonstrate severe impairment of normal work or avocational activities.
- Patients should not have another disease that would limit exercise even if revascularization were performed.
- The projected natural history of the patient should justify revascularization.
- Lesion morphology should predict a high probability of initial and long-term success.

Angioplasty is most effective in short-segment stenosis within large-caliber vessels, whereas surgical intervention (bypass) is favored for patients with distal, multilevel, or occlusive disease. Primary stenting is more effective in large inflow vessels (aortoiliac, common iliac, and external iliac arteries) but is not recommended in the femoral, popliteal, or tibial arteries as primary therapy. Preferred therapy for each arterial segment is summarized in **Table 40**.

Endovascular techniques are preferable to surgery in the treatment of obstructive aortoiliac disease, and primary stenting, which has an immediate procedural success rate of greater than 95%, is advocated. A meta-analysis of percutaneous transluminal angioplasty versus stent placement for occlusive aortoiliac disease demonstrated similar complication rates but higher technical success rates and lower long-term failure rates with primary stenting. Contraindications to aortoiliac endovascular therapy include lesions longer than 5 cm, aneurysmal disease, atheroembolic disease, and severe diffuse bilateral aortoiliac stenosis.

Compared with the aortoiliac arterial system, the femoral and popliteal arteries are smaller, have lower flow rates, and more commonly demonstrate complete occlusion. Disease involving the common femoral artery is best treated surgically using endarterectomy with patch angioplasty or iliofemoral bypass. Endovascular therapy for popliteal and infrapopliteal disease should be reserved for patients with severe claudication refractory to conservative management. Endovascular infrapopliteal intervention should be considered when outflow obstruction jeopardizes the success of a more proximal

TABLE 40 Preferred Interventional Therapy for Peripheral Arterial Disease by Arterial Segment

Arterial Segment	Preferred Interventional Therapy
Aortoiliac	Primary stenting
Common femoral artery	Endarterectomy and patch angioplasty, or iliofemoral bypass
Deep femoral artery	Endarterectomy and patch angioplasty, or bypass
Popliteal and tibial arteries	Bypass

intervention or when increased flow is essential to help with wound healing and infection.

> **KEY POINT**
>
> • Invasive management of peripheral arterial disease should be reserved for patients who face loss of a limb or have severe limitation despite conservative therapy.

Acute Limb Ischemia

Pathogenesis

Acute limb ischemia usually results from spontaneous or iatrogenic embolism or in situ thrombosis. Most patients present with the signs and symptoms listed in **Table 41**.

Spontaneous embolization may originate either within the heart or from an upstream vessel. The most common causes of cardiogenic embolization are chronic atrial fibrillation and ventricular aneurysm with mural thrombosis. In endocarditis, embolization of infected material (vegetation) may occur. Embolization may result from an abdominal aortic aneurysm as well, as thrombi are often present within these areas of abnormal blood flow.

Embolization may result from an invasive procedure such as angiography or cardiac catheterization whereby a mural thrombus is dislodged or cholesterol embolization is initiated through catheter manipulation. In situ thrombosis occurs more commonly within surgical bypass grafts or in patients with a severe underlying plaque. Less commonly, thrombosis may occur in patients with hypercoagulable states.

Cholesterol embolization may result in a systemic illness characterized by inflammation, renal failure, eosinophilia, livedo reticularis (**Figure 31**), and distal necrosis. Care is generally supportive.

Management

Three categories of acute limb ischemia have been established to help therapeutic decision-making (**Table 42**). Class I patients have moderate to severe claudication but no rest pain. Resting ankle pressure is generally greater than 50 mm Hg, but patients are unable to complete an exercise test and demonstrate a fall in post-exercise ankle pressure to below

50 mm Hg. Immediate initiation of antiplatelet therapy is warranted along with systemic anticoagulation with heparin. These patients require evaluation by a vascular specialist and angiography or invasive treatment within the next several days.

Class II patients have resting ischemic pain and ankle pressure below 40 mm Hg. Distal pulses may be absent or barely palpable. Class II patients require emergent hospitalization, consultation with a vascular specialist, and urgent intervention if the limb is to be salvaged. Patients with absent Doppler signals, transient sensory deficits, and no motor weakness are typically considered for intra-arterial thrombolytic therapy. Thrombolytic agents may take up to 24 hours to restore patency but are less disruptive to the underlying arterial architecture. Patients with motor weakness or persistent sensory loss generally require urgent endovascular or open surgical therapy for limb salvage. Parenteral use of prostaglandin E_1 may reduce ischemic pain and aid in wound healing; however, long-term use of oral iloprost (a prostacyclin analogue) has not been shown to reduce the risk of death or amputation.

Class III patients present with absent Doppler signals, muscle rigor, profound anesthesia, and paralysis. These patients have irreversible ischemia and require prompt amputation.

> **KEY POINTS**
>
> • Patients with acute limb ischemia with severe claudication but no rest pain (class I) should be treated with antiplatelet therapy and heparin.
>
> • Patients with acute limb ischemia with rest pain and transient or incomplete motor or sensory deficits (class IIb) require urgent medical or invasive revascularization.
>
> • Patients with acute limb ischemia, anesthesia, paralysis, absent Doppler signals, and muscle rigor (class III) require amputation.

TABLE 41 Signs and Symptoms of Critical Acute Limb Ischemia (the "Six P's")
Pulseless
Painful
Pallor
Paresthesia
Paralysis
Poikilothermy (cold)

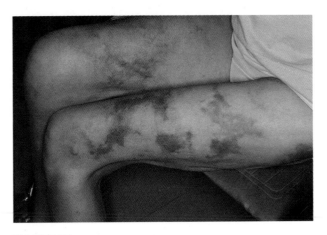

FIGURE 31.
Livedo Reticularis.

TABLE 42 Categories and Prognosis of Acute Limb Ischemia

Class	Sensory Loss	Muscle Weakness	Arterial Doppler Signals	Venous Doppler Signals	Prognosis
I	None	None	Audible	Audible	Not immediately threatened; viable
IIa	None to minimal (toes)	None	Inaudible	Audible	Salvageable with prompt treatment
IIb	More than toes	Mild to moderate	Inaudible	Audible	Salvageable only with immediate revascularization
III	Profound anesthesia	Profound; paralysis	Inaudible	Inaudible	Not viable; major tissue loss inevitable

Adapted from Rutherford RB, Baker JD, Ernst C, et al. Recommended standards for reports dealing with lower extremity ischemia: revised version [erratum in J Vasc Surg. 2001;33(4):805.]. J Vasc Surg. 1997;26(3):517-538. [PMID: 9308598] Copyright 1997, with permission from Elsevier.

Bibliography

Antithrombotic Trialists' Collaboration. Collaborative meta-analysis of randomised trials of antiplatelet therapy for prevention of death, myocardial infarction, and stroke in high-risk patients [erratum in BMJ. 2002;324(7330):141.]. BMJ. 2002;324(7329):71-86. [PMID: 11786451]

Bhatt DL, Flather MD, Hacke W, et al; CHARISMA Investigators. Patients with prior myocardial infarction, stroke, or symptomatic peripheral arterial disease in the CHARISMA trial. J Am Coll Cardiol. 2007;49(19):1982-1988. [PMID: 17498584]

CAPRIE Steering Committee. A randomised, blinded trial of clopidogrel versus aspirin in patients at risk of ischaemic events (CAPRIE). Lancet. 1996;348(9038):1329-1339. [PMID: 8918275]

Hirsch AT, Haskal ZJ, Hertzer NR, et al. ACC/AHA 2005 guidelines for the management of patients with peripheral arterial disease (lower extremity, renal, mesenteric, and abdominal aortic): executive summary: a collaborative report from the American Association for Vascular Surgery/Society for Vascular Surgery, Society for Cardiovascular Angiography and Interventions, Society for Vascular Medicine and Biology, Society of Interventional Radiology, and the ACC/AHA Task Force on Practice Guidelines (Writing Committee to Develop Guidelines for the Management of Patients With Peripheral Arterial Disease) endorsed by the American Association of Cardiovascular and Pulmonary Rehabilitation; National Heart, Lung, and Blood Institute; Society for Vascular Nursing; TransAtlantic Inter-Society Consensus; and Vascular Disease Foundation. J Am Coll Cardiol. 2006;47(6):1239-1312. [PMID: 16545667]

Mahmud E, Cavendish J, Salami A. Current treatment of peripheral arterial disease: role of percutaneous interventional therapies. J Am Coll Cardiol. 2007;50(6):473-490. [PMID: 17678729]

Mehler PS, Coll JR, Estacia R, Esler A, Schrier RW, Hiatt WR. Intensive blood pressure control reduces the risk of cardiovascular events in patients with peripheral arterial disease and type 2 diabetes. Circulation. 2003;107(5):753-756. [PMID: 12578880]

Pittler MH, Ernst E. Ginkgo biloba extract for the treatment of intermittent claudication: a meta-analysis of randomized trials. Am J Med. 2000;108(4):276-281. [PMID: 11014719]

Rutherford RB, Baker JD, Ernst C, et al. Recommended standards for reports dealing with lower extremity ischemia: revised version [erratum in J Vasc Surg. 2001;33(4):805.]. J Vasc Surg. 1997;26(3):517-538. [PMID: 9308598]

UK Prospective Diabetes Study (UKPDS) Group. Intensive blood-glucose control with sulfonylureas or insulin compared with conventional treatment and risk of complications in patients with Type II diabetes (UKPDS 33). [erratum in Lancet. 1999;354(9178):602.] Lancet. 1998;352(9131):837-853. [PMID: 9742976]

Yusuf S, Sleight P, Pogue J, Bosch J, Davies R, Dagenais G. Effects of an angiotensin-converting-enzyme inhibitor, ramipril, on cardiovascular events in high-risk patients. The Heart Outcomes Prevention Evaluation Study Investigators [erratum in N Engl J med. 2000;342(18):1376 and N Engl J Med. 2000;342(10):748.]. N Engl J Med. 2000;342(3):145-153. [PMID: 10639539]

Pregnancy and Cardiovascular Disease

Cardiovascular Changes with Pregnancy

Hemodynamic changes that occur during normal pregnancy include increased plasma volume and a lesser increase in erythrocyte mass, resulting in increased total blood volume and relative anemia. Changes in heart rate, systemic and pulmonary vascular resistance, and blood pressure also occur (**Table 43**). These changes cause a steady increase in cardiac output until the 32nd week, at which time cardiac output plateaus at approximately 40% above the prepregnancy level. At the time of delivery, cardiac output is as much as 80% above the prepregnancy level owing to increases in heart rate and blood pressure.

Prepregnancy Evaluation

A comprehensive prepregnancy evaluation is recommended for women with structural heart disease. A risk assessment to identify women with cardiovascular disease who are at high risk for cardiovascular complications during pregnancy is shown in **Table 44**. Prior cardiac events or arrhythmia, poor functional class or cyanosis, left heart obstruction, and left ventricular systolic dysfunction independently predict maternal cardiac complications. Women with severe pulmonary arterial hypertension are at very high risk, with an estimated maternal mortality rate of 30% to 50%. In the CARPREG study, pulmonary arterial hypertension was not an independent risk factor because of its

TABLE 43 Normal Versus Abnormal Cardiac Symptoms and Signs in Pregnancy

Symptom or Sign	Normal	Pathologic
Shortness of breath	Mild, with exertion	Orthopnea, PND, cough
Palpitations	Atrial and ventricular premature beats	Atrial fibrillation or flutter; ventricular tachycardia
Chest pain	No	Chest pressure, heaviness, or pain
Murmur	Basal systolic murmur grade 1/6 or 2/6 present in 80% of pregnant women	Systolic murmur ≥grade 3/6; any diastolic murmur
Tachycardia	Heart rate increased by 20%–30%	Heart rate >100/min
Low blood pressure	Blood pressure typically is unchanged	Low blood pressure associated with symptoms
Edema	Mild peripheral	Pulmonary edema
Gallop	S_3	S_4

PND = paroxysmal nocturnal dyspnea.

association with poor functional status and left heart obstruction. Ventricular systolic dysfunction (ejection fraction <40%) associated with New York Heart Association functional class III or IV heart failure carries a high risk of maternal and fetal complications and is generally considered a contraindication to pregnancy. Severe obstructive cardiac lesions are often associated with symptomatic deterioration during pregnancy; intervention prior to pregnancy is recommended.

KEY POINTS

- In women with cardiac disease, prior cardiac events or arrhythmia, left heart obstruction, and left ventricular systolic dysfunction independently predict maternal cardiac complications.

- Severe pulmonary arterial hypertension carries a maternal mortality rate of 30% to 50%; patients with this disorder should be counseled against pregnancy.

Management of Cardiovascular Disease During Pregnancy

There are no guidelines or official recommendations for the management of most cardiovascular conditions that occur during pregnancy. Recommendations regarding the management of pregnant women with cardiovascular disease are largely based on case series. Once a woman with cardiovascular disease becomes pregnant, special attention should be paid to her hemodynamic response. The time and route of delivery should be planned before spontaneous labor occurs. Vaginal delivery with a facilitated second stage (forceps delivery or vacuum extraction) is preferred for women with heart disease. Cesarean delivery should be performed when indicated for obstetrical reasons, in patients fully anticoagulated with warfarin, and in patients with pulmonary hypertension.

Peripartum Cardiomyopathy

Peripartum cardiomyopathy is ventricular dysfunction that occurs during the last trimester of pregnancy or up to 6 months postpartum in the absence of an identifiable cause. Peripartum cardiomyopathy occurs more frequently in multifetal pregnancies; multiparous women; women older than 30 years; black women; and in women with gestational hypertension, preeclampsia, or who are treated with tocolytic therapy.

Peripartum cardiomyopathy is the major cause of pregnancy-related death in North America; maternal death is related to heart failure, thromboembolic events, and arrhythmias. Left ventricular function improves within 6 months after delivery in approximately 50% of women with peripartum cardiomyopathy. Management includes early delivery (when peripartum cardiomyopathy is identified before parturition) and treatment for heart failure. Medical therapy for heart failure during pregnancy should include standard therapy for heart failure with β-blockers, digoxin, and diuretics, but excluding angiotensin-converting enzyme inhibitors and angiotensin receptor blockers until after delivery. Anticoagulation is recommended when left ventricular ejection fraction is less than 35%. Referral for transplantation should be considered for refractory ventricular systolic dysfunction.

Intravenous immune globulin and pentoxifylline should be considered when peripartum cardiomyopathy is diagnosed. An immune pathogenesis is supported by the frequent finding of lymphocytic myocarditis on endomyocardial biopsy and the fact that multiparity is a significant risk factor. Elevated levels of tumor necrosis factor α (TNF-α) have been noted in patients with peripartum cardiomyopathy, and the addition of pentoxifylline, which inhibits TNF-α, to conventional treatment has been shown to improve outcomes.

Recurrence of peripartum cardiomyopathy is common, and affected patients are at increased risk of reduction in ventricular function as well as morbidity and mortality with another pregnancy. Patients with peripartum cardiomyopathy should be counseled about the risks of subsequent pregnancies and those who have persistent ventricular dysfunction should be discouraged from becoming pregnant again.

TABLE 44 Predictors of Maternal Cardiac Events in Women with Congenital or Acquired Cardiac Disease

Risk Factor (Predictor)	Operational Definition
Prior cardiac event or arrhythmia	Heart failure, transient ischemic attack, stroke, arrhythmia
Baseline NYHA class >II or cyanosis	Mild symptoms (mild shortness of breath and/or angina pain) and slight limitation during ordinary activity
Left heart obstruction	Mitral valve area <2 cm^2; aortic valve area <1.5 cm^2 or peak left ventricular outflow tract gradient >30 mm Hg
Reduced left ventricular function	Ejection fraction <40%

Estimated Risk for Cardiac Events[a]

No. of Predictors	Estimated Risk (%)	Recommendation
0	4	Consideration of preconception cardiac intervention for specific lesions; increased frequency of follow-up; delivery at community hospital
1	31	Consideration of preconception cardiac intervention for specific lesions; referral to regional center for ongoing care
>1	69	Consideration of preconception cardiac intervention for specific lesions; referral to regional center for ongoing care

NYHA = New York Heart Association.

[a]Pulmonary edema, tachyarrhythmia, embolic stroke, cardiac death.

Data and recommendations from Siu SC, Sermer M, Colman JM, et al; Cardiac Disease in Pregnancy (CARPREG) Investigators. Prospective multicenter study of pregnancy outcomes in women with heart disease. Circulation. 2001;104(5):515-521. [PMID: 11479246]

Medication Use during Pregnancy

Most cardiovascular medications are not approved for use during pregnancy owing to limited data on their safety during pregnancy (**Table 45**). Although the desired therapeutic effect may outweigh the risk, these medications should be used only when necessary.

β-Blockers cross the placenta and are present in human breast milk, resulting in significant levels in the fetus and newborn. If these agents are used during pregnancy, fetal heart rate and newborn heart rate and blood glucose monitoring is indicated.

Low birth weight, early delivery, and small fetal size for gestational age have been associated with the use of atenolol, especially when initiated early in the pregnancy. In pregnant patients with supraventricular arrhythmias taking atenolol, metoprolol be considered as an alternative.

Angiotensin-converting enzyme inhibitors and angiotensin receptor blockers are contraindicated during pregnancy but can be restarted after delivery and are safe to use while breastfeeding.

Anticoagulation during Pregnancy

Pregnancy is a hypercoagulable state, and anticoagulation during pregnancy is suggested for patients with a mechanical valve prosthesis, atrial fibrillation in the setting of structural heart disease, paradoxical embolism, antiphospholipid antibody syndrome with recurrent spontaneous miscarriage, and venous or pulmonary thromboembolic disease.

Anticoagulation for atrial fibrillation during pregnancy can be accomplished safely with low-molecular-weight heparin; however, monitoring efficacy of therapy by measuring serum anti-Xa levels is recommended. Unfractionated heparin and warfarin can also be used for anticoagulation during pregnancy; meticulous monitoring and dose adjustment are recommended.

Pregnant women with mechanical prosthetic valves represent a high-risk subset with a substantial risk of valve thrombosis and increased fetal risk. Anticoagulation for the pregnant patient with a mechanical valve prosthesis is controversial. Continuous therapeutic levels of anticoagulation should be administered during pregnancy, and blood levels should be meticulously monitored.

Prolonged unfractionated heparin use in pregnant women with mechanical valve prostheses may increase the risk of thromboembolic complications, including fatal valve thrombosis. The dose of unfractionated heparin must be carefully monitored and adjusted to the activated partial thromboplastin time; the level of anticoagulation should be adjusted according to the type of valve prosthesis. Unfractionated heparin is the anticoagulant of choice around the time of delivery as it can be stopped or reversed should bleeding occur.

Warfarin crosses the placenta, increasing the risk of spontaneous abortion, prematurity, embryopathy, stillbirth, and fetal intracranial hemorrhage. Many centers outside the United States still recommend the standard approach of warfarin use throughout pregnancy until near term, however, which provides the lowest risk for maternal complications and death.

Low-molecular-weight heparins do not cross the placenta and are not teratogenic. However, prosthetic valve thrombosis has been reported in pregnant patients with valve prostheses. If these agents are used, serum anti-Xa levels must be carefully monitored.

The latest guidelines on management of anticoagulation during pregnancy conclude that unfractionated heparin, low-molecular-weight heparin, or warfarin may be used for anticoagulation of pregnant women with mechanical heart valves. Suggested approaches to anticoagulation in pregnant women with mechanical valves are shown in **Figure 32**.

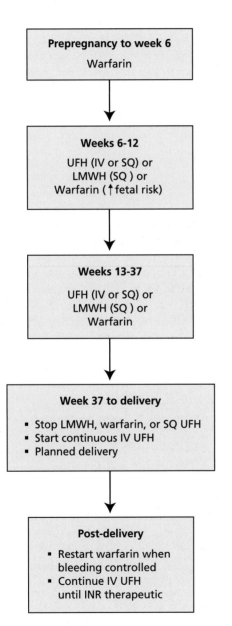

Anticoagulation must be continuously monitored as follows:

- UFH: aPTT at least twice control

- LMWH: anti Xa 0.7-1.2 U/mL 4-hour post-dose

- Warfarin: INR 3 (range 2.5-3.5)

FIGURE 32.
Anticoagulation for Prosthetic Valves in Pregnancy.

aPTT = activated partial thromboplastin time; IV = intravenous; LMWH = low-molecular-weight heparin; SQ = subcutaneous; UFH = unfractionated heparin.

Recommendations from Bonow RO, Carabello BA, Canu C, et al; American College of Cardiology/American Heart Association Task Force on Practice Guidelines; Society of Cardiovascular Anesthesiologists; Society for Cardiovascular Angiography and Interventions; Society of Thoracic Surgeons. ACC/AHA 2006 guidelines for the management of patients with valvular heart disease: report of the American College of Cardiology/American Heart Association Task Force on Practice Guidelines (Writing Committee to Develop Guidelines for the Management of Patients With Valvular Heart Disease). Circulation. 2006;114:457. [PMID: 16880336]

Pregnancy and Cardiovascular Disease

TABLE 45 Drugs for Cardiac Disorders in Pregnancy

Drug	Use Justified When Indicated[a]	Use Justified in Some Circumstances[b]	Use Rarely Justified[c]	Compatible with Breast Feeding	Comments
ACE inhibitors					
Captopril			√	Y	Teratogenic first trimester; cause fetal/neonatal renal failure with 2nd and 3nd trimester exposure; scleroderma renal crisis is only indication
Enalapril			√	Y	Same as above
Lisinopril			√	?	Same as above
ARBs			√	?	Teratogenic first trimester; cause fetal/neonatal renal failure with 2nd and 3nd trimester exposure
Adenosine	√				No change in fetal heart rate when used for supraventricular tachycardia
Amiodarone			√		Fetal hypothyroidism, prematurity
Antiplatelet agents					
Dipyridamole		√		?	No evidence of harm in animal studies; no human data
Clopidogrel		√		?	Same as above
Aspirin (≤81 mg)	√			Y	
β-Blockers					
Atenolol		√		N	Low birth weight, intrauterine growth restriction
Esmolol		√		?	More pronounced bradycardia
Labetalol	√			Y	Preferred drug in class
Metoprolol	√			Y	Shortened half-life
Propranolol		√		Y	Intrauterine growth restriction
Sotalol		√		?	Insufficient data; reserve use for arrhythmia not responding to alternative agent
Calcium channel blockers					
Diltiazem		√		Y	Maternal hypotension with rapid intravenous infusion; used for fetal supraventricular tachycardia
Verapamil		√		Y	Same as above
Digoxin		√		Y	Shortened half-life
Disopyramide		√			Case reports of preterm labor
Diuretics		√		Y	Use when needed for maternal volume overload only
Flecainide		√		?	Inadequate data but used for fetal arrhythmia; case report of fetal hyperbilirubinemia
Hydralazine	√			Y	Vasodilator of choice
Lidocaine	√			Y	Treatment of choice for ventricular arrhythmias
Nitroprusside			√	N	Potential fetal thiocyanate toxicity
Organic nitrates	√				No apparent increased risk

(Continued on next page)

TABLE 45 Drugs for Cardiac Disorders in Pregnancy *(continued)*

Drug	Use Justified When Indicated[a]	Use Justified in Some Circumstances[b]	Use Rarely Justified[c]	Compatible with Breast Feeding	Comments
Phenytoin			√	Y	Known teratogenicity and bleeding risk; last resort for arrhythmia
Procainamide	√			Y	Used for fetal arrhythmia as well
Propafenone		√		?	Used for fetal arrhythmia
Quinidine	√			Y	Preferred drug in class; increases digoxin levels

ACE = angiotensin-converting enzyme; ARB = angiotensin receptor blocker; N = no; Y = yes; ? = unknown.

[a]Data and/or extensive experience support the safety of the drug for the indication.

[b]Less extensive or desirable data are reported, but the drug is reasonable as a second-line agent or is indicated based on the severity of maternal disease.

[c]Use only when alternatives supported by experience and/or better safety data are not available or for life-threatening indications.

From Rosene-Montella K, Keely EJ, Lee RV, Barbour LA. Medical Care of the Pregnant Patient. 2nd Edition. Philadelphia, PA: American College of Physicians; 2007, page 356-357. Copyright 2007 American College of Physicians.

Bibliography

Blomström-Lundqvist C, Scheinman MM, Aliot EM, et al. ACC/AHA/ESC guidelines for the management of patients with supraventricular arrhythmias—executive summary. A report of the American college of cardiology/American heart association task force on practice guidelines and the European society of cardiology committee for practice guidelines (Writing committee to develop guidelines for the management of patients with supraventricular arrhythmias) developed in collaboration with NASPE-Heart Rhythm Society. J Am Coll Cardiol. 2003;42(8):1493-1531. [PMID: 14563598]

Bozkurt B, Villaneuva FS, Holubkov R, et al. Intravenous immune globulin in the therapy of peripartum cardiomyopathy. J Am Coll Cardiol. 1999;34(1):177-180. [PMID: 10400008]

Chan WS, Anand S, Ginsberg JS. Anticoagulation of pregnant women with mechanical heart valves: a systematic review of the literature. Arch Intern Med. 2000;160(2):191-196. [PMID: 10647757]

Elkayam U, Akhter MW, Singh H, et al. Pregnancy-associated cardiomyopathy: clinical characteristics and a comparison between early and late presentation. Circulation. 2005;111(16):2050-2055. [PMID: 15851613]

Fett JD, Christie LG, Murphy JG. Brief communication: Outcomes of subsequent pregnancy after peripartum cardiomyopathy: a case series from Haiti. Ann Intern Med. 2006;145(1):30-34. [PMID: 16818926]

Pearson GD, Veille JC, Rahimtoola S, et al. Peripartum cardiomyopathy: National Heart, Lung, and Blood Institute and Office of Rare Diseases (National Institutes of Health) workshop recommendations and review. JAMA. 2000;283(9):1183-1188. [PMID: 10703781]

Siu SC, Sermer M, Colman JM, et al; Cardiac Disease in Pregnancy (CARPREG) Investigators. Prospective multicenter study of pregnancy outcomes in women with heart disease. Circulation. 2001;104(5):515-521. [PMID: 11479246]

Siu SC, Sermer M, Harrison DA, et al. Risk and predictors for pregnancy-related complications in women with heart disease. Circulation. 1997;96(9):2789-2794. [PMID: 9386139]

Sliwa K, Fett J, Elkayam U. Peripartum cardiomyopathy. Lancet. 2006;368(9536):687-693. [PMID: 16920474]

Sliwa K, Skudicky D, Candy G, Bergemann A, Hopley M, Sareli P. The addition of pentoxifylline to conventional therapy improves outcome in patients with peripartum cardiomyopathy. Eur J Heart Fail. 2002;4(3):305-309. [PMID: 12034156]

Self-Assessment Test

This self-assessment test contains one-best-answer multiple-choice questions. Please read these directions carefully before answering the questions. Answers, critiques, and bibliographies immediately follow these multiple-choice questions. The American College of Physicians is accredited by the Accreditation Council for Continuing Medical Education (ACCME) to provide continuing medical education for physicians.

The American College of Physicians designates MKSAP 15 Cardiovascular Medicine for a maximum of 19 *AMA PRA Category 1 Credits*™. Physicians should only claim credit commensurate with the extent of their participation in the activity. Separate answer sheets are provided for each book of the MKSAP program. Please use one of these answer sheets to complete the Cardiovascular Medicine self-assessment test. Indicate in Section H on the answer sheet the actual number of credits you earned, up to the maximum of 19, in ¼-credit increments. (One credit equals one hour of time spent on this educational activity.)

Use the self-addressed envelope provided with your program to mail your completed answer sheet(s) to the MKSAP Processing Center for scoring. Remember to provide your MKSAP 15 order and ACP ID numbers in the appropriate spaces on the answer sheet. The order and ACP ID numbers are printed on your mailing label. If you have *not* received these numbers with your MKSAP 15 purchase, you will need to acquire them to earn CME credits. E-mail ACP's customer service center at custserv@acponline.org. In the subject line, write "MKSAP 15 order/ACP ID numbers." In the body of the e-mail, make sure you include your e-mail address as well as your full name, address, city, state, ZIP code, country, and telephone number. Also identify where you have made your MKSAP 15 purchase. You will receive your MKSAP 15 order and ACP ID numbers by e-mail within 72 business hours.

CME credit is available from the publication date of July 31, 2009, until July 31, 2012. You may submit your answer sheets at any time during this period.

Self-Scoring Instructions:
Cardiovascular Medicine

Compute your percent correct score as follows:

Step 1: Give yourself 1 point for each correct response to a question.

Step 2: Divide your total points by the total number of questions: 120.

The result, expressed as a percentage, is your percent correct score.

	Example	Your Calculations
Step 1	102	
Step 2	102 ÷ 120	÷ 120
% Correct	85%	%

Directions

*Each of the numbered items is followed by lettered answers. Select the **ONE** lettered answer that is **BEST** in each case.*

Item 1

A 52-year-old woman presents to the emergency department for ongoing substernal chest pressure associated with nausea, diaphoresis, and lightheadedness. Her symptoms began 3 hours ago. She has hypertension and hypercholesterolemia. Her daily medications are hydrochlorothiazide, pravastatin, and aspirin.

On physical examination, her blood pressure is 84/62 mm Hg, pulse is 88/min, and respiration rate is 20/min. Her BMI is 29. Cardiac auscultation reveals distant heart sounds with an S_4. The lungs are clear bilaterally; estimated central venous pressure is 9 cm H_2O. The extremities are cool.

Electrocardiogram with right-sided precordial leads is shown. (Leads V_1 through V_6 are recorded from the right side of the chest.)

Which of the following should be given next in the treatment of this patient?

(A) Dobutamine intravenously
(B) Metoprolol intravenously
(C) Nitroglycerin sublingually
(D) 0.9% saline intravenous bolus

Item 2

A 52-year-old man is evaluated regarding treatment of his coronary artery disease. He had a myocardial infarction 8 years ago and was treated with a coronary stent placed in his right coronary artery. Over the last 8 years he did well with medical therapy, with only mild episodes of exertional angina that resolved with rest or sublingual nitroglycerin. One month ago, he noted worsening of his exertional angina. Coronary angiography showed 50% stenosis of the left main coronary artery, severe disease (75% stenosis) of the left circumflex artery, severe disease (70% stenosis) of the proximal left anterior descending artery, and in-stent restenosis (80%) of the stent within the right coronary artery. Left ventricular systolic function is mildly reduced (ejection fraction, 50%). His medical therapy was increased, and he has remained pain-free with activity. He is active and is a construction worker.

Medical history is notable for diabetes mellitus, hyperlipidemia, and hypertension. Current medications are aspirin, ramipril, atorvastatin, metoprolol, isosorbide mononitrate, diltiazem, and metformin.

Physical examination shows a well-developed man who appears comfortable. Blood pressure is 110/60 mm Hg and heart rate is 60/min. BMI is 28. Neck examination demonstrates a right carotid bruit and no jugular venous distention. Cardiac examination reveals normal heart sounds and no murmurs. Lungs are clear bilaterally and there is no peripheral edema.

Which of the following is the most appropriate treatment for this patient?

(A) Coronary artery bypass graft surgery
(B) Enhanced external counterpulsation
(C) Percutaneous coronary intervention
(D) Start ranolazine

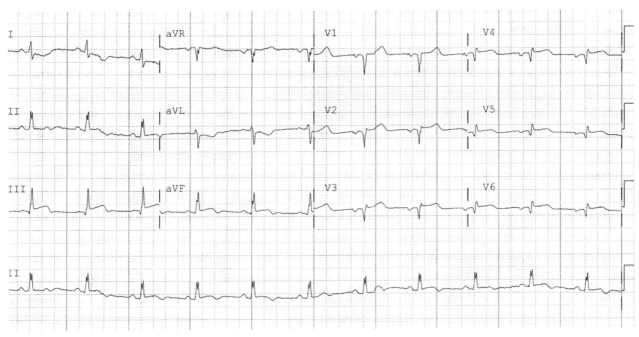

ITEM 1.

Item 3

A 60-year-old woman is evaluated for exertional dyspnea and shortness of breath. She reports no recent illnesses, fevers, chills, dental work, or sick exposures. She takes no medications.

On physical examination, temperature is normal, blood pressure is 122/80 mm Hg, and pulse is 86/min. Estimated central venous pressure is 12 cm H_2O. Cardiac examination reveals a loud S_1, normal S_2, and an opening snap. There is a regular rhythm with a grade 2/6 holosystolic murmur at the cardiac apex radiating to the axilla, and a low-pitched 3/6 middiastolic murmur following the opening snap that accentuates presystole. Lungs are clear to auscultation. There is 1+ bilateral pedal edema.

Transthoracic echocardiography demonstrates normal biventricular size and function. The left atrium is enlarged. There is mitral stenosis with a mean transvalvular gradient of 12 mm Hg and moderate mitral regurgitation. Pulmonary pressure estimates are 50 to 55 mm Hg.

Which of the following is the best treatment?

(A) Angiotensin-converting enzyme inhibitor therapy

(B) Mitral balloon valvuloplasty

(C) Mitral valve surgery

(D) No intervention, with follow-up in 1 year

Item 4

A 35-year-old black woman is evaluated for progressive dyspnea 3 weeks after delivery of her first child. Other than hypertension during pregnancy, the pregnancy and delivery were uncomplicated. She has no history of cardiovascular disease.

On physical examination, the blood pressure is 110/70 mm Hg in both upper extremities, the heart rate is 105/min and regular, and the respiratory rate is 28/min. The estimated central venous pressure is 10 cm H_2O and there are no carotid bruits. The apical impulse is displaced and diffuse. There is a grade 2/6 holosystolic murmur noted at the apex. Third and fourth heart sounds are also noted at the apex. There is dullness to percussion at the posterior lung bases bilaterally, and there are crackles extending up half of the lung fields. Lower extremity pulses are normal and without delay, but pedal edema is present.

The electrocardiogram demonstrates sinus tachycardia. There are no ST-segment or T-wave changes. The chest radiograph demonstrates bilateral pleural effusions and interstitial infiltrates. The aortic contour is unremarkable.

Which of the following is the most likely cause of the patient's current symptoms?

(A) Acute myocardial infarction

(B) Aortic dissection

(C) Coarctation of the aorta

(D) Peripartum cardiomyopathy

Item 5

A 72-year-old man is evaluated for fatigue and dyspnea. Over the last several months to a year, he has had increasing fatigue, exercise intolerance, and dyspnea on even mild exertion. He becomes short of breath walking across a room, although he is asymptomatic at rest. He denies chest pain, palpitations, syncope, orthopnea, and lower extremity edema. He has a history of coronary artery disease, with a myocardial infarction and four-vessel coronary artery bypass graft surgery 4 years ago. He also has hyperlipidemia and type 2 diabetes mellitus. Medications are aspirin, low-dose carvedilol, lisinopril, digoxin, spironolactone, furosemide, pravastatin, and glyburide.

On physical examination, his blood pressure is 92/57 mm Hg, pulse is 57/min, and respiration rate is 12/min. Cardiovascular examination reveals a point of maximal impulse that is displaced laterally. Rhythm is regular and bradycardic. S_1 and S_2 are normal, with a grade 2/6 to 3/6 holosystolic murmur at the apex. An S_3 is present. Estimated central venous pressure is 8 cm H_2O; there is no hepatojugular reflux. The lungs are clear. There is no ascites. The liver edge is palpable 1 cm below the right costal margin. The lower extremities are warm with decreased distal pulses bilaterally. There is no ankle edema.

Electrocardiogram demonstrates sinus rhythm with a rate of 55/min. PR interval is 180 msec, QRS width is 180 msec, and QT interval is 380 msec. Left bundle branch block is seen. A dobutamine stress echocardiogram reveals a left ventricular ejection fraction of 33% with a large anteroapical area of akinesis and no ischemia.

Which of the following is the most appropriate management option for this patient?

(A) Add amiodarone

(B) Biventricular pacemaker-defibrillator

(C) Dual-chamber pacemaker

(D) Implantable defibrillator

Item 6

A 70-year-old man with a history of a systolic murmur presents for further assessment of exertional dyspnea. He has had dyspnea his entire life, but has noted a recent deterioration in his exercise capacity. He has no other medical conditions and is on no medications.

On physical examination, his blood pressure is 120/70 mm Hg and pulse is 75/min and regular. The jugular venous pulse contour demonstrates a prominent a wave and the carotid pulses are normal. On cardiac examination, there is a parasternal impulse and a systolic thrill. The apical impulse is not displaced. An ejection click in close proximity to the S_1 is heard along the left sternal border and second left intercostal space, which decreases in intensity with inspiration. A grade 4/6 early systolic murmur that increases with inspiration is best heard in the second left intercostal space without radiation to the carotid arteries. No diastolic murmur is noted.

The electrocardiogram is shown. Chest radiograph demonstrates dilatation of the main pulmonary artery.

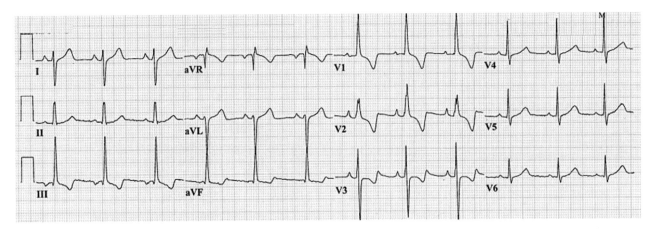

ITEM 6.

Which of the following is the most likely diagnosis in this patient?

(A) Aortic valve stenosis
(B) Atrial septal defect
(C) Mitral valve regurgitation
(D) Pulmonary valve stenosis
(E) Tricuspid valve regurgitation

Item 7

A 55-year-old man is evaluated for exertional dyspnea. He used to walk 2 to 3 miles several times per week. However, he has noted a progressive decline in exercise tolerance over the past 2 years and has had to discontinue exercise over time. His symptoms have been most pronounced over the past several months. The patient has a history of mitral valve prolapse. He smokes one pack of cigarettes. He drinks alcohol moderately and does not take illicit drugs. The patient has not noted any palpitations, syncope, presyncope, or edema. He has no other medical conditions and takes no medications.

On physical examination, his blood pressure is 126/80 mm Hg and his pulse is 62/min. BMI is 28. Carotid upstrokes are brisk. Central venous pressure is estimated at 7 cm H_2O. Cardiac auscultation reveals regular rhythm. Heart sounds are normal with no S_3 or S_4. A grade 3/6 late systolic apical murmur is heard that radiates toward the left axilla. Moving from a squatting position to a standing position increases murmur intensity. Following a Valsalva maneuver, the murmur intensity decreases. No diastolic murmur is heard. Lungs are clear to auscultation, but with an increased expiratory phase. There is no pedal edema. Distal pulses are 2+ and palpable.

Transthoracic echocardiogram demonstrates a myxomatous mitral valve with posterior leaflet prolapse. There is moderate mitral regurgitation.

Additional echocardiographic findings:

Left ventricular end-diastolic dimension	40 mm
Left ventricular end-systolic dimension	25 mm
Left ventricular ejection fraction	65%
Vena contracta width	6 mm
Regurgitant orifice area	0.4 cm²
Pulmonary arterial systolic pressure	30 mm Hg

A stress echocardiogram is performed. The patient exercised for 4 minutes and 30 seconds using a standard Bruce protocol and discontinued the study due to dyspnea. During stress, mitral regurgitation severity was comparable to images at rest, and pulmonary systolic pressure increased to 45 mm Hg (normal increase, between 10 and 25 mm Hg).

Which of the following is the most appropriate management?

(A) Mitral valve annuloplasty repair
(B) Pharmacologic afterload therapy
(C) Pulmonary function testing
(D) Right heart catheterization

Item 8

A 42-year-old man is hospitalized for progressively worsening dyspnea on exertion for 6 months, now occurring with minimal activities. He has had frequent episodes of dyspnea at rest, progressive fatigue, leg edema, and a 9.1-kg (20.0-lb) weight gain over the last 4 weeks. He reports symptoms of three-pillow orthopnea and nocturnal dyspnea but does not have chest pain, palpitations, syncope, or cough. There is no family history of sudden cardiac death. He has no other medical problems. His medications are metoprolol, disopyramide, and furosemide.

On physical examination, temperature is normal, blood pressure is 100/50 mm Hg, pulse is 48/min, and respiration rate is 28/min. Jugular venous distention is noted, with brisk carotid upstrokes. Estimated central venous pressure is 10 cm H_2O. Cardiac examination reveals an S_3 gallop at the apex and a grade 3/6 midsystolic murmur along the lower left sternal border that accentuates with a Valsalva maneuver and diminishes with a hand-grip maneuver. Pulmonary examination discloses dullness to percussion in the posterior lung fields at the bases, crackles in the basilar posterior lung fields, and no wheezing. The lower extremities show 3+ edema.

Laboratory studies:

Hemoglobin	13.5 g/dL (135 g/L)
Leukocyte count	8300/μL (8.3 × 10⁹/L) with normal differential
Creatinine	2.2 mg/dL (167.9 μmol/L)
Blood urea nitrogen	50 mg/dL (17.9 mmol/L)
Albumin	4.0 g/dL (40 g/L)
Iron	Normal
Ferritin	Normal
Thyroid-stimulating hormone	2.5 μU/mL (2.5 mU/L)
B-type natriuretic peptide	2045 pg/mL

Twelve-lead electrocardiogram shows sinus bradycardia, left atrial enlargement, and left ventricular hypertrophy. Echocardiogram shows hyperdynamic left ventricular systolic function, a left ventricular ejection fraction of 80%, asymmetric septal hypertrophy, left ventricular dynamic outflow obstruction with a peak gradient of 144 mm Hg, left ventricular diastolic dysfunction, and left atrial enlargement. Septal thickness is 26 mm. Chest radiograph discloses no infiltrates, an enlarged cardiac silhouette, and small pleural effusions.

Which of the following is the most appropriate treatment?

(A) Carvedilol
(B) Implantable cardioverter-defibrillator
(C) Permanent pacemaker
(D) Surgical septal myectomy

Item 9

A 66-year-old man is evaluated in the emergency department for left-sided chest pain that began at rest, lasted for 15 minutes, and has since resolved. A similar episode occurred at rest yesterday, and multiple similar episodes that were associated with exertion have occurred over the past 2 weeks. Pertinent medical history includes hypertension and type 2 diabetes mellitus. Family history is notable for his father undergoing coronary artery bypass graft surgery at age 69 years and his brother undergoing coronary artery bypass graft surgery at age 54 years. Current medications are amlodipine, glyburide, and aspirin.

On physical examination blood pressure is 125/65 mm Hg, heart rate is 70/min, and respiratory rate is 12/min. Estimated central venous pressure is 6 cm H_2O, carotid upstroke is normal, there are no cardiac murmurs, and the lung fields are clear. Extremities show no edema, and peripheral pulses are normal bilaterally.

Laboratory findings include a serum troponin I level of 1.2 ng/mL (1.2 μg/L), and a creatinine level of 1.4 mg/dL (106.8 μmol/L). Electrocardiogram shows 1-mm ST-segment depression in leads aVL, V_5, and V_6. Chest radiograph shows a normal cardiac silhouette, with no infiltrates and no pleural effusions.

The patient is treated with aspirin, intravenous nitroglycerin, unfractionated heparin, metoprolol, and pravastatin.

Which of the following should be the next step in this patient's management?

(A) Coronary angiography
(B) Obtain B-type natriuretic peptide level
(C) Pharmacologic stress testing
(D) Thrombolytic therapy

Item 10

A 70-year-old man is evaluated for two fainting spells last week; episodes occurred while sitting, without either prodrome or post-event symptoms. He is otherwise feeling well with no chest pain or palpitations. He has good functional status, walking several times a week for exercise. He had a cardiac transplant 10 years ago for ischemic cardiomyopathy. He has a history of hypertension, dyslipidemia, and chronic kidney disease (baseline serum creatinine 1.5 mg/dL [114.5 μmol/L], glomerular filtration rate 50 mL/min/1.73 m²) related to immunosuppression medications. He quit smoking 10 years ago, prior to the transplantation. He takes aspirin, pravastatin, lisinopril, cyclosporine, and mycophenolate mofetil. He was weaned off corticosteroids 5 years ago.

On physical examination, he is afebrile. Blood pressure is 130/80 mm Hg, pulse is 50/min, and respiration rate is 16/min. There is no jugular venous distention. Cardiac examination discloses a regular rate and rhythm with normal S_1 and S_2 and no S_3 or S_4. The lungs are clear bilaterally. The abdomen is soft, and there is no peripheral edema. Neurologic examination is unremarkable.

Laboratory evaluation is unremarkable and unchanged from previous evaluations. Electrocardiogram is unchanged from the previous one, and shows first-degree atrioventricular block and incomplete right bundle branch block.

Which of the following is the most likely diagnosis?

(A) Cardiac transplant rejection
(B) Central nervous system lymphoma
(C) Coronary artery disease
(D) Cyclosporine side effect

Item 11

A 52-year-old woman is evaluated during a routine follow-up examination for ischemic cardiomyopathy. She sustained a large inferoposterior myocardial infarction 2 years ago, which was treated acutely with percutaneous intervention and stent placement. Her ejection fraction was 37% six months ago. She has mild exercise limitations due to dyspnea with moderate exertion. She denies chest pain, orthopnea, paroxysmal nocturnal dyspnea, and edema. She has no palpitations, lightheadedness, or syncope. She has hyperlipidemia. She has a 31 pack-year history of smoking cigarettes, but quit smoking 2 years ago. Medications include aspirin, carvedilol, enalapril, and atorvastatin.

On physical examination, her blood pressure is 115/65 mm Hg and her pulse is 65/min. Cardiac auscultation reveals regular rate and rhythm with no murmurs or gallops.

The point of maximal impulse is slightly displaced laterally. Estimated central venous pressure is 5 cm H_2O. The lungs are clear and there is no edema. Her ejection fraction is 30%.

Which of the following is the most appropriate management for this patient?

(A) Add amiodarone

(B) Add furosemide

(C) Add spironolactone

(D) Implantable cardioverter-defibrillator placement

Item 12

A 70-year-old woman is evaluated for a 1-month history of dyspnea on exertion and fatigue. She can still perform activities of daily living, including vacuuming, grocery shopping, and ascending two flights of stairs carrying laundry. She has a history of hypertension, mild chronic obstructive pulmonary disease, and smoking. Her medications are lisinopril, hydrochlorothiazide, and albuterol as needed.

On physical examination, she is afebrile. Blood pressure is 110/80 mm Hg and pulse is 70/min. Jugular veins are not distended. There is a grade 2/6 holosystolic murmur at the left sternal border that radiates to the axilla, which was not noted during an examination 1 year ago. Rate and rhythm are regular, S_1 and S_2 are normal, and there is no S_3. The lung sounds are distant but clear without wheezing, and there is no edema. Laboratory studies show normal hemoglobin and thyroid-stimulating hormone levels. Electrocardiogram shows low voltage and left axis deviation. Echocardiogram shows an ejection fraction of 35%, global hypokinesis, and mild mitral regurgitation. Chest radiograph shows flattening of the diaphragms but is otherwise normal.

Which of the following is the most appropriate treatment?

(A) Amlodipine

(B) Carvedilol

(C) Digoxin

(D) Losartan

(E) Spironolactone

Item 13

A 37-year-old woman with a history of peripartum cardiomyopathy several years ago is evaluated 12 weeks into her second pregnancy. She became pregnant despite the use of a combination oral contraceptive and plans to proceed with the pregnancy. She is currently asymptomatic but leads a sedentary lifestyle. She is taking no medications.

On physical examination, the blood pressure is 110/70 mm Hg and the heart rate is 80/min and regular. The estimated central venous pressure is 3 cm H_2O and there are no carotid bruits. The cardiac and pulmonary examinations are normal. Lower extremity pulses are normal and there is no edema.

The electrocardiogram demonstrates sinus rhythm but is otherwise unremarkable. An echocardiogram is performed and demonstrates mild left ventricular enlargement with a calculated ejection fraction of 40%. The valves and pulmonary pressures are normal.

Which of the following medications should be initiated at this time?

(A) Digoxin

(B) Furosemide

(C) Hydralazine

(D) Lisinopril

(E) Metoprolol

Item 14

A 26-year-old woman who is 25 weeks pregnant is evaluated in the emergency department for palpitations and episodic lightheadedness. She has no history of cardiovascular disease or tachycardia.

On physical examination, her blood pressure is 100/70 mm Hg and her pulse is 175/min. The estimated central venous pressure is normal and there are no carotid bruits. The apical impulse is not displaced. There are no murmurs or abnormal heart sounds detected. The examination is otherwise unremarkable.

A Valsalva maneuver is performed by the patient and carotid sinus massage is performed by the attending physician, but the tachycardia continues. The electrocardiogram is shown.

Which of the following is the most appropriate intravenous medication to administer at this time?

(A) Adenosine

(B) Amiodarone

(C) Digoxin

(D) Diltiazem

(E) Metoprolol

Item 15

A 67-year-old business man is evaluated during a routine health examination. He has a 30 pack-year history of smoking, but quit 5 years ago. He consumes two or more alcoholic beverages on most days. He is asymptomatic, but performs no regular physical exercise. He takes no medications.

On physical examination, his blood pressure is 148/92 mm Hg and heart rate is 78/min and regular. His pulses are full, he has no bruits, and results of his lung, heart, abdominal, and rectal examinations are unremarkable.

Total serum cholesterol is 240 mg/dL (6.2 mmol/L), HDL cholesterol is 40 mg/dL (1.0 mmol/L), and triglyceride level is 100 mg/dL (1.1 mmol/L). Results of other serum laboratory studies are normal.

An abdominal ultrasound for screening purposes demonstrates an infrarenal abdominal aortic aneurysm measuring 4 cm in diameter.

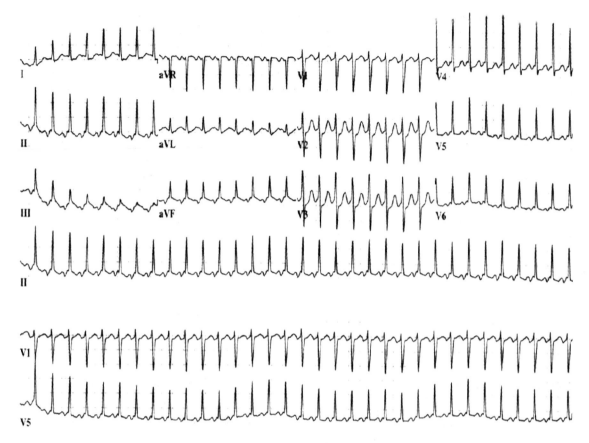

ITEM 14.

In addition to treatment of this patient's hyperlipidemia and hypertension and discussion about his at-risk drinking, which of the following is the best management option?

(A) Abdominal CT with intravenous contrast
(B) Antithrombotic therapy
(C) Follow-up ultrasound in 6 to 12 months
(D) Placement of an endovascular stent graft

Item 16

A 54-year-old woman is evaluated in the emergency department for jaw and shoulder pain that has occurred intermittently for the past week. The symptoms occur with activity and are relieved by rest. Medical and family history are unremarkable. She is not taking any medications.

Physical examination shows a blood pressure of 130/68 mm Hg and a pulse of 90/min. There is no jugular venous distention and carotid upstrokes are normal. There are no cardiac murmurs and the lung fields are clear. Extremities show no edema and peripheral pulses are normal bilaterally.

Laboratory studies:

Hematocrit	42%
Platelet count	220,000/µL (200×10^9/L)
Troponin I	9.0 ng/mL (9.0 µg/L)
Creatinine	1.0 mg/dL (76.3 µmol/L)

Electrocardiogram shows 1.0-mm ST-segment depression in leads V_1 through V_4 with T-wave inversions.

The patient is given aspirin, intravenous nitroglycerin, low-molecular-weight heparin, metoprolol, and atorvastatin. The pain subsides after approximately 20 minutes, and she is admitted to the coronary care unit. One hour later, she has recurrent jaw and shoulder pain. She denies chest pain. A repeat electrocardiogram is unchanged.

Which of the following is the most appropriate immediate treatment for this patient?

(A) Discontinue metoprolol and start verapamil
(B) Discontinue low-molecular-weight heparin and start unfractionated heparin
(C) Start enalapril
(D) Start a glycoprotein IIb/IIIa inhibitor

Item 17

A 75-year-old woman is evaluated in the emergency department for chest pain that has been present for 1 hour. The pain is located in the mid-chest area, and she describes it as a heavy weight. She has not experienced any previous episodes. Medical history is notable for hypertension and chronic kidney disease. Current medications are lisinopril and furosemide.

Physical examination shows blood pressure of 150/70 mm Hg and heart rate of 65/min. Jugular venous pulsations are normal, and no murmurs, extra sounds, or rubs are heard on cardiac auscultation. The lungs are clear, there is no peripheral edema, and distal pulses are normal bilaterally.

Laboratory findings include serum troponin I, 2.0 ng/mL (2.0 μg/L); creatinine, 2.0 mg/dL (152.6 μmol/L); and potassium, 4.6 meq/L (4.6 mmol/L). Her estimated glomerular filtration rate is less than 30 mL/min/1.73 m². Electrocardiogram shows T-wave inversions in leads V_4 through V_6.

Her chest pain resolves after one sublingual nitroglycerin tablet and supplemental oxygen.

Which of the following is the best anticoagulation management for this patient?

(A) Low-dose unfractionated heparin
(B) Full-dose unfractionated heparin
(C) Low-dose low-molecular-weight heparin
(D) Full-dose low-molecular-weight heparin

Item 18

A 58-year-old woman is hospitalized for acute left-sided flank pain. She has had fever and night sweats for 1 month and a 9.1-kg (20-lb) weight loss over 6 months.

On physical examination, temperature is 37.7 °C (99.8 °F), blood pressure is 135/88 mm Hg, pulse is 88/min, and respiration rate is 18/min. Heart sounds are normal. There is an early diastolic low-pitched sound after the S_2 with a diastolic murmur at the apex. There is tenderness of the left costophrenic angle. The abdomen is soft with normal bowel sounds and no tenderness. She does not have rash or petechiae, splinter hemorrhages, or Janeway lesions. Funduscopic examination is normal.

Laboratory studies:

Leukocyte count	14,000/uL (14.0 × 10⁹/L) with no left shift
Creatinine	1.3 mg/dL (99.2 μmol/L)
Blood urea nitrogen	14 mg/dL (5.0 mmol/L)
Urinalysis	Microscopic hematuria, no crystals, negative for protein

Twelve-lead electrocardiography shows normal sinus rhythm. Echocardiogram shows a 5- by 4-cm left atrial echogenic mobile globular mass attached to the atrial septum with diastolic protrusion into the left ventricle. Abdominal radiograph shows a normal gas pattern and no renal calculi. Contrast-enhanced CT scan of the abdomen and pelvis shows a wedge-shaped hypoperfusion defect in the upper pole of the left kidney. Mean transmitral valve inflow gradient is 15 mm Hg. Three sets of blood cultures are negative for growth after 5 days.

Which of the following is the most appropriate treatment?

(A) Cardiac surgery for resection of mass
(B) Mitral valve replacement
(C) Systemic anticoagulation with heparin
(D) Vancomycin and tobramycin

Item 19

A 78-year-old man is evaluated in an urgent care clinic for new-onset chest pain. The pain, which he describes as "crushing," is in the left substernal area, is nonradiating, and has been present for 14 hours. He has had no prior episodes of similar symptoms. His medical history is notable for hypertension and hyperlipidemia. Current medications include aspirin, hydrochlorothiazide, and atorvastatin.

On physical examination, blood pressure is 100/70 mm Hg in the right arm and 105/72 mm Hg in the left arm, pulse is 100/min, and respiration rate is 16/min. There is no jugular venous distention and no cardiac murmurs or rubs. The lungs are clear and there is no peripheral edema.

Laboratory results are notable for a platelet count of 120,000/μL (120 × 10⁹/L); serum creatine kinase, 450 U/L; and troponin I, 60 ng/mL (60 μg/L). Initial electrocardiogram shows ST-segment elevation of 2 mm in leads II, III, and aVF, and ST-segment depression in leads V_2 and V_3. Chest radiograph is normal.

Which of the following is the best management for this patient?

(A) Chest CT with contrast
(B) Echocardiogram
(C) Primary percutaneous coronary intervention
(D) Thrombolytic therapy

Item 20

A 22-year-old man is evaluated in the emergency department for fever and dyspnea. He reports a 3-week history of flu-like symptoms with decreased appetite and recurrent fevers as high as 39.4 °C (103.0 °F). He injects heroin, and his last use was 3 days ago. He has no other medical conditions and takes no medications. Blood cultures are drawn and intravenous vancomycin and gentamicin are started.

On physical examination, he appears uncomfortable. His temperature is 39.6 °C (103.2 °F), blood pressure is 80/50 mm Hg, and pulse is 110/min. Oxygen saturation on ambient air is 91%. Jugular venous distention is increased to the jaw line. Heart rhythm is regular with a summation gallop. A grade 4/6 continuous murmur is heard over the precordium that accentuates during diastole. There are bibasilar crackles on lung auscultation. He has 2+ bilateral pedal edema. Laboratory findings include a leukocyte count of 19,000/μL (19.0 × 10⁹/L) with a left shift.

Transesophageal echocardiography demonstrates normal left ventricular size with hyperdynamic systolic function. There is a prominent aortic right coronary sinus with color Doppler evidence of flow between the aorta and the right ventricle. An echolucency (fluid) is noted around the aortic valve annulus. There are multiple, mobile echodensities on the aortic valve, with moderate aortic valvular regurgitation. No abnormalities are seen on the other cardiac valves. Blood cultures are positive for *Staphylococcus aureus*.

Which of the following is the most appropriate management?

(A) Aortic valve replacement and aortic repair

(B) Aspirin

(C) Broaden antibiotic coverage

(D) Coronary angiography

(E) Intra-aortic balloon placement

Item 21

A 60-year-old man with type 2 diabetes mellitus and hypertension visits the office to establish medical care. He reports monitoring his blood pressure and blood glucose measurements at home with good results. He had a cholesterol panel checked approximately 5 years ago, at which time he was instructed by his prior physician to exercise, lose weight, and reduce his intake of dietary cholesterol. He has made some lifestyle changes, which he believes have helped his blood pressure and glucose control. His hypertension has been treated for 15 years and his diabetes for 5 years. His daily medications include lisinopril, amlodipine, metformin, and aspirin.

On physical examination, blood pressure is 128/65 mm Hg and pulse is 76/min. BMI is 26. The remainder of the physical examination is normal.

Laboratory studies:

Total cholesterol	215 mg/dL (5.6 mmol/L)
Triglycerides	185 mg/dL (2.1 mmol/L)
HDL cholesterol	39 mg/dL (1.0 mmol/L)
LDL cholesterol	145 mg/dL (3.8 mmol/L)
Hemoglobin A_{1c}	6.5%

Which of the following medications is the best choice for reducing this patient's risk of cardiovascular disease?

(A) Colestipol

(B) Ezetimibe

(C) Niacin

(D) Simvastatin

Item 22

A 54-year-old man is evaluated for right-sided chest pain that is described as sharp, begins following large meals, lasts for several minutes, and usually resolves spontaneously. The episodes are not clearly related to activity, nor are they relieved by rest. He has been experiencing the pain for about 4 months. Several of the episodes have resolved with antacids. The most recent episode, which occurred yesterday while walking, lasted 20 minutes and resolved.

Pertinent medical history includes hypertension and hyperlipidemia. Family history is notable for a brother who had coronary stent placement at the age of 43 years. Current medications are aspirin, atenolol, and atorvastatin.

Physical examination is notable for estimated central venous pressure of 6 cm H_2O; normal carotid upstroke; and no cardiac murmurs, rubs, or S_3. Lung fields are clear. Extremities show no edema, and peripheral pulses are normal bilaterally.

Laboratory findings include hematocrit, 44%; serum troponin I at presentation is 0.0 ng/mL (0.0 µg/L); troponin I at 4 hours is 0.0 ng/mL (0.0 µg/L); creatine kinase, 50 U/L. Electrocardiogram shows normal sinus rhythm and no ST- or T-wave changes. Chest radiograph shows a normal cardiac silhouette, no infiltrates, and no pleural effusions.

Which of the following is the best diagnostic option?

(A) Coronary angiography

(B) Esophagogastroduodenoscopy

(C) Exercise stress test

(D) Empiric treatment with a proton pump inhibitor

Item 23

A 40-year-old black man is hospitalized for heart failure. He has had fatigue and progressive dyspnea on exertion for 12 months, pedal edema for 6 months, paroxysmal nocturnal dyspnea for 3 months, and recent onset of orthostatic lightheadedness. These symptoms have worsened over the past week, prompting the hospitalization. He has a history of sickle cell anemia with frequent painful hemolytic crises and numerous blood transfusions. Medications are furosemide, metolazone, diltiazem, lisinopril, hydroxyurea, and folic acid.

On physical examination, temperature is normal, blood pressure is 115/70 mm Hg supine and 80/50 mm Hg standing, pulse is 90/min supine and 122/min standing, and respiration rate is 30/min. Oxygen saturation on ambient air is 95%. There is jugular venous distention that worsens with inspiration. Cardiac examination discloses a right-sided S_4 gallop, no pericardial friction rub, and a grade 2/6 holosystolic murmur at the lower left sternal border. Pulmonary auscultation reveals normal breath sounds and faint bibasilar crackles. The abdomen is distended with shifting dullness. There is 3+ lower extremity edema to the level of the knees.

Laboratory studies:

Hemoglobin	8 g/dL (80 g/L)
Ferritin	650 ng/mL (650 mg/L)
Iron	512 µg/dL (91.7 µmol/L)
Fasting transferrin saturation	78%

Twelve-lead electrocardiogram shows normal sinus rhythm and normal QRS voltage. Echocardiogram shows severe biatrial enlargement, normal left ventricular wall thickness, a left ventricular ejection fraction of 70%, normal ventricular cavity size, and restrictive left ventricular filling without respiratory variation in peak filling velocity. Endomyocardial biopsy is positive for iron deposits.

Which of the following is the most appropriate treatment?

(A) Heart transplant

(B) Increase the dosage of furosemide

(C) Iron chelation

(D) Phlebotomy

Item 24

A 65-year-old woman who recently moved to the area presents for an evaluation to establish care. Her medical history is significant for an occasional sensation of "single skipped heart beats." These palpitation episodes occur once or twice per year and have not increased in intensity or frequency over the past several years. They are not associated with syncope or presyncope. She is active and swims laps three or four times per week. She does not smoke. She takes no medications.

On physical examination, her blood pressure is 118/60 mm Hg. There are no carotid bruits. There is a normal S_1 and a physiologically split S_2. There is a grade 2/6 midsystolic murmur that does not radiate, heard best at the second right intercostal space. The rest of the physical examination is unrevealing. Electrocardiogram is normal.

Which of the following is the most appropriate management?

(A) Antibiotic endocarditis prophylaxis
(B) 24-Hour ambulatory electrocardiographic monitoring
(C) Transthoracic echocardiography
(D) Treadmill stress echocardiography
(E) No further intervention

Item 25

A 45-year-old man is evaluated in the emergency department for a 2-day history of substernal sharp intermittent chest pain that is aggravated by deep breaths. He began experiencing severe chest pain 4 hours prior to his emergency department visit. He has a 3-day history of nonproductive cough, sore throat, myalgias, and malaise. He has had hypertension for 12 years. His medications are hydrochlorothiazide and amlodipine.

On physical examination, temperature is 37.8 °C (100.0 °F), blood pressure is 168/100 mm Hg, pulse is 110/min, and respiration rate is 26/min. Oxygen saturation on ambient air is 96%. The patient's face and chest appear diaphoretic. The oropharynx is erythematous. There is no jugular venous distention and no hepatojugular reflux. Cardiac examination discloses a two-component rub that is loudest at the apex, distant heart sounds, and no murmurs. Pulmonary examination discloses normal breath sounds and no crackles. There is no palpable chest wall tenderness. Laboratory studies show a leukocyte count of 12,300/μL (12.3 × 10⁹/L) with 50% polymorphonuclear cells, 30% lymphocytes, and no band forms. Initial serum troponin T level is 0.6 ng/mL (0.6 μg/L). Twelve-lead electrocardiogram shows sinus tachycardia and concave upward ST-segment elevation in leads V_1 through V_6. Chest radiograph shows no infiltrates and a normal cardiac silhouette.

Which of the following is the most likely diagnosis?

(A) Acute myocardial infarction
(B) Acute viral pericarditis
(C) Costochondritis
(D) Pleuritis
(E) Pulmonary embolism

Item 26

A 60-year-old man was hospitalized 3 days ago with an acute anterior ST-elevation myocardial infarction. He underwent primary percutaneous coronary intervention with stent placement in his mid left anterior descending coronary artery. His course was uncomplicated. Echocardiogram performed the day of admission revealed anterior and anteroseptal hypokinesis with an ejection fraction of 30% to 35%. He also has hypertension and hypercholesterolemia, and he is a smoker. Current medications include aspirin, clopidogrel, carvedilol, captopril, and atorvastatin.

On physical examination, his blood pressure is 135/77 mm Hg and his pulse is 65/min. Estimated central venous pressure is 6 cm H_2O. Cardiac auscultation reveals a regular S_1 and S_2 without murmurs or gallops. The point of maximal impulse is within normal limits. The lungs are clear. The lower extremities are warm, well perfused, and without edema.

In addition to counseling for smoking cessation, which of the following is the most appropriate management for this patient?

(A) Add eplerenone
(B) Add valsartan
(C) Implantable cardioverter-defibrillator placement
(D) Repeat echocardiogram at follow-up

Item 27

A 59-year-old man is evaluated for chest pain that is sometimes accompanied by a burning sensation. The pain episodes began 4 weeks ago. The pain comes on during periods of both exertion and rest. He has a history of hypertension, for which he currently takes nifedipine. The patient recently sustained a knee injury that has prevented him from walking without the aid of a cane.

On physical examination, the patient is afebrile. Blood pressure is 138/86 mm Hg, pulse is 74/min, and respiration rate is 16/min. BMI is 28. The patient does not show signs of heart failure.

Laboratory studies:

Total cholesterol	210 mg/dL (5.4 mmol/L)
LDL cholesterol	140 mg/dL (3.6 mmol/L)
HDL cholesterol	40 mg/dL (1.0 mmol/L)
Creatinine	1.2 mg/dL (91.6 μmol/L)

The results of cardiac enzyme studies are negative. An electrocardiogram shows left ventricular hypertrophy with sinus rhythm, with no change from a previous electrocardiogram.

Which of the following is the most appropriate test to perform next in this patient?

(A) Adenosine positron emission tomography stress test
(B) Cardiac catheterization with coronary angiography
(C) Coronary artery calcium score
(D) CT coronary angiography
(E) Nuclear perfusion imaging stress test

Item 28

A 74-year-old man is evaluated for continued chest pain that occurs on a daily basis with minimal activity and is resolved with rest or sublingual nitroglycerin. He has an extensive history of coronary artery disease. Twenty years ago, and again 8 years ago, he underwent coronary artery bypass graft surgery. Over the past 5 years, he has undergone multiple coronary artery stent procedures. He is on maximal medical therapy, including ranolazine. Because of continued symptoms, coronary angiography was performed 3 months ago, but no targets were identified for percutaneous revascularization. He was seen by a cardiothoracic surgeon, who recommended no additional surgery because of extensive scar tissue in the anterior mediastinum and a patent saphenous vein graft to the left anterior descending artery.

Current medications are aspirin, metoprolol, isosorbide dinitrate, pravastatin, diltiazem, and ranolazine.

On physical examination, blood pressure is 100/60 mm Hg and heart rate is 48/min. There is no jugular venous distention. Cardiac examination reveals no murmurs, the lungs are clear, and there is no peripheral edema.

Which of the following should be the next step in this patient's management?

(A) Add ticlopidine
(B) Add nifedipine
(C) External enhanced counterpulsation
(D) Increase metoprolol

Item 29

A 54-year-old man is evaluated for recurrent arrhythmia. He was diagnosed with atrial flutter with a rapid ventricular response 6 weeks ago. Rate control was initially difficult to achieve; he underwent cardioversion and was started on metoprolol. He has had general fatigue since initiation of metoprolol. Two days ago, he had a recurrence of his arrhythmia; his fatigue worsened, and he began experiencing dyspnea on exertion. He denies chest pain, lightheadedness, and heart racing. He has no other medical problems, and his only other medication is daily aspirin.

On physical examination, his blood pressure is 123/65 mm Hg and his pulse is 50/min. BMI is 24. Cardiac examination reveals bradycardia with an irregular rhythm, normal S_1 and S_2, and no murmurs or gallops. Lungs are clear to auscultation.

The electrocardiogram shows atrial flutter with a 6:1 block and a ventricular rate of 50/min.

Which of the following is the most appropriate management for this patient?

(A) Add amiodarone
(B) Add digoxin
(C) Discontinue metoprolol; initiate flecainide
(D) Radiofrequency ablation

Item 30

A 68-year-old woman is evaluated in the emergency department for the sudden onset of severe pain, which began 3 hours ago. The pain is in the middle of her chest and radiates to her back. Medical history includes hypertension treated with hydrochlorothiazide and lisinopril.

On physical examination, the patient is afebrile. Her blood pressure is 190/110 mm Hg, pulse is 108/min and regular, and respiration rate is 18/min. An S_4 gallop is auscultated. No pericardial rub or murmur is present. Distal pulses are equal, full, and symmetric. Neurologic examination is normal. Laboratory results include normal serum cardiac troponin and serum creatinine levels. Oxygen saturation is 99% while breathing ambient air.

Electrocardiogram shows tachycardia but is otherwise normal. CT scan of the chest with intravenous contrast demonstrates a crescent-shaped density within the media of the aorta, arising just distal to the origin of the left subclavian artery and extending to just above the celiac axis. Contrast dye is not present within this crescent.

In addition to analgesia and intravenous β-blockade, which of the following is the most appropriate treatment?

(A) Endovascular repair
(B) Intravenous sodium nitroprusside
(C) Intravenous unfractionated heparin
(D) Urgent surgical repair

Item 31

A 76-year-old man is evaluated during a routine follow-up examination for hypertension, and he mentions having had a syncopal event a few weeks earlier. He was standing in line at the grocery store and lost consciousness without any preceding symptoms. He estimates that the duration of the episode was less than a minute, and he drove himself home. He has had two other syncopal events in the last 3 years, one while sitting, and one during a walk. He has never injured himself seriously during an event. He has intermittent episodes of lightheadedness that do not have obvious triggers and are not related to positional changes. He is otherwise asymptomatic, with no chest pain, dyspnea, orthopnea, edema, or palpitations. He is healthy and active, playing golf nearly every day. His only daily medication is lisinopril.

On physical examination, his blood pressure is 140/85 mm Hg without orthostatic changes and his pulse is 82/min. Cardiac auscultation reveals regular rate and rhythm without murmurs or gallops. There are no carotid bruits and no peripheral edema. Carotid pressure does not result in bradycardia or hypotension. The lungs are clear.

The electrocardiogram and echocardiogram are both normal.

Exercise stress testing is performed, using the Bruce protocol, with an exercise duration of 9 minutes. Peak heart rate is 90% of the maximal predicted value. Blood pressure increase with exercise is normal, and there are no ischemic changes on the electrocardiogram.

Which of the following diagnostic tests is most likely to yield useful results for this patient?

(A) 24-Hour ambulatory monitoring
(B) Event monitoring
(C) Implantable loop recorder
(D) Electrophysiology study

Item 32

A 65-year-old woman is evaluated in the hospital 36 hours after presenting in the emergency department with midsternal chest pain. Electrocardiogram on presentation demonstrated no ST-segment shifts, but T-wave inversion was present in leads V_3 and V_4. She was given nitroglycerin, unfractionated heparin, and a glycoprotein IIb/IIIa inhibitor and was admitted to the hospital. She has a history of hypertension and hyperlipidemia and is a prior smoker. Her medications prior to admission were metoprolol, 25 mg twice daily; atorvastatin, 80 mg/d; and aspirin, 325 mg/d.

On physical examination, the patient is afebrile. Blood pressure is 132/82 mm Hg, pulse is 68/min and regular, and respiration rate is 16/min. BMI is 25. There is no jugular venous distention, and no crackles are auscultated. Heart sounds are normal. There is no rub, murmur, or gallop. Her serum cardiac troponin I level rose to a peak of 4.2 ng/mL (4.2 µg/L) at 24 hours following the index event. Results of a basic metabolic profile, including blood glucose levels, are normal.

Coronary angiography demonstrates diffuse, mild luminal irregularities in all coronary arteries, along with diffuse severe disease in the distal left anterior descending coronary artery not amenable to percutaneous coronary intervention. Left ventriculography demonstrates a left ventricular ejection fraction of 55% with a small focal region of hypokinesis in the apex. The left ventricular end-diastolic pressure is 12 mm Hg.

The glycoprotein IIb/IIIa inhibitor is discontinued.

Which one of the following agents should be added to this patient's medication regimen?

(A) Verapamil
(B) Clopidogrel
(C) Eplerenone
(D) Warfarin

Item 33

A 30-year-old woman who recently immigrated to the United States from Mexico is evaluated in the emergency department for shortness of breath, paroxysmal nocturnal dyspnea, palpitations, and pedal edema. She is gravida 1, para 0, and she is 30 weeks pregnant. She has not received prenatal care until this point. She reports no recent illnesses, fevers, chills, dental work, or sick exposures. She has no significant past medical history.

On physical examination, she is afebrile, blood pressure is 112/80 mm Hg, and pulse is 96/min. The patient appears uncomfortable and is sitting upright to breathe. There is jugular venous distention to her jaw line while sitting upright. Cardiac auscultation demonstrates an irregularly irregular rhythm, a loud S_1, normal S_2, and an opening snap. A grade 2/6 holosystolic murmur is heard at the cardiac apex radiating to the axilla, and a low-pitched diastolic murmur is heard following the opening snap. Bibasilar crackles are present. There is 3+ bilateral pitting pedal edema. Oxygen saturation is 91% on ambient air.

Transthoracic echocardiography demonstrates normal biventricular size and function. The left atrium is moderately enlarged. There is mitral stenosis with a mean transvalvular gradient of 15 mm Hg and mild mitral regurgitation. Pulmonary pressure is increased (45-50 mm Hg).

In addition to intravenous diuretic therapy, which of the following is the best immediate management option?

(A) Direct-current cardioversion
(B) Intravenous β-blocker therapy
(C) Percutaneous mitral balloon valvuloplasty
(D) Pregnancy induction and delivery

Item 34

A 34-year-old woman is evaluated for sharp intermittent pleuritic chest pain that has persisted for 1 week. The pain is worse when she lies down in the supine position. She has had no fever, chills, cough, or weight loss. She had acute viral pericarditis 6 months ago that was treated initially with ibuprofen, but when she failed to respond after 3 days, a 10-day tapering dosage of prednisone was instituted, leading to resolution of clinical symptoms. She has a 10-year history of essential hypertension, and she takes hydrochlorothiazide and potassium chloride.

On physical examination, temperature is normal, blood pressure is 98/54 mm Hg, pulse is 99/min, and respiration rate is 20/min. Cardiac examination discloses a pericardial friction rub at the lower left sternal border but no gallops. Pulmonary auscultation reveals normal breath sounds and no crackles. There is no jugular venous distention and no chest-wall tenderness. Laboratory studies reveal a serum creatinine level of 1.0 mg/dL (76.3 µmol/L). Electrocardiogram is shown. Chest radiograph shows a normal-sized cardiac silhouette and clear lung fields.

Which of the following is the most appropriate treatment?

(A) Colchicine
(B) High-dose aspirin
(C) High-dose ibuprofen
(D) Prednisone

Item 35

A 30-year-old man is evaluated in the emergency department for dull substernal chest pressure for 1 hour with diaphoresis, mild nausea, palpitations, and dyspnea. The pain began approximately 6 hours after inhaling cocaine. He is a cigarette smoker with a 12 pack-year history. There is no history of premature coronary artery disease in his family, and he has no other medical problems and takes no medications.

On physical examination, blood pressure is 154/88 mm Hg and equal in both arms, pulse is 95/min, respiration rate is 20/min, and BMI is 23. Cardiac examination reveals a rapid regular rhythm, normal heart sounds, and a grade 1/6 early systolic murmur at the upper left sternal border. The electrocardiogram demonstrates sinus

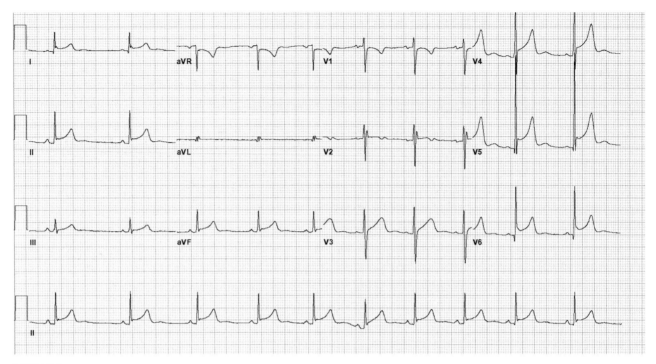

ITEM 34.

tachycardia, without ST-segment or T-wave abnormalities, with a rate of 100/min.

Which of the following is the most appropriate management for this patient?

(A) Coronary angiography
(B) Heparin intravenously
(C) Metoprolol intravenously
(D) Nitroglycerin sublingually

Item 36

A 25-year-old man is evaluated during a routine examination. He has a history of aortic coarctation repaired in childhood. He has not had regular cardiovascular follow-up and is entirely asymptomatic.

On physical examination, his blood pressure is 150/40 mm Hg and his heart rate is 80/min. Estimated central venous pressure is normal. The carotid upstroke is brisk and collapses quickly. The apical impulse is displaced. There is a grade 2/6 early systolic murmur noted at the second right intercostal space. A grade 3/6 high-pitched decrescendo diastolic murmur is noted along the left sternal border and toward the apex. There is evidence of nailbed pulsation. Femoral pulsations are full, collapse quickly, and there is no lag between the radial and femoral pulsations.

Which of the following is the most likely cause of this patient's cardiovascular findings?

(A) Ascending aortic aneurysm
(B) Bicuspid aortic valve with aortic valve regurgitation
(C) Mitral valve prolapse with mitral regurgitation
(D) Recoarctation with associated systemic hypertension

Item 37

A 65-year-old man is evaluated during a routine follow-up examination for coronary artery disease. He was diagnosed with a myocardial infarction 5 years previously, and was started on medical therapy with aspirin, metoprolol, atorvastatin, lisinopril, and sublingual nitroglycerin. He was asymptomatic until 3 months ago, when he noted progressive exertional angina after walking two blocks. He now uses sublingual nitroglycerin on a daily basis. He has not had any episodes of pain at rest or prolonged chest pain that were not relieved by sublingual nitroglycerin. He has hyperlipidemia and hypertension.

Physical examination shows a well-developed man who appears comfortable. Blood pressure is 140/60 mm Hg and heart rate is 85/min. Carotid upstrokes are normal with no bruits. Cardiac examination reveals no murmurs. The lungs are clear. Peripheral pulses are equal throughout and there is no peripheral edema.

His electrocardiogram is unchanged since the last visit, with no evidence of acute changes.

In addition to adding a long-acting nitrate, which of the following is the most appropriate management for this patient?

(A) Add ranolazine
(B) Increase metoprolol
(C) Coronary angiography
(D) Exercise treadmill stress testing

Item 38

A 50-year-old woman with unrepaired congenital heart disease and long-standing cyanosis is evaluated for recent-onset fatigue and exertional dyspnea. She has a history of an unrepaired ventricular septal defect with associated Eisenmenger syndrome. She has had no cardiovascular concerns, but has recently experienced exertional dyspnea and fatigue. The remainder of her general medical history and review of systems is significant for menorrhagia.

On physical examination, her blood pressure is 120/70 mm Hg and her heart rate is 70/min and regular. The jugular venous pulse contour demonstrates a prominent a wave. The carotid examination is normal. The cardiac apex is not displaced. There is a +2 parasternal impulse. The pulmonic component of the S_2 is accentuated. There is no S_3 or S_4. A soft systolic murmur is noted at the left sternal border, and an ejection click is noted at the second left intercostal space. No diastolic murmur is noted. Digital clubbing and cyanosis are present.

Laboratory results include a hematocrit of 47% and hemoglobin level of 13.5 g/dL (135 g/L). Serum creatinine concentration is 1.3 mg/dL (99.2 μmol/L). The fasting plasma glucose level is normal.

The electrocardiogram demonstrates right axis deviation and right ventricular hypertrophy. The chest radiograph demonstrates prominent central pulmonary arteries with reduced vascularity in the lung fields.

Which of the following is the most appropriate treatment at this time?

(A) Blood transfusion
(B) Low-dose iron therapy
(C) Pulmonary vasodilator therapy
(D) Observation and follow-up

Item 39

A 62-year-old woman is evaluated for pain and cramping in her buttocks and thighs. She works as a clerk at a supermarket, and experiences the pain after standing at work for several hours. The discomfort also sometimes occurs when walking, especially downhill. The pain began about 4 months ago. She has hypertension treated with extended-release verapamil and is a current smoker with a 20-pack-year history. Her father, who had diabetes mellitus and was a smoker, had a myocardial infarction at age 54 years.

On physical examination, temperature is normal, blood pressure is 128/72 mm Hg, pulse is 68/min, and respiration rate is 16/min. BMI is 26. There are no abdominal or femoral bruits. The distal pulses are full and symmetric. Ankle-brachial index is 1.0. No skin or hair changes are noted in the lower extremities. Deep tendon reflexes are decreased at the ankle but normal at the knee. The remainder of the neurologic examination is normal. Laboratory findings include total serum cholesterol, 180 mg/dL (4.7 mmol/L); HDL cholesterol, 60 mg/dL (1.6 mmol/L); and plasma glucose, 82 mg/dL (4.6 mmol/L).

Which of the following diagnostic tests should be performed next?

(A) Exercise ankle-brachial index
(B) Lower-extremity CT angiography
(C) MRI of the lumbosacral spine
(D) Segmental limb plethysmography

Item 40

A 60-year-old woman is evaluated in the emergency department for an episode of syncope that occurred 2 hours ago while she was seated at the table eating dinner. There was no warning prodrome, and she experienced total loss of consciousness for 20 seconds with no jerking motions. There were no symptoms of confusion or loss of bowel or bladder continence after the episode. She currently feels well. She had two episodes of syncope last week, once while seated watching television and once while walking. Idiopathic cardiomyopathy was diagnosed 1 month ago, with an ejection fraction of 20% at that time. She has been feeling well and without symptoms since initiation of medical therapy. She has been able to continue exercising by walking and slow jogging regularly. Current medications are enalapril, carvedilol, and furosemide.

On physical examination, she is afebrile. In a supine position, blood pressure is 100/70 mm Hg and pulse is 55/min. In a standing position, blood pressure is 95/65 mm Hg and pulse is 60/min. There is no jugular venous distention. Cardiac examination shows a regular rate and rhythm, normal S_1 and S_2, and no S_3 or murmurs. The lungs are clear. There is no edema, and a neurologic examination is normal. Serum troponin level is within normal limits.

Electrocardiogram is shown. Telemetry monitoring shows no arrhythmias.

Which of the following is the most appropriate management?

(A) Amiodarone
(B) Event monitor
(C) Implantable cardioverter-defibrillator
(D) Midodrine
(E) Pacemaker

Item 41

A 76-year-old woman residing in an independent living facility is evaluated during a routine examination. She ambulates well, using a cane because of hip pain, but does not exercise regularly and takes public transportation to complete her daily shopping. She does not have exertional chest discomfort, dizziness, palpitations, dyspnea, or fatigue. She has hypertension. There is no known history of coronary artery disease. She does not smoke. Medications are hydrochlorothiazide and low-dose aspirin.

On physical examination, temperature is normal and blood pressure is 150/80 mm Hg. BMI is 22. Cardiac examination reveals a sustained apical impulse; normal S_1; and a single, soft S_2. An S_4 is present. There is a grade 3/6 early-onset systolic, late-peaking murmur that is heard best at the right upper sternal border and radiates to the left carotid artery. Carotid pulses are delayed. There is trace pedal edema.

Transthoracic echocardiography demonstrates severe aortic stenosis. No other valvular abnormalities are seen. Biventricular function is normal. There is concentric left ventricular hypertrophy. Pulmonary pressures are at the upper limits of normal.

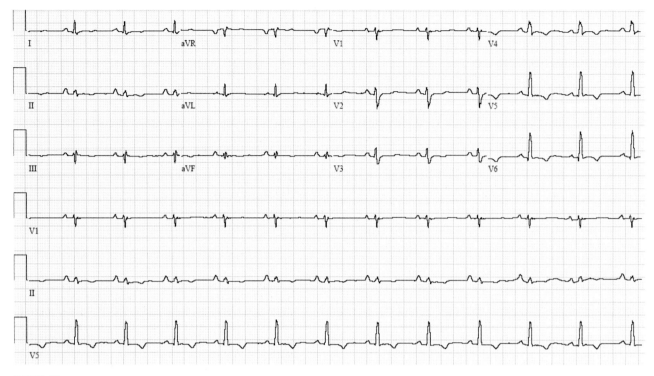

ITEM 40.

Which of the following is the most appropriate test to perform next?

(A) Cardiac CT angiography
(B) Coronary angiography
(C) Exercise treadmill stress testing
(D) Transesophageal echocardiography
(E) No diagnostic testing at this time

Item 42

A 72-year-old man is evaluated in the emergency department after experiencing shocks from his implanted cardioverter-defibrillator (ICD) three times during the past 24 hours. He is active, has had no recent illnesses, and denies chest pain, dyspnea, palpitations, syncope, or other symptoms of coronary insufficiency. He has heart failure (New York Heart Association class II) and coronary artery disease, treated with coronary artery bypass grafting. He has no history of arrhythmia, and the ICD was placed 2 years ago for primary prevention of sudden cardiac death. He has hypertension and hypercholesterolemia. Medications include metoprolol, aspirin, lisinopril, and pravastatin.

On physical examination, his temperature and respiration rate are normal. His blood pressure is 140/82 mm Hg and his pulse is 88/min. He appears anxious and is slightly tachycardic. The ICD pocket shows no evidence of infection or hematoma formation. During the examination, he receives an ICD shock while in sinus rhythm. The lungs are clear and no murmurs or gallops are heard. Estimated central venous pressure is 6 cm H_2O; there is no peripheral edema or other signs of heart failure. The electrocardiogram demonstrates sinus rhythm and evidence of an old anteroseptal myocardial infarction. Chest radiograph reveals no evidence of lead fracture or dislodgement.

Which of the following is the most appropriate management for this patient?

(A) Add amiodarone
(B) Add verapamil
(C) Substitute atenolol for metoprolol
(D) Temporary disabling of the ICD

Item 43

A 45-year-old man is evaluated in the emergency department for a 3-day history of progressively worsening dyspnea on exertion to the point that he is unable to walk more than one block without resting. He has had sharp intermittent pleuritic chest pain and a nonproductive cough with myalgias and malaise for 7 days and has had orthostatic dizziness for 2 days. He is taking no medications.

On physical examination, temperature is 37.7 °C (99.9 °F), blood pressure is 88/44 mm Hg, pulse is 125/min, and respiration rate is 29/min; BMI is 27. Oxygen saturation on ambient air is 95%. Pulsus paradoxus is 15 mm Hg. Estimated central venous pressure is 10 cm H_2O. Cardiac examination discloses muffled heart sounds with no rubs. Lung auscultation reveals normal breath sounds and no crackles. There is 2+ pedal edema. Blood pressure and heart rate are unchanged after a 500-mL intravenous normal saline challenge.

Laboratory studies:

Prothrombin time	12 s
Activated partial thromboplastin time	28 s
Creatinine	1.3 mg/dL (99.2 µmol/L)
Blood urea nitrogen	26 mg/dL (9.3 mmol/L)

Twelve-lead electrocardiogram shows sinus tachycardia, diffuse low voltage, and no ST-segment shifts. Echocardiogram shows a large circumferential pericardial effusion, right ventricular and atrial free wall diastolic collapse, normal left ventricular systolic function, and an ejection fraction of 70%. Chest radiograph shows an enlarged cardiac silhouette and no pulmonary infiltrates.

Which of the following is the most appropriate treatment?

(A) Dobutamine
(B) Levofloxacin and tobramycin
(C) Pericardiocentesis
(D) Surgical pericardiectomy

Item 44

A 65-year-old man is evaluated for 2 months of central chest pain with exertion and relief with rest, exertional dyspnea, orthopnea, and lower-extremity edema. He has a 25-year history of hypertension and a 44-year history of smoking. His only medication is hydrochlorothiazide.

On physical examination, he is afebrile. Blood pressure is 118/80 mm Hg, pulse is 95/min, and respiration rate is 16/min. There is mild jugular venous distention. Cardiac examination reveals a regular rate and rhythm, normal S_1 and S_2, and no murmurs or S_3. Crackles are heard at both lung bases. There is mild bilateral edema at the ankles. Laboratory studies show a serum troponin T level of less than 0.01 ng/mL (0.01 µg/L). Electrocardiogram is normal. Echocardiogram shows an ejection fraction of 40%, global hypokinesis, and mild left ventricular hypertrophy.

Which of the following is the most appropriate diagnostic test?

(A) Cardiac catheterization
(B) Cardiac MRI
(C) Radionuclide ventriculography
(D) Nuclear medicine stress test
(E) Standard exercise stress test

Item 45

A 50-year-old man is evaluated after an episode of joint pain, confusion, headache, nausea, vomiting, and seizure that occurred shortly after scuba diving. The incident was felt to be related to decompression illness and gas embolization. He has otherwise been in excellent health and has no history of cardiovascular disease.

On examination, he is post-ictal without evidence of a neurologic deficit. His blood pressure is 110/70 mm Hg and the heart rate is 125/min and irregular. Oxygen saturation on ambient air is 97%. Cardiac and pulmonary examinations are unremarkable. There is no clubbing or cyanosis. The electrocardiogram shows atrial fibrillation that spontaneously converts to normal sinus rhythm with a heart rate of 100/min. Chest radiograph is normal.

He is treated with hyperbaric oxygen therapy in a recompression chamber and makes an uneventful recovery.

Which of the following is the most appropriate test to perform next in this patient?

(A) Cardiac catheterization
(B) Cardiac magnetic resonance imaging
(C) Intracardiac echocardiography
(D) Transesophageal echocardiography

Item 46

A 67-year-old woman is evaluated in the emergency department for substernal chest pressure that has lasted for just over 3 hours. The pressure has not remitted despite administration of one dose of sublingual nitroglycerin on the way to the hospital. The emergency department is in a community hospital that does not have percutaneous coronary intervention (PCI) capability. The nearest hospital with PCI capability is 45 minutes away.

The patient has a history of hypertension and hyperlipidemia. There is no history of recent surgery or bleeding diathesis. Current medications include lisinopril, hydrochlorothiazide, and simvastatin. She has no known drug allergies. Aspirin and sublingual nitroglycerin are administered upon arrival.

On physical examination, her temperature is 37.2 °C (99.0 °F), blood pressure is 146/92 mm Hg, pulse is 104/min and regular, and respiration rate is 18/min. The patient appears uncomfortable. Crackles are heard at the bases of both lung fields. The S_1 is normal; the S_2 is paradoxically split. No murmur or gallop is present. Results of a complete blood count, basic metabolic profile, and clotting studies are normal. Initial serum troponin I level is 0.5 ng/mL (0.5 µg/L). A stool sample tests negative for occult blood. An electrocardiogram demonstrates normal sinus rhythm with a left bundle branch block. No prior tracing is available for comparison. Intravenous heparin, β-blockers, and morphine are administered.

Which of the following is the most appropriate next step in the management of this patient?

(A) Administer thrombolytic therapy
(B) Administer a glycoprotein IIb/IIIa inhibitor
(C) Obtain serial cardiac enzyme measurements
(D) Transfer to the nearest hospital with PCI capability

Item 47

A 72-year-old man is evaluated in the emergency department for dyspnea. One week ago, an episode of severe dyspnea awoke him from sleep. His wife described audible wheezing. Over the next several days, he felt easily fatigued, but his dyspnea stabilized. On the morning of admission, the patient noted a sudden increase in dyspnea and called emergency medical services. His medical history is significant for hypertension, hyperlipidemia, and chronic obstructive pulmonary disease. He currently takes simvastatin, aspirin, lisinopril, and ipratropium and salmeterol metered-dose inhalers.

On physical examination, he is afebrile, blood pressure is 86/52 mm Hg, pulse is regular at 110/min, and respiration rate is 24/min. Oxygen saturation is 92% on 6 L of oxygen. The patient appears uncomfortable, sitting up with labored breathing. Estimated central venous pressure is 14 cm H_2O. Cardiac examination reveals a grade 2/6 holosystolic murmur at the cardiac apex radiating toward the left axilla. Bibasilar crackles are present. There is trace pitting pedal edema.

An electrocardiogram is shown. Transthoracic echocardiogram reveals hypokinesis of the inferior wall and a left ventricular ejection fraction of 50%. There is severe mitral regurgitation due to posteromedial papillary muscle rupture. The pulmonary arterial systolic pressure is 55 mm Hg. A chest radiograph shows pulmonary vascular congestion.

Which of the following is the best management option?

(A) Chest CT
(B) Percutaneous coronary intervention
(C) Transesophageal echocardiography
(D) Urgent mitral valve surgery

Item 48

A 67-year-old man is evaluated for 2 days of intermittent fever to 38.7 °C (101.7 °F). He was treated with a 7-day course of ciprofloxacin that ended 5 days ago for a urinary tract infection, and urinary symptoms have resolved. He has anorexia and fatigue, but no nausea, vomiting or diarrhea. He denies symptoms of upper respiratory tract infection, cough, or dyspnea. He has sick sinus syndrome, with a pacemaker placed 3 years ago. He also has type 2 diabetes mellitus and obesity. Medications are aspirin and metformin.

On physical examination, his temperature is 38.3 °C (101.0 °F). Blood pressure is 137/80 mm Hg, pulse is 85/min, and respiration rate is 14/min. BMI is 34. Heart sounds are normal, with no extra sounds or murmurs. There are no stigmata of endocarditis, and the pacemaker pocket is benign. The lungs are clear. Laboratory findings are significant for a leukocyte count of 14,000/µL (14.0 × 10^9/L). Pacemaker interrogation shows normal lead and battery parameters.

Which of the following is the most appropriate next step in the management of this patient?

(A) Blood and urine cultures
(B) Pacemaker pocket aspiration
(C) Repeat a course of ciprofloxacin
(D) Vancomycin plus gentamicin

Item 49

A 31-year-old black woman is evaluated for painless, bilateral lower extremity edema of 4 weeks' duration. She denies chest pain, dyspnea, orthopnea, and paroxysmal nocturnal

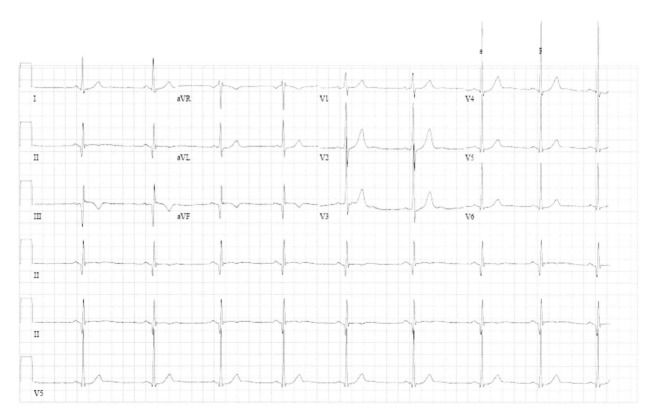

ITEM 47.

dyspnea. She has hypertension, which has been treated for 2 years with hydrochlorothiazide. At age 5 years, she had acute lymphoblastic leukemia, which was treated with vincristine, doxorubicin, and dexamethasone. She is currently on no medications other than hydrochlorothiazide.

On physical examination, her blood pressure is 138/92 mm Hg, pulse is 90/min, and respiration rate is 18/min. Her BMI is 27. Her estimated central venous pressure is 10 cm H_2O. Cardiac examination reveals a nondisplaced apical impulse, normal heart sounds, and no murmurs or extracardiac sounds. Pulmonary examination is normal. There is bilateral lower extremity edema to the knees. Laboratory results include normal levels of sodium, potassium, blood urea nitrogen, and creatinine. Urinalysis is normal and there is no evidence of proteinuria.

Electrocardiogram demonstrates sinus rhythm (88/min) and left bundle branch block.

Which of the following is the most appropriate management for this patient?

(A) Adenosine nuclear perfusion imaging study
(B) Bilateral lower extremity venous duplex ultrasound
(C) Change hydrochlorothiazide to furosemide
(D) Transthoracic echocardiography

Item 50

A 45-year-old man is evaluated for a 6-month history of progressive dyspnea on exertion and lower-extremity edema. He can now walk only one block before needing to rest. He reports orthostatic dizziness in the last 2 weeks. He denies chest pain, palpitations, or syncope. He was diagnosed 15 years ago with non-Hodgkin lymphoma, which was treated with chest irradiation and chemotherapy and is now in remission. He also has type 2 diabetes mellitus. He takes furosemide (80 mg, 3 times daily), glyburide, and low-dose aspirin.

On physical examination, he is afebrile. Blood pressure is 125/60 mm Hg supine and 100/50 mm Hg standing; pulse is 90/min supine and 110/min standing. Respiration rate is 23/min. BMI is 28. There is jugular venous distention and jugular venous engorgement with inspiration. Estimated central venous pressure is 15 cm H_2O. Cardiac examination discloses diminished heart sounds and a prominent early diastolic sound but no gallops or murmurs. Pulmonary auscultation discloses normal breath sounds and no crackles. Abdominal examination shows shifting dullness, and lower extremities show 3+ pitting edema to the level of the knees. The remainder of the physical examination is normal.

Laboratory studies:

Creatinine	2 mg/dL (152.6 μmol/L)
Blood urea nitrogen	40 mg/dL (14.3 mmol/L)
Cholesterol, total	300 mg/dL (7.8 mmol/L)
Albumin	3.0 g/dL (30 g/L)
Alanine aminotransferase	130 U/L
Aspartate aminotransferase	112 U/L
Urinalysis	Negative for protein

Which of the following is the most likely diagnosis?

(A) Cirrhosis
(B) Constrictive pericarditis
(C) Nephrotic syndrome
(D) Systolic heart failure

Item 51

A 43-year-old man is evaluated for discomfort and fatigue in his left arm with exertion, particularly with lifting, for the past 3 months. He has no history of chest pain or dyspnea with walking several flights of stairs. He has hypertension and hypothyroidism. At age 16 years, he had Hodgkin disease, which was treated with mantle radiation and chemotherapy. His daily medications are amlodipine and levothyroxine.

On physical examination, his blood pressure is 105/58 mm Hg in the left arm and 130/74 mm Hg in the right arm, pulse is 82/min, and respiration rate is 16/min. His BMI is 23. Cardiac examination reveals a grade 2/6 early peaking systolic murmur at the right upper sternal border and the left clavicular region that does not radiate to the right clavicle or neck. The S_2 is normal; carotid upstrokes are normal bilaterally; there is no jugular venous distention and no edema. The left brachial and radial pulses are diminished compared to the right. Electrocardiogram reveals sinus rhythm with a rate of 78/min and no ST-segment or T-wave abnormalities.

Which of the following is the most likely diagnosis?

(A) Cardiac tamponade
(B) Coronary artery disease
(C) Left ventricular systolic dysfunction
(D) Severe aortic stenosis
(E) Subclavian steal syndrome

Item 52

A 67-year-old man is evaluated for follow-up for an asymptomatic large pericardial effusion that has persisted for 4 months. He denies chest pain, dyspnea, fever, chills, cough, edema, and weight loss. He has a 30-year history of hypertension for which he takes amlodipine. A chest radiograph performed 4 months ago to evaluate chronic cough demonstrated an enlarged cardiac silhouette. Laboratory results at that time included normal complete blood count and serum electrolytes, creatinine, blood urea nitrogen, and thyroid-stimulating hormone levels. An antinuclear antibody assay and tuberculin skin test both were negative. Chest CT scan was normal. Echocardiography performed 4 and 2 months ago showed a moderate pericardial effusion, no evidence of tamponade, and normal left and right ventricular function and size.

On physical examination, temperature is normal, blood pressure is 135/75 mm Hg, pulse is 76/min, and respiration rate is 16/min. Estimated central venous pressure is less than 5 cm H_2O. Cardiac examination reveals muffled heart sounds, an absent apical impulse, and no pericardial friction rub. Pulmonary auscultation reveals normal breath sounds.

Echocardiogram shows a large circumferential pericardial effusion and no findings of tamponade, and is otherwise without change from 4 and 2 months ago.

Which of the following is the most appropriate next step in management?

(A) Colchicine
(B) Indomethacin
(C) Pericardiectomy
(D) Pericardiocentesis
(E) Prednisone

Item 53

A 52-year-old man is evaluated for right shoulder pain and weakness associated with a job injury 2 weeks ago, in which he tripped and fell onto his outstretched right arm. He takes NSAIDs frequently, and his symptoms are not responsive to rest or application of heat. The pain is making it difficult to work. He complains of anterior shoulder pain and weakness aggravated by reaching, pulling, or lifting with the arm above shoulder level. He has a pacemaker because of chronotropic incompetence. He has no other medical problems and is on no medications.

On physical examination, blood pressure is 130/70 mm Hg and pulse is 75/min. Examination of his right arm demonstrates weakness of external rotation and abduction. There is subacromial tenderness. No atrophy of the infraspinatus or supraspinatus muscles is noted in the scapular fossa.

Conventional radiography of the right shoulder is normal. The pacemaker leads are in stable position. Interrogation

of his pacemaker reveals normal lead and battery parameters, without evidence of fracture or dislodgement.

Which of the following diagnostic tests of the shoulder is indicated in this patient?

(A) CT
(B) CT arthrography
(C) MRI
(D) MRI arthrography

Item 54

A 32-year-old woman presents for evaluation of a murmur recently heard on physical examination. She has noted mild reduction in exercise capacity over the past 6 to 12 months. She has no known history of cardiovascular disease, although a murmur was reported early in life.

On physical examination, the blood pressure is 100/70 mm Hg and the pulse is 68/min and regular. The estimated central venous pressure is mildly elevated; the jugular venous pulse contour demonstrates equal *a* and *v* waves. The apical impulse is not displaced. There is an impulse noted along the left sternal border. The S_1 is normal. The S_2 is split throughout the respiratory cycle. A grade 2/6 midsystolic murmur is noted at the second left intercostal space. There is a grade 2/6 diastolic rumble noted at the lower left sternal border. Both of these murmurs increase with inspiration. The remaining findings on physical examination are unremarkable.

An electrocardiogram demonstrates normal sinus rhythm with normal axis and intervals. The chest radiograph images are shown.

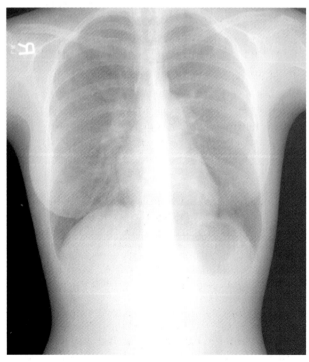

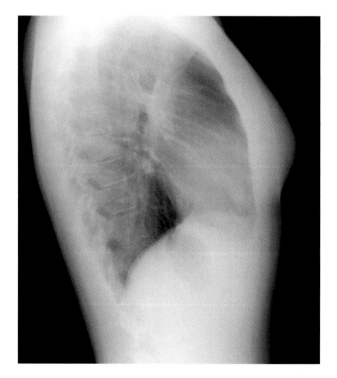

ITEM 54.

Which of the following is the most likely diagnosis in this patient?

(A) Atrial septal defect
(B) Hypertrophic cardiomyopathy
(C) Left atrial myxoma
(D) Pulmonary arterial hypertension
(E) Rheumatic mitral stenosis

Item 55

A 58-year-old man presents to the emergency department within 4 hours of worsening pleuritic chest pain, which has become progressively more severe. Ten days ago, he had an acute anterior ST-elevation myocardial infarction and underwent successful thrombolytic therapy within 2 hours of the onset of symptoms. He has a history of hypertension. Medications include metoprolol, clopidogrel, simvastatin, aspirin, and isosorbide mononitrate.

On physical examination, temperature is 37.9 °C (100.2 °F), blood pressure is 110/70 mm Hg, pulse is 60/min, and respiration rate is 18/min. There is no jugular venous distention. Cardiac examination discloses a two-component pericardial friction rub but no murmurs or gallops. Crackles are heard on pulmonary auscultation. There is no pedal edema.

Laboratory studies:

Erythrocyte sedimentation rate	60 mm/h
Leukocyte count	12,000/μL (12.0 × 10⁹/L)
Creatinine	1.0 mg/dL (76.3 μmol/L)
Blood urea nitrogen	15 mg/dL (5.4 mmol/L)

Twelve-lead electrocardiogram during an episode of chest pain shows normal sinus rhythm with diffuse, concave, upward 1.0- to 1.5-mm ST-segment elevation and 1-mm PR-segment depression in leads II, III, and aVF.

Which of the following is the most appropriate treatment at this point?

(A) Colchicine
(B) High-dose aspirin
(C) High-dose ibuprofen
(D) Prednisone

Item 56

A 43-year-old man is evaluated during a routine examination. He has a history of a cardiac murmur diagnosed during childhood. He exercises regularly without restriction to activity and has no history of syncope, presyncope, palpitations, or edema. He is on no medications.

On physical examination, he is afebrile, blood pressure is 120/64 mm Hg, pulse is 80/min and regular, and respiration rate is 16/min. BMI is 25. He appears well. Cardiac examination reveals a normal S_1 and a physiologically split S_2. There is a grade 2/6 decrescendo diastolic murmur at the left sternal border. Distal pulses are brisk. There is no pedal edema.

A transthoracic echocardiogram demonstrates normal ventricular size and function, with ejection fraction of 60% to 65%. There is a bicuspid aortic valve with moderate regurgitation. The proximal ascending aorta diameter measures 4.2 cm. Pulmonary pressure estimates are in the normal range.

Which of the following is the most appropriate management option for this patient?

(A) Antibiotic prophylaxis prior to dental procedures
(B) Clinical follow-up in 1 year
(C) Surgical referral for aortic valve replacement
(D) Transesophageal echocardiography

Item 57

A 65-year-old woman is evaluated in the office for chest discomfort. The discomfort is located at the left side of the chest and usually occurs with activity but may occur when lying down after a large meal. The pain is frequently, but not consistently, relieved with rest. It has been present for 3 months and is gradually worsening. She also has reactive airways disease; degenerative arthritis of the knees, which limits ambulation; hypertension; and hyperlipidemia. Her father had coronary artery disease treated with coronary stent placement. She is a current smoker (40 pack-year history). Current medications are albuterol metered-dose inhaler, an inhaled corticosteroid, lisinopril, atorvastatin, and acetaminophen.

Physical examination shows a thin, ill-appearing woman. She is afebrile, blood pressure is 130/80 mm Hg, pulse is 80/min, and respiration rate is 18/min. Neck veins are not distended, heart sounds are distant, lung sounds have mild diffuse wheezing, and there is no peripheral edema.

Electrocardiogram shows no Q waves and nonspecific ST-segment and T-wave changes.

Which of the following is the most appropriate diagnostic test to assess this patient's symptoms?

(A) Adenosine nuclear stress testing
(B) Coronary angiography
(C) Coronary artery calcium scan
(D) Dobutamine echocardiographic stress testing
(E) Exercise treadmill stress testing

Item 58

A 60-year-old woman is evaluated during a routine follow-up appointment after a diagnosis of heart failure due to nonischemic cardiomyopathy 1 month ago. At that time, her ejection fraction was 40% by echocardiogram, and she was started on 2.5 mg of enalapril once daily and 6.25 mg of carvedilol twice daily. She is currently feeling well with no shortness of breath, orthopnea, or lightheadedness. She is on no other medications.

On physical examination, she is afebrile. Blood pressure is 120/80 mm Hg and pulse is 65/min. The jugular veins are not distended, and the lungs are clear. Cardiac examination discloses a regular rate and rhythm with no S_3 or murmurs. There is no edema.

Laboratory studies:

	Current	1 Month Ago
Potassium	5.7 meq/L (5.7 mmol/L)	4.5 meq/L (4.5 mmol/L)
Creatinine	1.8 mg/dL (137.3 µmol/L)	1.0 mg/dL (76.3 µmol/L)

In addition to stopping the enalapril, which of the following agents should be added to her regimen?

(A) Candesartan

(B) Digoxin

(C) Eplerenone

(D) Hydralazine and a nitrate

Item 59

A 67-year-old man presented to the emergency department 2 days ago with an acute ST-elevation myocardial infarction. During the initial evaluation, he became unresponsive due to ventricular fibrillation. He was successfully resuscitated and taken to the cardiac catheterization lab, where a 100% occlusion of his proximal left anterior descending artery was stented. His postinfarction course was notable for mild heart failure, which has now resolved. He is now stable on his current medical regimen. Current medications include aspirin, metoprolol, atorvastatin, clopidogrel, and lisinopril.

On physical examination, his blood pressure is 115/72 mm Hg, his pulse is 65/min, and his respiration rate is 12/min. There is no jugular venous distention, crackles, murmur, or S_3. Transthoracic echocardiogram reveals mild hypokinesis of the anterior wall and a left ventricular ejection fraction of 42%.

Which of the following is the best management option at this time?

(A) Add amiodarone

(B) Continue medical management

(C) Implantable cardioverter-defibrillator placement

(D) Order electrophysiology study

Item 60

A 68-year-old man is evaluated during a routine examination to establish care. He feels well overall, has no limitations to daily activities, walks several times a week, and has no chest pain. He has a history of coronary artery disease and had a myocardial infarction 3 months ago treated with percutaneous coronary intervention with placement of a drug-eluting stent. His last measured left ventricular ejection fraction (2 weeks ago) was 25%. Current medications are aspirin, lisinopril, metoprolol, clopidogrel, eplerenone, furosemide, and simvastatin.

On physical examination, he is afebrile. Blood pressure is 95/65 mm Hg and pulse is 60/min. Jugular veins are not distended. Cardiac examination reveals a regular rate and rhythm and normal S_1 and S_2. Chest is clear. There is no edema. Electrocardiogram shows normal sinus rhythm and a normal QRS complex.

Which of the following is the most appropriate management option?

(A) Biventricular pacemaker-defibrillator placement

(B) Coronary angiography

(C) Implantable cardioverter-defibrillator placement

(D) Treadmill exercise stress test

(E) Warfarin

Item 61

A 57-year-old woman is evaluated for dyspnea on exertion and fatigue. She has known of a cardiac murmur for many years, but has no other medical conditions and is on no medications.

On physical examination, her blood pressure is 120/70 mm Hg and her heart rate is 75/min and regular. The jugular venous pulse contour demonstrates a prominent *a* wave. The carotid pulse is normal. On cardiac examination, there is a parasternal impulse and the cardiac apex is not displaced. A palpable early systolic murmur is noted over the second left intercostal space. There is a grade 4/6 midsystolic murmur noted at the left sternal border. The pulmonic component of the S_2 is not audible. No diastolic murmur is noted.

A transthoracic echocardiogram demonstrates a right ventricular systolic pressure of 100 mm Hg and a peak right ventricular outflow tract gradient of 85 mm Hg at valve level. Systolic doming is present. There is mild pulmonary valve regurgitation. Left ventricular and right ventricular systolic function is normal. Right ventricular hypertrophy is present. No additional cardiovascular abnormalities are identified.

Which of the following is the most appropriate treatment option at this time?

(A) Angiotensin-converting enzyme inhibitor

(B) Pulmonary balloon valvuloplasty

(C) Surgical intervention

(D) Close clinical follow-up

Item 62

A 45-year-old woman is admitted to the hospital for evaluation of a 6-week history of progressive, dull chest pressure associated with mild dyspnea and nausea. At onset, the chest pain occurred during physical exertion (housework) and was relieved by rest within 5 minutes. For the past several days, the patient has had similar episodes that occurred with minimal activity, such as walking, and also at rest, including an episode this morning, which she described as 8/10 in severity of the pain and lasted for 10 to 15 minutes. The chest discomfort is not pleuritic or positional and is not related to eating. She has hypertension, treated for the past 6 years, and systemic lupus erythematosus for 24 years, with a history of pericarditis, arthritis, and a photosensitive facial rash. Her medications include prednisone, hydroxychloroquine, aspirin, and enalapril.

On physical examination, she is afebrile, blood pressure is 132/78 mm Hg, pulse is 86/min, and respiration rate is 18/min. Oxygen saturation on ambient air is 98%. BMI is 25. Her lungs are clear to auscultation. Estimated central venous pressure is normal; there is no Kussmaul sign or hepatojugular reflux. Cardiac auscultation reveals regular rhythm with normal S_1 and S_2 and no murmur, rub, or gallop.

Laboratory studies

Erythrocyte sedimentation rate	39 mm/h
Creatine kinase	65 U/L
Creatine kinase MB fraction	3%
Troponin T	0.04 ng/mL (0.04 µg/L)

Electrocardiogram demonstrates sinus rhythm, with a rate of 92/min. There are symmetric T-wave inversions in leads V_1 through V_4; there is no ST-segment depression or elevation. Chest radiograph shows a normal cardiac silhouette with no infiltrate or edema.

Which of the following diagnostic tests is most appropriate at this time?

(A) Coronary angiography
(B) Exercise stress echocardiogram
(C) High-sensitivity C-reactive protein level
(D) Transthoracic echocardiography

Item 63

A 56-year-old man is evaluated in the emergency department for chest discomfort that began 3 hours ago. He describes the pain, which is well localized to the left chest, as pressure. He denies prior episodes. Medical history is notable for type 2 diabetes mellitus and hyperlipidemia. Medications include aspirin, metformin, and atorvastatin.

On physical examination, he is diaphoretic and in moderate distress owing to the chest pain. Blood pressure is 95/60 mm Hg and heart rate is 110/min. There is jugular venous distention, with an estimated central venous pressure of 14 cm H_2O. An S_3 is heard on cardiac auscultation, but no murmurs are present. The lung fields are clear and there is no peripheral edema.

The electrocardiogram shows sinus tachycardia, 2-mm ST-segment elevation in leads II, III, and aVF, and 0.5-mm ST-segment elevation in lead V_1. He is given aspirin, metoprolol, unfractionated heparin, and thrombolytic therapy. Twenty minutes later, he has continued chest pain and sublingual nitroglycerin is given. Blood pressure falls to 70 mm Hg systolic and he remains tachycardic, with a heart rate of 100/min.

Which of the following is the most likely cause of hypotension in this patient?

(A) Pericardial tamponade
(B) Right ventricular infarction
(C) Increased vagal tone
(D) Ventricular septal defect

Item 64

A 22-year-old woman is evaluated for symptoms of a "racing heart," which she has experienced since her teenage years. Previously, episodes were short and resolved spontaneously or would terminate with deep breathing. In the last few months, however, the episodes have been more frequent—up to two or three times a week—and sustained. Longer episodes (over 5 minutes) have been associated with dizziness, but no syncope has occurred. She denies chest discomfort, but does experience mild dyspnea and neck pounding. Episodes are triggered by caffeine, dehydration, and bending over. She is active and runs competitively. She is on no medications.

On examination, her blood pressure is 92/56 mm Hg without orthostatic changes, and her pulse is 50/min. An electrocardiogram demonstrates normal intervals and no preexcitation.

Which of the following is the most appropriate management option for this patient?

(A) Atenolol
(B) 24-Hour ambulatory monitoring
(C) Loop recorder monitoring
(D) Sertraline
(E) No further testing

Item 65

A 78-year-old man is admitted to the hospital for treatment of a myocardial infarction. Medical history includes hypertension and type 2 diabetes mellitus.

Physical examination shows blood pressure of 140/60 mm Hg and a pulse of 65/min. Estimated central venous pressure is 6 cm H_2O. There are no murmurs or extra heart sounds, the lung fields are clear, and there is no peripheral edema.

Initial electrocardiogram shows 3-mm ST-segment elevations in leads V_1 through V_6 and ST-segment depression in leads II, III, and aVF. Chest radiograph shows increased pulmonary vascular markings.

The hospital does not have a cardiac catheterization laboratory, and the patient receives thrombolytic therapy and unfractionated heparin. His pain subsides 40 minutes after the initiation of reteplase. Metoprolol, nitroglycerin, and captopril are started. Three hours later, he develops respiratory distress in the absence of chest pain. Repeat physical examination shows blood pressure of 125/70 mm Hg, pulse of 110/min, and respiration rate of 20/min. Estimated central venous pressure is now 15 cm H_2O. There is an S_3 but no murmurs. Crackles are heard throughout both lung fields. A repeat electrocardiogram shows 0.5-mm ST-segment elevation in leads V_1 through V_6.

Which of the following is the best immediate treatment?

(A) Increase metoprolol
(B) Intravenous dobutamine
(C) Intravenous furosemide
(D) Repeat administration of thrombolytic therapy

Item 66

An 82-year-old woman is evaluated at the hospital after tripping and falling. She has sustained a right hip fracture and needs urgent hip replacement. She reports no angina, chest discomfort, syncope, or presyncope. She has had no signs or symptoms of heart failure. Prior to her fall, she was active and walked daily.

On physical examination, temperature is normal, blood pressure is 164/82 mm Hg, and pulse is 96/min. BMI is 26. Point of maximal impulse is undisplaced. There is a normal S_1 and a single S_2. There is a grade 3/6 systolic ejection murmur on examination heard at the right upper sternal border that radiates to the left carotid artery. Carotid pulses are delayed.

Transthoracic echocardiogram demonstrates severe aortic stenosis and normal left ventricular size and function. Pulmonary pressures are normal.

Which of the following is the best perioperative management option?

(A) Aortic balloon valvuloplasty

(B) Aortic valve replacement

(C) Intra-aortic balloon placement

(D) Intravenous afterload reduction (nitroprusside)

(E) Proceed directly to hip replacement

Item 67

A 22-year-old female student is evaluated for a rapid heartbeat that builds over the course of the day and is not associated with chest pain or shortness of breath. She adds that she has been drinking a lot of coffee lately to finish term papers and study for finals. She is one of the best players on an intramural soccer team. The patient's medical history is significant for tetralogy of Fallot repair that she underwent at age 2 years. She received a patch closure of the ventricular septal defect and a transannular patch to relieve pulmonic stenosis. She last saw her pediatric cardiologist 4 years ago, who told her everything was "OK."

On physical examination, she is afebrile, her blood pressure is 110/60 mm Hg, pulse is 92/min, and respiration rate is 16/min. Estimated central venous pressure is 8 cm H_2O. She has a mild right ventricular heave, a single S_2, and a soft diastolic murmur at the base that increases in intensity with inspiration. She has clear lungs and no peripheral edema. The results of a hematocrit and thyroid function tests are within normal limits.

An echocardiogram shows a repaired tetralogy of Fallot and a mildly enlarged aorta and no residual ventricular septal defect. Left ventricular systolic function is normal. The right ventricle is moderately enlarged with normal systolic function. The pulmonic valve is not easily viewed, but regurgitation is present.

Which of the following is the most appropriate management option?

(A) Cardiac magnetic resonance imaging

(B) Chest CT

(C) Counsel her to avoid pregnancy

(D) Endocarditis prophylaxis for dental procedures

(E) Reassurance

Item 68

A 47-year-old woman is evaluated for a 4-month history of a sensation of "thumping" in her chest and feeling as if her heart stops. The symptoms occur frequently throughout the day; they interrupt her thinking, concentration, and sleep. She feels them particularly at night when lying on her left side. Symptoms appear to decrease with exercise. She denies chest pain, dyspnea, orthopnea, or edema. She is healthy and active and on no medications.

On physical examination, her blood pressure is 110/67 mm Hg and her pulse is 72/min with occasional ectopy. Cardiac auscultation is normal except for occasional ectopy in the cardiac rhythm associated with jugular cannon waves, with no murmurs, gallops, or clicks. Estimated central venous pressure is 5 cm H_2O. The lungs are clear to auscultation. Point of maximal impulse is undisplaced.

Electrocardiogram demonstrates sinus rhythm with normal intervals and occasional premature ventricular contractions of varying morphologies, which correspond with her symptoms of palpitations. Echocardiogram reveals a structurally normal heart with normal left ventricular, right ventricular, and valvular function.

Which of the following is the most appropriate treatment for this patient?

(A) Amiodarone

(B) Metoprolol

(C) Pacemaker

(D) Radiofrequency ablation

Item 69

A 65-year-old black man is evaluated during a routine annual visit. Over the past year he has had a progressive decline in functional status. Last year he could exercise by walking several blocks at a time, and now he gets tired after one block at most; sometimes he gets short of breath with dressing and showering. He reports no symptoms of orthopnea or paroxysmal nocturnal dyspnea and has had no change in medications since last year. He has a 25-year history of hypertension, a 5-year history of ischemic cardiomyopathy, and received an implantable cardioverter-defibrillator 1 year ago. An echocardiogram done 6 months ago showed an ejection fraction of 20%. He takes aspirin, enalapril, metoprolol, spironolactone, furosemide, digoxin, pravastatin, and isosorbide dinitrate.

On physical examination, he is afebrile. Blood pressure is 100/70 mm Hg and pulse is 70/min. There is no jugular venous distention and the lungs are clear. Cardiac examination discloses a regular rate and rhythm with no S_3 or murmurs. There is no edema.

Laboratory studies:

Hemoglobin	11 g/dL (110 g/L) (unchanged from 1 year ago)
Creatinine	1.5 mg/dL (114.5 µmol/L) (unchanged from 1 year ago)
Thyroid-stimulating hormone	Normal

Digoxin   0.8 µg/L (1.0 nmol/L)
               (therapeutic range, 0.8-1.5 µg/L
               [1.0-1.9 nmol/L])

Electrocardiogram shows sinus rhythm.

Which of the following is the most appropriate adjustment to this patient's treatment?

(A) Add hydralazine
(B) Increase digoxin
(C) Increase furosemide
(D) Stop metoprolol

Item 70

A 42-year-old man is evaluated for recurrent, highly symptomatic paroxysmal atrial fibrillation. He was initially diagnosed 6 months ago. His evaluation revealed no underlying cause and his resting electrocardiogram and echocardiogram were normal. Despite treatment with metoprolol, episodes occur 3 to 4 times daily and last from a few minutes to several hours. During events, he feels drained and unable to concentrate, with a sensation of an irregular heartbeat. He experiences dyspnea on exertion and lightheadedness, but denies chest discomfort and syncope. Episodes are triggered by activity, caffeine, and alcohol (both of which he discontinued upon diagnosis). He takes no medications other than the metoprolol.

On physical examination, blood pressure is 130/60 mm Hg and pulse is 70/min and regular. S_1 and S_2 are normal and there is no murmur or extra heart sounds. Estimated central venous pressure is 5 cm H_2O, and the lungs are clear. There is no edema. The remainder of the physical examination is normal.

Which of the following is the most appropriate management for this patient?

(A) Add amiodarone
(B) Add digoxin
(C) 24-Hour ambulatory monitoring
(D) Implanted loop recorder

Item 71

A 48-year-old man is evaluated in the emergency department for sudden onset of severe discomfort in the chest and between the shoulder blades. The pain was maximal in intensity at its onset 90 minutes ago and is unaffected by position or breathing. He has a history of hypertension, for which he takes hydrochlorothiazide, 25 mg/d; and lisinopril, 40 mg/d.

On physical examination, his temperature is normal, blood pressure is 200/120 mm Hg, pulse is 100/min, and respiration rate is 20/min. An S_4 gallop is present. No cardiac murmur or pericardial rub is present. The lungs are clear to auscultation. Distal pulses are equal and symmetric. Results of a neurologic examination are normal. A urine toxicology screen is positive for cocaine. Serum creatinine level is 2.2 mg/dL (167.9 µmol/L). His creatinine level was 0.8 mg/dL (61.0 µmol/L) at the time of his last office

evaluation. Oxygen saturation is 98% on ambient air. Serum cardiac troponin and myoglobin levels are normal. An electrocardiogram reveals left ventricular hypertrophy with a secondary repolarization abnormality and sinus tachycardia. Chest radiograph is normal.

In addition to emergently lowering the blood pressure and heart rate, which of the following diagnostic tests should be performed next?

(A) CT scan of chest with intravenous contrast
(B) Nuclear myocardial perfusion scan
(C) Transesophageal echocardiogram
(D) Ventilation-perfusion lung scan

Item 72

A 26-year-old woman recently diagnosed with an ostium secundum atrial septal defect is evaluated to determine a treatment plan. She has no symptoms, but an exercise stress test demonstrates reduced exercise tolerance at 70% of predicted functional aerobic capacity. An electrocardiogram demonstrates normal sinus rhythm, first-degree atrioventricular block, and an incomplete right bundle branch block. A transthoracic echocardiogram demonstrates a 1.5-cm ostium secundum atrial septal defect with evidence of moderate right-sided cardiac chamber enlargement. There is no evidence of pulmonary hypertension by clinical evaluation or Doppler echocardiography.

Which of the following is the most appropriate next step in the management of this patient?

(A) Re-evaluate in 12 months
(B) Recommend endocarditis prophylaxis
(C) Refer for atrial septal defect closure
(D) Start warfarin anticoagulation

Item 73

A 40-year-old man presents to the office for evaluation of his risk for cardiovascular disease. He has not seen a physician for many years. He works in a business office and is inactive outside of work. He has no cardiac history and no chest pain or dyspnea during his normal activities. His family history is negative for premature coronary artery disease. The patient is a current smoker with a 10 pack-year history.

On physical examination, he is an obese man in no distress. Temperature is normal, blood pressure is 138/75 mm Hg, pulse is 74/min, and respiration rate is 16/min. BMI is 39, and waist circumference is 92 cm. Cardiac examination shows a regular rhythm with distant heart sounds but no murmur or gallop.

Laboratory studies:

Total cholesterol	216 mg/dL (5.6 mmol/L)
HDL cholesterol	38 mg/dL (1.0 mmol/L)
LDL cholesterol	142 mg/dL (3.7 mmol/L)
Triglycerides	180 mg/dL (2.0 mmol/L)
Glucose (fasting)	105 mg/dL (5.8 mmol/L)

Electrocardiogram shows sinus rhythm and nonspecific T-wave abnormalities.

Based on his systolic blood pressure, triglyceride level, and HDL cholesterol level, the patient meets the criteria for the diagnosis of metabolic syndrome. Based on the Framingham score, he is estimated to have an 11% 10-year risk of a coronary artery disease event.

Which of the following is the most appropriate next step in the management of this patient?

(A) Initiate antihypertensive therapy
(B) Initiate lifestyle modifications
(C) Initiate statin therapy
(D) Obtain serum lipoprotein(a) and homocysteine levels
(E) Order exercise stress treadmill testing

Item 74

A 32-year-old woman is hospitalized for 2 days of malaise, fatigue, frequent chest pain without particular exacerbating or relieving factors, subjective fevers, and shortness of breath with exertion that is improved by rest. Her medical history is unremarkable, she does not smoke or use illicit drugs, and she is on no medications. She has no history of arthralgias, arthritis, photosensitivity, pleuritis, or pericarditis. Both of her parents are alive and well.

On physical examination, temperature is 38.1 °C (100.6 °F), blood pressure is 110/75 mm Hg, and pulse is 120/min. She is oriented and alert. There is mild jugular venous distention. Cardiac examination discloses a regular tachycardic rate and rhythm, a soft S_1 and S_2, and an S_3. The

lungs are clear. There is no hepatosplenomegaly, no rash, and no edema. Chest radiograph shows pulmonary congestion and cardiomegaly.

Laboratory studies:

Hemoglobin	14.0 g/dL (140 g/L)
Leukocyte count	8500/µL (8.5×10^9/L)
Platelet count	158,000/µL (158×10^9/L)
Creatinine	0.9 mg/dL (68.7 µmol/L)
Troponin	5 ng/mL (5 µg/L)
Liver chemistry tests	Normal
Antinuclear antibody test	Negative
Thyroid-stimulating hormone	3 µU/mL (3 mU/L)

Electrocardiogram is shown. Echocardiogram shows an ejection fraction of 30%, global hypokinesis, and minimal pericardial effusion. There is no evidence of valvular heart disease.

Which of the following is the most appropriate treatment?

(A) Amiodarone
(B) Captopril and carvedilol
(C) Methylprednisolone
(D) Tissue plasminogen activator
(E) Vancomycin and ceftriaxone

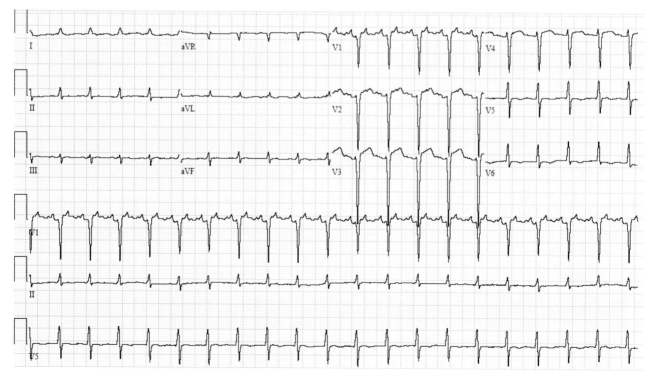

ITEM 74.

Item 75

A 68-year-old woman is evaluated during a follow-up visit after coronary bare metal stent placement 2 weeks ago for unstable angina. She did well following coronary stent placement and has not experienced any recurrent chest pain. Medical history is notable for hypertension. Current medications are aspirin, clopidogrel, metoprolol, atorvastatin, and sublingual nitroglycerin.

Physical examination shows a blood pressure of 110/60 mm Hg and a heart rate of 60/min. Jugular venous pulsations are normal, and there no murmurs or rubs on cardiac auscultation. The lungs are clear and there is no peripheral edema.

Which of the following is the correct approach to antiplatelet therapy in this patient?

(A) Continue clopidogrel and aspirin for a minimum of 2 more weeks
(B) Continue clopidogrel and aspirin indefinitely
(C) Continue clopidogrel for a minimum of 2 more weeks and aspirin indefinitely
(D) Stop clopidogrel now and continue aspirin indefinitely

Item 76

A 69-year-old woman is evaluated in the emergency department for chest pain. The pain, which she describes as uncomfortable, begins in the mid-chest region and radiates to the left arm. It occurs with activity, and symptoms have been present for 2 weeks with increasing severity and duration. Before being brought to the emergency department, a prolonged episode occurred at rest for the first time and resolved after 20 minutes. Medical history is notable for oxygen-dependent chronic obstructive pulmonary disease, hypertension, and hyperlipidemia. Her last FEV_1 was less than 30% of predicted. Current medications are simvastatin, lisinopril, albuterol metered-dose inhaler, ipratropium metered-dose inhaler, and prednisone.

Physical examination shows a frail elderly woman who appears uncomfortable because of wheezing and shortness of breath. Blood pressure is 160/60 mm Hg and heart rate is 110/min. Neck examination shows normal carotid upstrokes. Estimated central venous pressure is 10 cm H_2O. Cardiac examination reveals distant heart sounds and an S_4. Examination of the lungs is notable for diminished breath sounds bilaterally and end-expiratory wheezes without crackles. There is 1+ pretibial edema, and pulses are equal bilaterally.

Electrocardiogram shows normal sinus rhythm, with T-wave inversions in the inferior and lateral leads and no Q waves. Serum troponin I level is 0.4 ng/mL (0.4 µg/L). Chest radiograph shows changes consistent with chronic obstructive pulmonary disease without evidence of heart failure.

In addition to aspirin and low-molecular-weight heparin, which of the following is the most appropriate treatment for this patient?

(A) Diltiazem

(B) Labetalol
(C) Metoprolol
(D) Ranolazine

Item 77

A 40-year-old woman is evaluated for 2 months of progressive dyspnea on exertion, orthopnea, and lower extremity edema. She has no other medical problems and takes no medications, including over-the-counter drugs, and she does not use illicit drugs. She does not smoke cigarettes and rarely drinks alcohol. There is no family history of heart disease.

On physical examination, she is afebrile. Blood pressure is 120/80 mm Hg and pulse is 80/min. Estimated central venous pressure is 8 cm H_2O. The lungs are clear. Cardiac examination reveals a regular rhythm, an S_3, and no murmurs. There is mild ankle edema. Chest radiograph shows mild vascular congestion. Electrocardiogram shows normal sinus rhythm. Initial laboratory evaluation reveals a normal hemoglobin level and metabolic profile, including thyroid studies.

Which of the following is the most appropriate initial diagnostic test?

(A) B-type natriuretic peptide level
(B) Echocardiography
(C) Radionuclide ventriculography
(D) Stress test

Item 78

A 48-year-old woman is evaluated in the emergency department 3 hours after the sudden onset of chest pain and dyspnea. The pain follows a waxing and waning pattern and is focused in the midsternal area without radiation. The patient describes the pain as grade 3 on a scale of 1 to 10. There is consistent chest pressure, tightness, and dyspnea. Her last menstrual period was 2 weeks ago. She is not on any medications.

On physical examination, the patient is afebrile. Her blood pressure is 144/76 mm Hg bilaterally, pulse is 118/min, and respiration rate is 18/min. BMI is 29. She is tachypneic and tachycardic. Estimated central venous pressure is 15 cm H_2O. There are no murmurs, rubs, or gallops on cardiac auscultation. Her lungs are clear. There is mild pedal and lower leg edema that is more pronounced on the right side.

The electrocardiogram shows ST-segment depression in the lateral leads. The chest radiograph is normal. Handheld echocardiography shows a small, hyperdynamic left ventricle with normal regional wall motion.

Which of the following is the best diagnostic test to perform next in this patient?

(A) Cardiac MRI
(B) CT pulmonary angiography
(C) Coronary angiography

(D) Radionuclide perfusion imaging

(E) Transesophageal echocardiography

Item 79

A 32-year-old woman is evaluated for exertional dyspnea that has developed within the last few months. She reports a lifelong history of a heart murmur, but has had no other cardiovascular symptoms and has not had prior cardiac testing. She recently moved to the United States from North Africa, and she did not receive regular health care prior to moving to the United States. She is not on any medications.

On physical examination, her blood pressure is 130/40 mm Hg and her heart rate is 70/min and regular. The jugular venous pulse contour demonstrates prominent a waves and the carotid pulses are bounding. The cardiac apex is displaced to the anterior axillary line of the sixth intercostal space, and a parasternal impulse is present. There is a systolic and diastolic murmur palpable over the left chest. A continuous grade 4/6 systolic and diastolic murmur is noted over the left side of the chest and primarily over the second left intercostal space. There is no S_3 or S_4. No additional sounds are noted. There is no evidence of digital clubbing or cyanosis.

Electrocardiogram demonstrates bi-atrial enlargement and features of left ventricular hypertrophy. Chest radiograph demonstrates cardiomegaly.

Which of the following is the most likely diagnosis?

(A) Atrial septal defect with associated pulmonary valve stenosis

(B) Eisenmenger syndrome

(C) Mitral stenosis and regurgitation

(D) Patent ductus arteriosus

(E) Ventricular septal defect

Item 80

A 56-year-old woman is evaluated during a routine follow-up examination. She has a history of aortic stenosis due to a bicuspid aortic valve. Six months ago, she underwent valve replacement with a mechanical prosthesis after she had developed exertional dyspnea and a decline in exercise tolerance. Her initial postoperative course was uneventful. She describes fatigue and mild exertional dyspnea, but this is improved over her preoperative symptoms. She reports no palpitations, fevers, chills, weight loss, dental procedures, or sick contacts. She has been compliant with her medical regimen and reports therapeutic INR levels since hospital discharge.

On physical examination, blood pressure is 126/70 mm Hg and pulse is 72/min. Her cardiac examination reveals a normal S_1 and mechanical S_2 without an S_3 or S_4. There is a nonradiating grade 2/6 midpeaking systolic murmur heard best at the lower left sternal border. There is no jugular venous distention or pedal edema. Lung fields are clear. The rest of her physical examination is unremarkable.

Laboratory studies:

Leukocyte count	Normal
Hematocrit	31%
Platelet count	144,000/µL (144 × 10⁹/L)
INR	2.6
Serum creatinine	1.3 mg/dL (99.2 µmol/L)
Serum lactate dehydrogenase	440 U/L
Serum haptoglobin	8 mg/dL (80 mg/L)

The blood smear demonstrates normocytic erythrocytes with schistocytes. Reticulocyte count is 6% of erythrocytes.

Postoperative echocardiogram demonstrates normal left ventricular size and function. There is a mechanical aortic prosthesis with paravalvular regurgitation that is mild in severity. The valve leaflets appear to move normally. The transaortic velocity is 3.4 m/s with an aortic valve area of 1.5 cm². Pulmonary pressures are in the normal range.

Which of the following is the most likely cause of her persistent exertional dyspnea?

(A) Endocarditis

(B) Hemolytic anemia

(C) Pannus formation

(D) Prosthesis mismatch

Item 81

A 40-year-old man visits the office to discuss his risk of cardiovascular disease. He is concerned because he recently turned 40 years old, and his father died at age 42 years of a heart attack. The patient recently had a high-sensitivity C-reactive protein blood test performed and was told that the results indicated that he was at higher than average risk of future cardiovascular disease. He has been concerned about his risk of heart disease for many years. He reports that his diet is mostly vegetarian and that he exercises about 4 days per week on a treadmill or stationary bicycle for 30 to 40 minutes. He has a history of cigarette smoking (1 pack per day for 4 years) but stopped at age 22 years.

On physical examination, his blood pressure is 122/68 mm Hg, pulse is 74/min, and respiration rate is 14/min. His BMI is 24. The remainder of his cardiovascular and general physical examination is normal.

Laboratory studies:

Total cholesterol	190 mg/dL (4.9 mmol/L)
HDL cholesterol	72 mg/dL (1.9 mmol/L)
LDL cholesterol	88 mg/dL (2.3 mmol/L)
Triglycerides	150 mg/dL (1.7 mmol/L)

An electrocardiogram demonstrates sinus rhythm, with a rate of 64/min.

Which of the following is the most appropriate management for this patient?

(A) Begin aspirin

(B) Begin simvastatin

(C) Order exercise electrocardiographic stress test

(D) No further diagnostic testing or treatment at this time

Item 82

An 18-year-old woman is evaluated for recurrent syncope. She has experienced four syncopal episodes in her lifetime, all of which occurred during activity. The most recent was last week, when she dove into a pool and had a brief loss of consciousness. Episodes have no prodrome, and she has had no dizziness. She is healthy and active, without cardiopulmonary complaints, and takes no medications. Her maternal cousin drowned at age 10 years, and her mother has been diagnosed with a seizure disorder.

On physical examination, her blood pressure is 112/65 mm Hg and her pulse is 67/min and regular. The cardiopulmonary and general physical examinations are normal. Electrocardiogram is shown.

Which of the following is the most likely diagnosis?

(A) Brugada syndrome
(B) Long QT syndrome
(C) Short QT syndrome
(D) Wolff-Parkinson-White syndrome

Item 83

A 40-year-old man is admitted to the hospital after an episode of syncope at work. He has had a 1-week history of progressive shortness of breath, orthopnea, and fatigue. On admission he is found to be hypotensive and is started on intravenous dopamine. Echocardiogram shows dilated left and right ventricles with a left ventricular ejection fraction of 10% and no regional wall motion abnormalities. Telemetry shows frequent and prolonged runs of nonsustained ventricular tachycardia. He has no other medical problems and takes no medications.

On physical examination, he is afebrile. Blood pressure is 70 mm Hg systolic, pulse is 110/min, and respiration rate is 20/min. The jugular veins are distended. Heart rate is regular, and a summation gallop is noted. There is no rash or skin lesions. Extremities are cool with no edema.

Laboratory studies show a serum troponin level of 5 ng/mL (5 µg/L). Chest radiograph shows mild cardiomegaly and pulmonary edema and no other abnormalities. Electrocardiogram shows sinus tachycardia, normal QRS duration, and frequent premature ventricular complexes. Cardiac catheterization after admission shows normal coronary arteries.

Which of the following is the most appropriate management step?

(A) Biventricular pacemaker placement
(B) Cardiac MRI
(C) Endomyocardial biopsy
(D) Implantable defibrillator placement

Item 84

A 62-year-old man is evaluated for hypertension. In home blood pressure measurements over the past 2 weeks, his average blood pressure has been 128/90 mm Hg. He has type 2 diabetes mellitus and had an inferior myocardial infarction 5 years ago, which was treated with placement of a bare metal stent in the right coronary artery. His current medications include lisinopril (10 mg/d), metoprolol (50 mg twice daily), aspirin, pravastatin, and glipizide. He tolerates his medication without side effects.

On physical examination, his blood pressure is 130/95 mm Hg, pulse is 56/min, and respiration rate is 14/min. BMI is 28. Cardiac auscultation reveals an S_4.

Laboratory testing reveals normal serum electrolyte, creatinine, and blood urea nitrogen levels. Hemoglobin A_{1c} concentration is 6.8% and urine albumin/creatinine ratio is 10 mg/g.

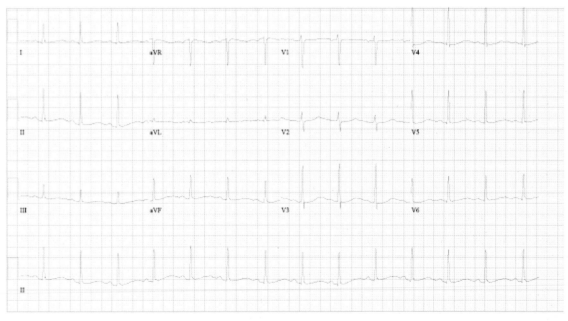

ITEM 82.

Electrocardiogram reveals sinus rhythm with a rate of 60/min with first-degree atrioventricular block; Q waves in leads II, III, and aVF; and nonspecific T-wave abnormalities.

Which of the following is the most appropriate treatment for this patient's hypertension?

(A) Increase metoprolol dosage
(B) Increase lisinopril dosage
(C) Add losartan
(D) Substitute losartan for lisinopril
(E) Make no changes at this time

Item 85

A 40-year-old man with a history of a cardiac murmur is evaluated during a routine examination. He has no history of chest discomfort, palpitations, shortness of breath, or syncope. He is active and cycles three or four times per week.

On physical examination, temperature is normal, blood pressure is 132/50 mm Hg, and pulse is 80/min. There is no jugular venous distention. Cardiovascular examination reveals a point of maximal impulse that is displaced laterally 1 cm from the midclavicular line and is diffuse. There is a grade 3/6 early decrescendo diastolic murmur heard at the left parasternal third intercostal space that does not radiate. Lungs are clear. There are brisk, prominent distal pulses throughout the extremities, with a "pistol shot" sound heard when auscultating over the peripheral arteries. There is no pedal edema.

A transthoracic echocardiogram demonstrates a bicuspid aortic valve and severe aortic regurgitation.

Additional echocardiographic findings:

Left ventricular end-diastolic dimension	75 mm
Left ventricular end-systolic dimension	60 mm
Ejection fraction	50%
Vena contracta width	6 mm
Proximal ascending aorta diameter	50 mm (normal <35 mm)
Pulmonary pressures	35-40 mm Hg

Which of the following is the best management option?

(A) Aortic valve replacement
(B) Digoxin and diuretic therapy
(C) Treadmill stress echocardiogram
(D) No intervention at this time

Item 86

A 62-year-old man with coronary artery disease is evaluated for angina. He was diagnosed with coronary artery disease 4 years ago, when he developed exertional chest pain and underwent an exercise treadmill stress test. Medical therapy was started with aspirin, metoprolol, isosorbide mononitrate, and sublingual nitroglycerin. He was asymptomatic until 8 months ago, when he noted exertional angina; his dosages of metoprolol and isosorbide mononitrate were increased and long-acting diltiazem was added, resulting in control of his symptoms. However, over the past 2 months, he has had gradually increasing symptoms, and currently he

requires daily nitroglycerin for angina relief during exercise. He has not had any episodes of angina at rest. He has hyperlipidemia treated with pravastatin.

Physical examination shows a well-developed man who appears comfortable. Blood pressure is 110/60 mm Hg and heart rate is 48/min. Carotid upstroke is normal with no bruits. Cardiac examination reveals no murmurs, and the lungs are clear. Peripheral pulses are equal throughout and there is no peripheral edema.

An electrocardiogram shows no acute ischemic changes.

Which of the following should be the next step in this patient's management?

(A) Add ranolazine
(B) Coronary angiography
(C) Exercise treadmill stress testing
(D) Intravenous heparin and nitroglycerin

Item 87

An asymptomatic 25-year-old man is evaluated for hypertension diagnosed during a recent pre-employment physical examination. He does not remember being told about hypertension in the past, and he has no family history of hypertension. He is not taking any medications.

On physical examination, his blood pressure is 170/60 mm Hg in both upper extremities. The heart rate is 65/min and regular. Carotid examination is normal; estimated central venous pressure is not elevated. The apical impulse is displaced and sustained. An ejection click is noted at the apex and left sternal border. There is a grade 2/6 early systolic murmur noted at the second right intercostal space. No diastolic murmur is noted over the anterior precordium. Systolic and diastolic murmurs are noted over the patient's back. There is no bruit noted over the abdomen. The lower extremity pulses are reduced and delayed.

A chest radiograph is shown.

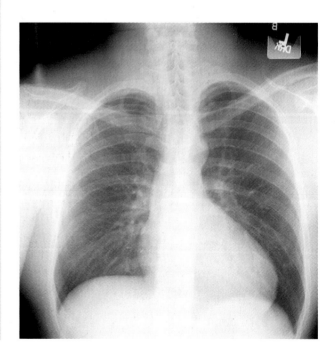

Which of the following is the most likely diagnosis in this patient?

(A) Coarctation of the aorta

(B) Essential hypertension

(C) Pheochromocytoma

(D) Renal artery stenosis

Item 88

A 31-year-old woman is evaluated for fatigue and exertional dyspnea. She reports no chest pain, palpitations, or syncope. She has no symptoms of collagen vascular disease. She has had no recent fevers, sick contacts, or weight gain. She smokes one pack of cigarettes per day and denies illicit drug use. Her family history is significant for a mother with mitral valve prolapse. She is on no medications and has never taken oral contraceptives.

On physical examination, temperature is normal, blood pressure is 122/60 mm Hg, and pulse is 80/min. BMI is 23. Cardiac examination reveals a point of maximal impulse that is undisplaced. A grade 2/6 lower left parasternal systolic murmur is heard that increases with inspiration but does not radiate. There are prominent jugular venous pulsations. There is 1+ pedal edema.

Leukocyte count is normal. An electrocardiogram shows evidence of right ventricular hypertrophy. A chest radiograph shows enlarged pulmonary arteries, right atrium, and right ventricle. A transthoracic echocardiogram demonstrates normal left ventricular size and function. The right ventricle is moderately enlarged. Aortic and mitral valve function are normal. There is moderate tricuspid regurgitation. No evidence of an interatrial shunt is seen by color Doppler imaging or following agitated saline contrast. Pulmonary pressure estimates are 60 to 65 mm Hg.

Which of the following is an appropriate next diagnostic test?

(A) Cardiac magnetic resonance imaging

(B) Stress echocardiogram

(C) Transesophageal echocardiogram

(D) Ventilation-perfusion lung scan

Item 89

A 57-year old man is evaluated for cramping discomfort in the right thigh, which occurs when walking two blocks and is relieved quickly with rest. The patient is a house painter who goes up and down ladders frequently in the course of his work. He is a current smoker with a 40-pack-year history. His brother has coronary artery disease, and his mother died at age 65 of a heart attack. He is taking no medications.

On physical examination, his temperature is normal, pulse is 72/min and regular, and his respiration rate is 16/min. The blood pressure in his right and left arms is 140/84 mm Hg and 140/82 mm Hg. His highest right ankle/foot systolic pressure is 138 mm Hg, and his highest left ankle/foot systolic pressure is 142 mm Hg. Examination of his lower extremities reveals scant hair present below mid-shin level. There is no abdominal or femoral bruit. Distal pulses are present but diminished. Capillary refill in the toes is intact, and there is no pedal edema, varicosities, skin breakdown, or ulceration. Results of a neurologic examination are normal.

Which of the following is the most appropriate management option for this patient?

(A) MRI of the lumbosacral spine

(B) Measurement of ankle-brachial index with exercise

(C) Treatment with ibuprofen

(D) Venous duplex ultrasonography of the lower extremities

Item 90

A 23-year-old woman is evaluated for management of pulmonary arterial hypertension. She is minimally symptomatic (New York Heart Association functional class I-II). She was diagnosed with idiopathic pulmonary arterial hypertension several months ago and is on no pulmonary vasodilator therapy at this time. She inquires about pregnancy.

Which of the following options regarding management of pregnancy is most appropriate for this patient?

(A) Addition of bosentan prior to proceeding with pregnancy

(B) Admission to a high-risk pregnancy unit at 30 weeks

(C) Cesarean delivery at 34 weeks

(D) Recommend avoiding pregnancy

(E) Treatment with low-molecular-weight heparin and aspirin beginning at conception

Item 91

A 61-year-old man is evaluated during a routine blood pressure monitoring visit. He has hypertension, treated with enalapril, and hyperlipidemia. The patient was previously taking simvastatin but had an adverse reaction of muscle pains and an elevated serum creatine kinase level, which resolved when the medication was ceased. He then was treated briefly with lovastatin, but muscle pain recurred, and it also was discontinued. He has never smoked cigarettes and has a sedentary lifestyle. He states that recently he has not been compliant with his low-fat diet.

On physical examination, his blood pressure is 148/88 mm Hg, and pulse is 76/min. BMI is 25. Results of the cardiac examination are normal. Laboratory results include total serum cholesterol, 190 mg/dL (4.9 mmol/L); LDL cholesterol, 140 mg/dL (3.6 mmol/L); and HDL cholesterol, 35 mg/dL (0.9 mmol/L). Serum creatinine is 1.3 mg/dL (99.2 µmol/L).

Which of the following is the most appropriate test for further stratifying this patient's cardiovascular risk?

(A) High-sensitivity C-reactive protein level

(B) CT coronary angiography

(C) Echocardiography

(D) Exercise stress test

Item 92

A 72-year-old man is admitted to the hospital after experiencing the acute onset of right-sided weakness and difficulty speaking that completely resolved after 2 hours. He is a prior smoker and has hypertension, for which he takes hydrochlorothiazide and irbesartan.

On physical examination, the patient is afebrile. His blood pressure is 138/84 mm Hg, pulse is 78/min and regular, and respiration rate is 16/min. Cardiac examination reveals a grade 3/6 early systolic murmur at the cardiac base with radiation to the carotid arteries. The S_2 is diminished and there is an S_4. Ophthalmologic and neurologic examinations are normal and speech fluency is intact.

Electrocardiogram demonstrates normal sinus rhythm. A transesophageal echocardiogram demonstrates no left atrial or atrial appendage thrombi and normal left ventricular function. A small patent foramen ovale is documented by color flow, but no right-to-left shunting is documented. Moderate to severe calcific aortic stenosis without regurgitation is present. Mild mitral annular calcification is present. A mobile, 5-mm echo-bright density is present in the ascending aorta associated with diffuse, mild, sessile atheromas. Carotid duplex imaging demonstrates less than 50% stenosis of the right internal carotid artery and less than 25% stenosis of the left internal carotid artery.

In addition to statin therapy, which of the following is the most appropriate treatment for this patient?

(A) Aortic valve and root replacement
(B) Carotid endarterectomy
(C) Percutaneous closure of the patent foramen ovale
(D) Warfarin

Item 93

A 29-year-old woman with a mechanical mitral valve prosthesis presents for pregnancy counseling. She has a history of mitral regurgitation and had mitral valve replacement for progressive left ventricular enlargement several years ago. She recently married and would like to start a family. She is asymptomatic and has been on a stable dose of warfarin (4 mg/d) for the past 2 years.

On physical examination, her blood pressure is 120/70 mm Hg. The estimated central venous pressure is 3 cm H_2O. There is a crisp, mechanical S_1. No murmurs are detected. The remainder of the examination is unremarkable.

Which of the following is the most appropriate anticoagulation regimen for this patient if she becomes pregnant?

(A) Continue warfarin, adjusted to INR
(B) Stop warfarin; start aspirin and clopidogrel
(C) Stop warfarin; start fondaparinux
(D) Stop warfarin; start weight-based low-molecular-weight heparin

Item 94

A 48-year-old man is evaluated in the emergency department for dyspnea on exertion and paroxysmal nocturnal dyspnea for 3 days. He has a history of type 2 diabetes mellitus and hypertension but no other medical problems. He does not smoke cigarettes. He currently takes metformin, lisinopril, and low-dose aspirin.

On physical examination, he is afebrile. Blood pressure is 130/80 mm Hg, pulse is 100/min, and respiration rate is 20/min; BMI is 40. Jugular veins are distended. Cardiac examination reveals a normal S_1 and S_2, the presence of an S_3, and a regular rate and rhythm with no murmurs. The point of maximal impulse is not displaced, and there are no heaves. Pulmonary auscultation discloses crackles at the bilateral lung bases. There is mild bilateral edema to the shins. Laboratory studies reveal a serum creatinine level of 1.0 mg/dL (76.3 µmol/L) and a B-type natriuretic peptide level of 100 pg/mL. Electrocardiogram is shown. Chest radiograph is pending.

Which of the following is the most likely diagnosis?

(A) Acute heart failure
(B) Acute pulmonary embolism
(C) Cor pulmonale
(D) Recent myocardial infarction

Item 95

An 89-year-old woman is evaluated during a routine examination. She maintains her exercise regimen, which includes walking three or four times per week, but notes that she is more easily fatigued than she used to be. It takes her almost an hour to walk her current route, which took 25 to 30 minutes a year ago, and she occasionally has to pause to catch her breath. She denies angina, presyncope, syncope, or pedal edema. The patient's medical history is significant for hypertension and osteoporosis. She is currently taking hydrochlorothiazide, lisinopril, alendronate, calcium, and a multivitamin.

On physical examination, the patient's temperature is normal, blood pressure is 148/90 mm Hg, and pulse is 82/min. Estimated central venous pressure is 4 cm H_2O. There is a sustained apical impulse. S_1 is normal. There is a single S_2 and an S_4 but no S_3. A grade 3/6 late-peaking systolic murmur is heard best at the right second intercostal space, with radiation into the right carotid artery. Carotid artery upstrokes are delayed. Lungs are clear.

Transthoracic echocardiogram shows concentric left ventricular hypertrophy and normal systolic function. There is a trileaflet aortic valve with heavy calcification. Aortic jet velocity is 4.8 m/s, peak transaortic gradient is 92 mm Hg, and valve area is 0.7 cm^2.

Which of the following is the best management option?

(A) Aortic balloon valvuloplasty
(B) Aortic valve replacement
(C) Discontinue hydrochlorothiazide and begin furosemide
(D) Clinical follow-up in 1 year

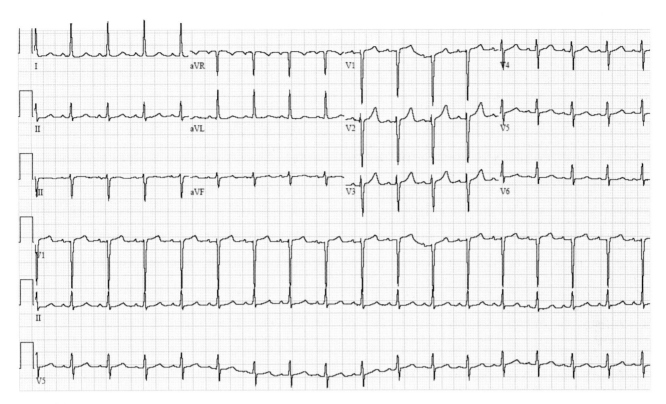

ITEM 94.

Item 96

A 49-year-old woman is evaluated for a routine physical examination. She has no prior cardiac history. She is frustrated by her inability to lose weight, and has tried a number of diets without significant or sustained weight loss. She has a sedentary lifestyle and does not exercise. With her usual activities, she has not experienced chest pain or dyspnea. She is a current smoker with a 32 pack-year history. She has perimenopausal symptoms and has taken estrogen (0.625 mg/d) for the past 4 years. Her father had a myocardial infarction and bypass surgery at age 58 years.

On physical examination, her blood pressure is 132/85 mm Hg and her pulse is 86/min. Her BMI is 31. The remainder of the physical examination is normal.

Laboratory studies:

Total cholesterol	180 mg/dL (4.7 mmol/L)
HDL cholesterol	50 mg/dL (1.3 mmol/L)
LDL cholesterol	92 mg/dL (2.4 mmol/L)
Triglycerides	190 mg/dL (2.1 mmol/L)

Which of the following lifestyle modifications is most important in reducing this patient's risk of future cardiovascular disease?

(A) Aerobic exercise 30 minutes 3 or 4 days weekly
(B) Cessation of cigarette smoking
(C) Discontinuation of hormone replacement therapy
(D) Sodium-restricted diet
(E) Weight loss to BMI below 25

Item 97

A 35-year-old black woman is admitted to the hospital after experiencing two episodes of syncope in the same day. The episodes were brought on by standing, with abrupt loss of consciousness for 5 minutes. There were no prodromal symptoms and the episodes were nonexertional. She had no associated nausea, vomiting, diaphoresis, or postictal confusion. She has had a 12-month history of chest pain, cough, and dyspnea. Exercise thallium stress testing done 2 months ago demonstrated patchy uptake of radionuclide throughout the ventricular myocardium and no demonstrable ischemia. Her mother died suddenly at age 45 years.

On physical examination, the patient is afebrile, blood pressure is 110/60 mm Hg without orthostasis, pulse is 65/min, and respiration is unlabored at a rate of 16/min. Yellowish-brown maculopapular lesions are present around the lips and eyelids. Jugular veins are distended. Pulmonary auscultation reveals faint scattered expiratory wheezes. Cardiac examination discloses normal heart sounds with no murmurs or gallops. Trace pedal edema is noted.

Twelve-lead electrocardiogram shows sinus rhythm, first-degree atrioventricular block, and left bundle branch block. Chest radiograph shows hilar lymphadenopathy and scattered interstitial infiltrates. Twenty-four-hour electrocardiographic monitoring shows frequent premature ventricular ectopic beats and nonsustained ventricular tachycardia. Endomyocardial biopsy discloses noncaseating granulomata.

Which of the following is the most appropriate management option?

(A) Amiodarone
(B) Cardiac magnetic resonance imaging
(C) Electrophysiologic study
(D) Implantable cardioverter-defibrillator placement
(E) Implantation of permanent pacemaker

Item 98

A 22-year-old man is evaluated in the emergency department with intermittent palpitations and dizziness for the past week. He has not experienced chest pain, dyspnea, or orthopnea. He has no prior medical history and is healthy and active. He reports being ill 6 to 8 weeks ago with fever, fatigue and myalgias, and a gradually expanding, flat, erythematous rash on his abdomen measuring a minimum of 5 cm at widest point. He works as a forester in Massachusetts and has not traveled out of the area recently.

On physical examination, his temperature is normal, blood pressure is 120/70 mm Hg, and pulse is 45/min. There is no edema or rash, and results of cardiac and pulmonary auscultation are normal.

An electrocardiogram demonstrates sinus rhythm with a rate of 90/min with complete heart block and a junctional escape rate of 50/min.

In addition to admitting the patient to the hospital for cardiac monitoring, which of the following is the most appropriate management for this patient?

(A) Electrophysiology study
(B) Intravenous ceftriaxone
(C) Intravenous erythromycin
(D) Permanent pacemaker placement
(E) Temporary pacemaker placement

Item 99

A 68-year-old woman is evaluated for atypical chest pain of 3 months' duration. She describes the pain as a left-sided burning that occurs both at rest and when she exercises. It lasts for about 10 minutes, and is relieved by rest and eating.

The patient has no history of cardiac disease. She has hypertension, for which she currently takes hydrochlorothiazide. She is a smoker and she has asthma, for which she takes inhaled corticosteroids and frequently uses inhaled bronchodilators. If she pretreats herself with the inhaled bronchodilator, she can walk long distances at a brisk pace.

On physical examination, she is afebrile, her blood pressure is 158/84 mm Hg, her pulse is 64/min, and her respiration rate is 18/min. Estimated central venous pressure is 5 cm H_2O. On cardiac examination, no murmurs, rubs, or extra heart sounds are noted. The lungs are clear to auscultation. There is trace peripheral edema. Laboratory findings include total cholesterol, 200 mg/dL (5.2 mmol/L); LDL cholesterol, 140 mg/dL (3.7 mmol/L); and HDL cholesterol, 50 mg/dL (1.3 mmol/L). The results of an electrocardiogram are normal.

Which of the following is the most appropriate diagnostic test for this patient?

(A) Adenosine nuclear perfusion stress test
(B) Coronary angiography
(C) Coronary artery calcium score
(D) Dobutamine stress echocardiography
(E) Exercise treadmill stress test

Item 100

A 35-year-old woman is evaluated for gradually progressive exertional dyspnea. She has a history of congenital heart disease with previous surgical intervention, including an atrial septal defect closure in childhood. She has not had regular cardiovascular follow-up since childhood.

On physical examination, her blood pressure is 120/60 mm Hg and her heart rate is 70/min and regular. The jugular venous pulse contour demonstrates a normal wave form. The carotid examination is normal. The cardiac apex is displaced to the sixth intercostal space at the midclavicular line. There is no parasternal impulse. There is no S_3 or S_4. A grade 3/6 holosystolic murmur is noted at the apex that radiates to the axilla and is best heard during expiration. No clicks are identified. A diastolic murmur is not noted. There is no evidence of digital clubbing or cyanosis. Peripheral arterial examination is normal.

The electrocardiogram is shown.

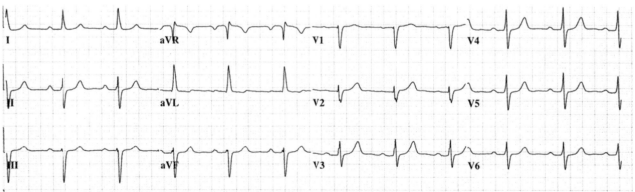

ITEM 100.

Which of the following is the most likely diagnosis?

(A) Aortic valve stenosis
(B) Mitral valve regurgitation
(C) Pulmonary valve stenosis
(D) Residual atrial septal defect

Item 101

A 75-year-old woman is evaluated during a follow-up examination after being hospitalized 2 weeks ago for heart failure exacerbation. Her furosemide dose was increased at the time of discharge. Since then, she has had increasing fatigue and a 2.3-kg (5-lb) weight loss. She has a 3-year history of idiopathic cardiomyopathy (her last ejection fraction 1 month ago was 36%) and a 6-month history of chronic atrial fibrillation. She currently takes lisinopril, metoprolol, and furosemide.

On physical examination, she is afebrile. Blood pressure is 100/50 mm Hg (120/70 mm Hg at hospital discharge) and pulse is 95/min (85/min at discharge). Jugular veins are flat. Cardiac examination reveals an irregularly irregular rhythm, soft heart sounds, variable intensity of S_1, and no murmurs. The lungs are clear. There is no edema.

Laboratory studies:

	Current	1 Month Ago
Creatinine	2.6 mg/dL (198.4 µmol/L)	1.5 mg/dL (114.5 µmol/L)
Blood urea nitrogen	60 mg/dL (21.4 mmol/L)	30 mg/dL (10.7 mmol/L)
Potassium	5.0 meq/L (5.0 mmol/L)	4.0 meq/L (4.0 mmol/L)
B-type natriuretic peptide	200 pg/mL	—

Electrocardiogram shows atrial fibrillation.

Which of the following is the most appropriate treatment?

(A) Intravenous diltiazem
(B) Intravenous normal saline
(C) Milrinone
(D) Nesiritide

Item 102

A 68-year-old man is evaluated for left calf pain that occurs after walking 2 to 3 blocks and is relieved with rest; he has had the pain for about 6 months. He has a history of coronary artery disease with depressed left ventricular systolic function (left ventricular ejection fraction, 30%) treated with coronary artery bypass grafting 2 years ago and subsequent implanted cardiac defibrillator placement for primary prevention purposes. He has hypertension and hyperlipidemia, and is a prior cigarette smoker. His medications include atorvastatin, aspirin, metoprolol, and lisinopril.

On physical examination, blood pressure is 110/70 mm Hg, pulse is 68/min and regular, and respiration rate is 16/min. Peripheral pulses are diminished. There is no skin breakdown or ulceration and no abdominal or femoral bruits. Ankle-brachial index is 0.7 on the left and 1.0 on the right. Segmental plethysmography demonstrates a pressure drop of 20 mm Hg below the left knee.

Which of the following is the most appropriate treatment for this patient?

(A) Femoral-popliteal bypass
(B) Medical treatment with cilostazol
(C) Percutaneous intervention
(D) Supervised exercise program

Item 103

A 33-year-old woman is brought to the emergency department by her boyfriend. She is confused and unable to answer questions. Her boyfriend relays a recent history of progressive fatigue and dyspnea over the past 2 to 3 weeks. As a child, she was diagnosed with congenital aortic stenosis and underwent aortic valve replacement with a bileaflet mechanical prosthesis. Her boyfriend denies illicit drug use on her part and states she has been compliant with warfarin.

On physical examination, temperature is 39.1 °C (102.4 °F), blood pressure is 78/31 mm Hg, and pulse is 112/min. Oxygen saturation is 91% on ambient air. The patient appears disoriented. Central venous pressure is estimated at 12 cm H_2O. Cardiac examination reveals a soft S_1 and mechanical S_2. There is a grade 3/6 early systolic murmur heard throughout the precordium and a grade 2/6 diastolic murmur. Lungs have bibasilar crackles. Her extremities are warm to the touch, and there is trace pedal edema.

Laboratory results include a leukocyte count of 19,000/µL (19×10^9/L) with a left shift. Hematocrit is 32% and the INR is 3.2. Serum haptoglobin and lactate dehydrogenase concentrations are normal. The rest of the laboratory evaluation is unremarkable.

Transthoracic echocardiography demonstrates hyperdynamic left ventricular function without regional wall motion abnormalities. There is a mechanical aortic valve with severe regurgitation. No obvious vegetations are seen. Pulmonary pressures are 45 to 50 mm Hg.

Which of the following is the best treatment option?

(A) Aortic valve replacement
(B) Intra-aortic balloon pump
(C) Intravenous inotropic therapy
(D) Thrombolytic therapy

Item 104

A 62-year-old woman is brought to the emergency department by paramedics for chest pain that has been present for 5 hours. Medical history is notable for type 2 diabetes mellitus, hypertension, and a stroke 1 year ago. Medications include glyburide, lisinopril, atorvastatin, and aspirin.

On physical examination, she appears comfortable. She is afebrile, blood pressure is 190/90 mm Hg, pulse rate is 88/min and respiration rate is 16/min. Cardiac examination shows no murmurs, extra sounds, or rubs. The lungs are clear and pulses are equal bilaterally. Neurologic examination is normal.

The electrocardiogram shows 2-mm ST-segment elevation in leads II, III, and aVF.

A coronary catheterization laboratory is not available, and the nearest hospital with percutaneous intervention capability is 1 hour away.

Which of the following is the best management option for this patient?

(A) Aggressive medical therapy without reperfusion attempt
(B) Immediate thrombolytic therapy
(C) Transfer for coronary artery bypass graft surgery
(D) Transfer for percutaneous coronary intervention

Item 105

A 60-year-old white woman is evaluated for dyspnea with mild activity (ascending less than one flight of stairs, walking less than one block on level ground) that has been stable for the past year. She has a history of nonischemic cardiomyopathy (last ejection fraction 20%). Her current medications are lisinopril, carvedilol, digoxin, and furosemide. She had an implantable cardioverter-defibrillator placed 1 year ago.

On physical examination, she is afebrile. Blood pressure is 95/75 mm Hg, and pulse rate is 70/min. Jugular veins are not distended, and the lungs are clear. Cardiac examination discloses a regular rate and rhythm, no murmurs, normal S_1 and S_2, and no S_3. There is no edema. Laboratory studies show a serum potassium level of 4.7 meq/L (4.7 mmol/L) and a creatinine level of 1.8 mg/dL (137.3 µmol/L), which has been stable for the past year.

Which of the following is the most appropriate addition to her treatment?

(A) Angiotensin receptor blocker
(B) Hydralazine
(C) Metolazone
(D) Spironolactone

Item 106

A 30-year-old woman is hospitalized for a 3-day history of progressive fatigue, dyspnea, nausea, and early satiety. She has a history of viral cardiomyopathy that was diagnosed 3 years ago. Her last ejection fraction was 20% by echocardiogram done 3 months ago. An implantable defibrillator was placed 2 years ago for primary prophylaxis of sudden death. Medications are metoprolol and enalapril.

On physical examination, she is afebrile and slightly lethargic. Blood pressure is 80/60 mm Hg, pulse is 110/min, and respiration rate is 20/min. Estimated central venous pressure is 5 cm H_2O. Heart sounds are soft and regular. The lungs are clear. There is mild right upper quadrant abdominal tenderness without rebound or guarding. No edema is noted.

Laboratory findings are as follows: hemoglobin, 10 g/dL (100 g/L) (down from 12 g/dL [120 g/L] 1 month ago); leukocyte count, 9000/µL (9.0×10^9/L); creatinine, 2.8 mg/dL (213.6 µmol/L) (up from 1.3 mg/dL (99.2

µmol/L) 1 month ago); alanine aminotransferase (ALT), 500 U/L; and aspartate aminotransferase (AST), 860 U/L. (Both ALT and AST were normal 1 month ago.)

Electrocardiogram shows sinus tachycardia. She is admitted to the intensive care unit and a pulmonary artery catheter is placed to manage hypotension and for assessment of volume status.

Pulmonary artery catheterization measurements:

Central venous pressure	5 mm Hg
Pulmonary artery pressure	25/14 mm Hg
Pulmonary capillary wedge pressure	14 mm Hg
Cardiac output	2.54 L/min
Cardiac index	1.48 L/min/m²

In addition to stopping the metoprolol, which of the following is the most appropriate treatment?

(A) Intravenous furosemide
(B) Intravenous milrinone
(C) Intravenous nesiritide
(D) Intravenous saline
(E) Packed erythrocyte transfusion

Item 107

A 72-year-old man is evaluated in the emergency department for acute severe pain during rest in the lower left leg that began 3 days ago. The patient has repeatedly used oxycodone/acetaminophen that he had at home for relief of pain. His pain is now much better, but he finds that he is having difficulty walking. He has had progressive exertional pain in the lower left leg over the past year. Five years ago, he had a left femoral popliteal bypass for occlusive peripheral arterial disease with distal ulceration. He has hypertension and hyperlipidemia. He has a 50 pack-year smoking history. Current daily medications include aspirin, lisinopril, hydrochlorothiazide, and simvastatin.

On physical examination, the patient's temperature is 37.8 °C (100.1 °F), blood pressure is 106/60 mm Hg, pulse is 100/min, and respiration rate is 20/min. The left lower extremity is pale and cool from the toes to the mid shin, and there is a small ulceration on the ball of the left foot. The left posterior tibialis and dorsalis pedis pulses are not palpable and cannot be identified by Doppler ultrasonography. Venous Doppler signals are audible. The left foot and calf feel stiff, and the patient can only weakly flex the foot. Toe movement on the left side is minimal, and sensation to light touch is absent.

Which of the following is the most appropriate treatment for this patient?

(A) Emergent surgical revascularization
(B) Intravenous heparin
(C) Intra-arterial thrombolytic therapy
(D) Prompt amputation

Item 108

A 77-year-old woman is admitted to the hospital for intermittent dizziness over the past few days. She does not have chest discomfort, dyspnea, palpitations, syncope, orthopnea, or edema. She underwent coronary artery bypass graft surgery 6 years ago after a myocardial infarction. She has hypertension, hyperlipidemia, and paroxysmal atrial fibrillation with a history of rapid ventricular response. She notes that over the past several years, she feels she has slowed down and has had problems with memory, which she attributes to aging. Medications are metoprolol, hydrochlorothiazide, pravastatin, lisinopril, aspirin, and warfarin.

On physical examination, her blood pressure is 137/88 mm Hg and her pulse is 52/min. Estimated central venous pressure is 7 cm H_2O. The point of maximal impulse is felt in the fifth intercostal space and at the midcostal line. Cardiac auscultation reveals bradycardia with regular S_1 and S_2, as well as an S_4. A grade 2/6 early systolic murmur is heard at the left upper sternal border. The lungs are clear to auscultation. Edema is not present.

On telemetry, she has sinus bradycardia with rates between 40/min and 50/min, with two symptomatic sinus pauses of 3 to 5 seconds each.

Which of the following is the most appropriate management for this patient?

(A) Add amiodarone
(B) Discontinue metoprolol
(C) Echocardiography
(D) Pacemaker implantation

Item 109

A 60-year-old woman is evaluated for follow-up after hospitalization 2 weeks ago for pulmonary edema and volume overload that readily resolved with intravenous diuretics. She is currently feeling well without edema or shortness of breath. A stress echocardiogram done in the hospital was negative for ischemia and showed an ejection fraction of 60% and no significant valvular abnormalities. She has a history of hypertension, hyperlipidemia, and chronic atrial fibrillation. She takes metoprolol (75 mg twice daily), hydrochlorothiazide, warfarin, aspirin, and pravastatin.

On physical examination, she is afebrile. Blood pressure is 150/90 mm Hg and pulse is 50/min. Jugular veins are not distended, and the lungs are clear. Cardiac examination shows an irregularly irregular rhythm with variable intensity of the S_1 with no murmurs. There is no edema.

Which of the following is the most appropriate adjustment to her treatment?

(A) Add candesartan
(B) Add digoxin
(C) Change hydrochlorothiazide to furosemide
(D) Increase metoprolol dosage

Item 110

A 68-year-old man presents to the emergency department at 2 AM for the evaluation of chest pain that has been present for 2 hours. He describes it as a "tight" pain that is located in the substernal area and radiates to his back. The pain began suddenly while sleeping. He denies prior episodes of similar pain. Medical history is notable for hypertension treated with diltiazem. Family history is notable for premature coronary artery disease in an older brother and younger sister.

Physical examination shows blood pressure of 190/65 mm Hg and heart rate of 100/min. The patient is in moderate distress owing to pain. There is no jugular venous distention. Cardiac examination reveals an early grade 2/6 diastolic decrescendo murmur heard best along the upper left sternal border. The lungs are clear bilaterally.

The electrocardiogram demonstrates sinus tachycardia, voltage criteria for left ventricular hypertrophy, and 0.5-mm ST-segment elevation in leads V_1 through V_3. Laboratory data are pending.

Which of the following is the most appropriate next step in management of this patient?

(A) Aspirin, intravenous heparin, and metoprolol
(B) Contrast-enhanced chest CT scan
(C) Thrombolytic therapy
(D) Transthoracic echocardiogram

Item 111

A 20-year-old female college student is evaluated at the student health center to establish care. She had no major medical problems prior to college, and there is no family history of cardiovascular disease.

On physical examination, blood pressure is 110/60 mm Hg and pulse is 70/min. S_1 and S_2 are normal and there is an S_4 present. There is a harsh grade 2/6 midsystolic murmur heard best at the lower left sternal border. The murmur does not radiate to the carotid arteries. A Valsalva maneuver increases the intensity of the murmur; moving from a standing position to a squatting position, performing a passive leg lift while recumbent, and performing isometric handgrip exercises decrease the intensity. Rapid upstrokes of the carotid pulses are present. Blood pressures in the upper and lower extremities are equal.

Which of the following is the most likely diagnosis?

(A) Aortic coarctation
(B) Bicuspid aortic valve
(C) Hypertrophic cardiomyopathy
(D) Mitral valve prolapse
(E) Ventricular septal defect

Item 112

A 32-year-old woman with repaired tetralogy of Fallot seeks counseling regarding potential pregnancy and the risk of having a child with congenital heart disease. She has no cardiovascular symptoms and takes no medications. She has no significant cardiac chamber enlargement and has had no arrhythmias. She has moderate pulmonary valve regurgitation.

On physical examination, the patient has dysmorphic features with low-set ears. The rest of the physical examination is unremarkable with the exception of a +1 parasternal impulse and an early diastolic murmur noted along the left sternal border that increases with inspiration. There is no digital clubbing or cyanosis.

The electrocardiogram demonstrates right bundle branch block with a QRS duration of 120 msec. The patient is in sinus rhythm. Chest radiograph demonstrates mild cardiomegaly. The echocardiogram demonstrates borderline right-sided cardiac chamber enlargement. On a Bruce protocol exercise test, the patient exercises at 98% of predicted capacity.

Which of the following is the greatest concern regarding pregnancy outcome in this patient?

(A) Fetal congenital heart disease
(B) Intrauterine growth retardation causing a low-birth-weight infant
(C) Maternal arrhythmia
(D) Maternal cardiovascular morbidity

Item 113

A 70-year-old man is evaluated in the emergency department for severe lower back pain that began suddenly 2 days ago and was associated with a syncopal episode. Since that time, he has had vague lower abdominal and back discomfort. There has been no change in bowel or urinary habits and no fever or chills. The patient has a 40 pack-year history of smoking cigarettes. He also has hypertension and hyperlipidemia. His daily medications are atorvastatin, aspirin, lisinopril, and hydrochlorothiazide.

On physical examination, his temperature is 37.7 °C (99.8 °F), blood pressure is 100/60 mm Hg, pulse is 98/min and regular, and respiration rate is 18/min. BMI is 31. Results of the cardiac and neurologic examinations are normal. Abdominal examination reveals normal bowel sounds and no hepatosplenomegaly. Rectal examination is unremarkable. There is moderate tenderness to palpation in the infra-umbilical and suprapubic regions, but without guarding or rebound tenderness.

Laboratory results include a hematocrit of 32% and a leukocyte count of 12,000/μL (12.0×10^9/L). Results of liver chemistry studies and urinalysis are normal. A stool sample tests negative for occult blood. Electrocardiogram shows normal sinus rhythm and meets criteria for left ventricular hypertrophy. A plain abdominal radiograph shows no free air or air-fluid levels.

Which of the following is the most likely diagnosis?

(A) Acute myocardial infarction
(B) Diverticulitis
(C) Nephrolithiasis/renal colic
(D) Ruptured abdominal aortic aneurysm

Item 114

An 85-year-old woman is admitted to the coronary care unit following successful thrombolytic therapy for an acute anterior wall ST-elevation myocardial infarction (STEMI). Prior to the myocardial infarction she had been active without any medical problems and was taking no medications. Blood pressure is 120/70 mm Hg and heart rate is 90/min. There is no jugular venous distention and no cardiac murmurs. The lung fields are clear and there is no peripheral edema. Medications started in the hospital are aspirin, low-molecular-weight heparin, intravenous nitroglycerin, and oral metoprolol. The electrocardiogram shows Q waves in the anterior leads with upsloping ST segments.

On hospital day 3, the patient experiences acute onset of respiratory distress, and her systolic blood pressure falls to 80 mm Hg. Her oxygen saturation remains at 80% despite the administration of 100% oxygen by face mask. She is given dopamine and intravenous furosemide. On physical examination, blood pressure is 96/40 mm Hg, pulse rate is 100/min, and respiration rate is 28/min. Findings include jugular venous distention, crackles throughout both lung fields, and a grade 4/6 systolic murmur associated with a thrill. A pulmonary artery catheter is placed via the right internal jugular vein. The pulmonary capillary wedge pressure tracing shows prominent *v* waves.

Pulmonary artery pressures:

Cardiac Chamber	Pressure (mm Hg)	Oxygen Saturation (%)
Right atrium	Mean 8	68
Right ventricle	50/06	82
Pulmonary artery	50/30	
Pulmonary capillary wedge	32; *v* waves to 45	

Which of the following is the best immediate treatment option?
(A) Mitral valve repair
(B) Pericardiocentesis
(C) Pulmonary artery thrombectomy
(D) Ventricular septal defect repair

Item 115

An 88-year-old man is evaluated for follow-up of persistent atrial fibrillation with a rapid ventricular response diagnosed several months ago. His initial diagnosis was made during evaluation prior to cataract surgery. He underwent transesophageal echocardiography–guided cardioversion after diagnosis, but the atrial fibrillation recurred within 2 weeks. He has been managed with warfarin, digoxin, and verapamil. He was initially prescribed atenolol, but discontinued it because of side effects of fatigue and impaired concentration and memory. He is entirely asymptomatic despite an inadequately controlled ventricular rate. He also has hypertension treated with valsartan. He states that he generally is averse to taking more medications.

On physical examination, his blood pressure is 140/80 mm Hg and his pulse is 147/min. Cardiac auscultation reveals an irregularly irregular rhythm and a grade 2/6 holosystolic murmur. Estimated central venous pressure is 6 cm H_2O. The lungs are clear to auscultation and there is no edema. Serum thyroid-stimulating hormone level is normal.

A 24-hour ambulatory monitor demonstrates a mean heart rate of 137/min, with a minimum rate of 70/min and a maximum rate of 170/min.

Which of the following is the most appropriate management for this patient?

(A) Amiodarone
(B) Atrioventricular node ablation and pacemaker placement
(C) Maze surgical procedure
(D) Radiofrequency ablation

Item 116

A 30-year-old woman is evaluated for management of new-onset atrial fibrillation. She has a history of tetralogy of Fallot that was repaired at age 18 months. She has had no cardiovascular concerns since that time and has not had regular follow-up since childhood.

On examination, her blood pressure is 120/70 mm Hg and her heart rate is 70/min and irregular. The estimated central venous pressure is 10 cm H_2O; the jugular venous pulse contour includes a prominent v wave. The carotid examination is normal. The apical impulse is normal and there is a parasternal impulse. A grade 2/6 holosystolic murmur is noted along the lower left sternal border that increases with inspiration. A grade 2/6 early decrescendo diastolic murmur is also noted at the second left intercostal space; this also increases with inspiration.

An electrocardiogram demonstrates right bundle branch block and atrial fibrillation. The heart rate is 90/ min.

Chest radiographs are shown.

Which of the following is the most likely cause of this patient's atrial fibrillation?

(A) Aortic and mitral valve regurgitation
(B) Pulmonary and tricuspid valve regurgitation
(C) Residual ventricular septal defect
(D) Right ventricular outflow tract obstruction

Item 117

A 60-year-old man is evaluated during a routine office visit. He has stable New York Heart Association functional class III symptoms, experiencing shortness of breath with minimal activity such as dressing or walking up less than one flight of stairs. He has a 2-year history of ischemic cardiomyopathy following a large anterior myocardial infarction. At the time of his myocardial infarction, he presented with chest pain and florid heart failure. During that episode, β-blocker therapy was initiated but had to be discontinued due to clinical deterioration. His last measured ejection fraction was 15% 1 year ago; at that time, he underwent implantable cardioverter-defibrillator placement. He currently takes lisinopril, spironolactone, digoxin, aspirin, and simvastatin.

On physical examination, he is afebrile. Blood pressure is 90/60 mm Hg, and pulse is 70/min. Jugular veins are not distended, and the lungs are clear. Cardiac auscultation discloses a regular rate and rhythm with no S_3. There is no edema. Electrocardiogram shows normal sinus rhythm.

Which of the following is the most appropriate addition to this patient's treatment?

(A) Candesartan

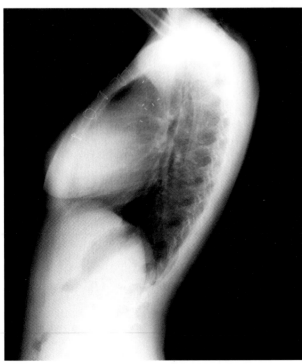

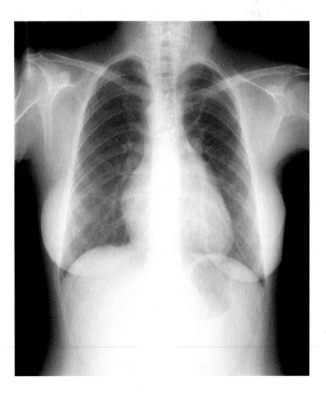

ITEM 116.

(B) Carvedilol

(C) Clopidogrel

(D) Warfarin

Item 118

A 42-year-old woman with a history of myxomatous mitral valve disease presents for routine follow-up after an echocardiogram performed 2 years ago demonstrated normal left ventricular size and function. There was bileaflet mitral valve prolapse with moderate regurgitation and normal pulmonary pressures. She admits to a sedentary lifestyle and does not exercise regularly. She does not describe a decline in her baseline exercise tolerance. The patient has no history of hypertension, dyslipidemia, or family history of premature coronary disease. She denies syncope, presyncope, palpitations, edema, or dyspnea.

On physical examination, blood pressure is 116/70 mm Hg and pulse is 70/min. BMI is 35. Central venous pressure is estimated at 5 cm H_2O. A cardiac examination reveals a regular rate and rhythm. S_1 is normal, S_2 is physiologically split, and there is no S_3 or S_4. She has a grade 3/6 holosystolic murmur heard best at the apex of the heart and radiates toward the left axilla and back. No diastolic murmur is heard. Carotid upstrokes are brisk. Lungs are clear to auscultation. Distal pulses are 2+ and palpable. There is trace pedal edema.

Transthoracic echocardiogram demonstrates myxomatous changes of the mitral valve with bileaflet prolapse. There is now a chordal rupture of the tip of the posterior mitral valve leaflet ("flail" tip) with severe mitral regurgitation.

Additional echocardiographic findings:

Left ventricular end-diastolic dimension	50 mm
Left ventricular end-systolic dimension	35 mm
Ejection fraction	65%
Vena contracta width	7 mm
Regurgitant orifice area	0.5 cm^2
Pulmonary arterial systolic pressure	35 mm Hg

Which of the following is the best management option?

(A) Coronary angiography

(B) Exercise treadmill echocardiogram

(C) Mitral valve surgical repair

(D) Mitral valve replacement

Item 119

A 45-year-old man with nonischemic cardiomyopathy presents to the emergency department with progressive shortness of breath and edema but no chest pain. He has been orthopneic for the past month. Previously, he was symptomatic with moderate activity (New York Heart Association class II heart failure). He has a dual-chamber implantable cardioverter-defibrillator. Current medications are lisinopril, furosemide, and carvedilol; however, he ran out of carvedilol 6 weeks ago. His most recent echocardiogram 3 months ago showed a left ventricular ejection fraction of 20%.

On physical examination, he is afebrile with blood pressure of 80/50 mm Hg, pulse of 115/min, and respiration rate of 16/min. He has jugular venous distention. Heart rhythm is regular, and an S_3 is heard. Lung examination reveals crackles. Edema is present. The extremities are cool, and mentation is intact.

Pertinent laboratory results include serum sodium, 130 meq/L (130 mmol/L); creatinine, 2.6 mg/dL (198.4 µmol/L) (was normal 1 month ago); and troponin, less than 0.01 ng/mL (0.01 µg/L). Electrocardiogram shows no acute ischemic changes; QRS duration is 100 msec.

Which of the following is the most appropriate treatment at this time?

(A) Intravenous dobutamine

(B) Intravenous furosemide

(C) Intravenous nesiritide

(D) Oral carvedilol

Item 120

A 78-year-old woman with a history of aortic stenosis presents for evaluation after undergoing aortic valve replacement with a bileaflet mechanical prosthesis 2 years ago. At the time of valve replacement she had diagnostic coronary angiography, which showed no significant coronary artery disease. She did well during her postoperative course, returning to her normal preoperative level of activity within 2 to 3 months. She now has symptomatic cholelithiasis and is scheduled for elective cholecystectomy. The patient reports no palpitations or syncope. There are no signs or symptoms of heart failurex. She has had no chest discomfort and has been able to maintain a normal level of daily activity. She currently takes warfarin, atorvastatin, and atenolol.

On physical examination, temperature is normal, blood pressure is 138/84 mm Hg, and pulse is 76/min. Cardiac examination reveals a mechanical S_2 and a normal S_1 without an S_3 or S_4. There is a nonradiating, midpeaking grade 2/6 early systolic murmur heard at the upper left sternal border. The rest of the physical examination is unremarkable.

In addition to withholding warfarin 5 days prior to surgery, which of the following is the best preoperative management option?

(A) Inpatient intravenous unfractionated heparin

(B) Oral vitamin K reversal

(C) Outpatient oral clopidogrel

(D) No other intervention prior to surgery

Answers and Critiques

Item 1   Answer: D
Educational Objective: Manage right ventricular myocardial infarction.

Volume expansion is the primary supportive treatment for the hemodynamic abnormalities of a right ventricular myocardial infarction. Although ischemia of the right ventricle may occur in a high percentage of patients with inferior ST-elevation myocardial infarction (STEMI), only 10% to 15% develop right ventricular myocardial infarction with hemodynamic abnormalities. These patients have a significantly higher in-hospital mortality rate (25%-30%) compared with patients with inferior STEMI without right ventricular infarction, and thus these patients should receive reperfusion therapy.

The physical examination findings of hypotension, clear lung fields, and elevated estimated central venous pressure represent the classic triad of right ventricular myocardial infarction. However, the most predictive finding is ST-segment elevation on right-sided electrocardiographic lead V_4R. Therefore, all patients with an inferior STEMI should have a right-sided electrocardiogram performed at the time of presentation. This patient's electrocardiogram shows ST-segment elevation in frontal inferior leads II, III, and aVF and 1-mm ST-segment elevation in right-sided precordial lead V_4R. These findings indicate inferior and right ventricular injury in the setting of an inferior STEMI, likely related to a right coronary artery occlusion.

In the setting of right ventricular myocardial infarction, right ventricular contractility is reduced, resulting in higher right ventricular diastolic pressure, lower right ventricular systolic pressure, and reduced preload or filling of the left ventricle. Volume expansion improves the hemodynamic abnormalities of right ventricular myocardial infarction because the gradient of pressure from the right atrium to the left atrium maintains filling of the left ventricle. In addition to reperfusion therapy for STEMI, the acute treatment of right ventricular myocardial infarction is supportive.

Inotropic support, specifically using intravenous dobutamine, is appropriate treatment in patients with right ventricular myocardial infarction whose hypotension is not corrected after 1 L of saline infusion. However, volume expansion should be tried before giving inotropic agents.

Bradycardia, potentially caused by increased vagal activity or sinoatrial node ischemia, exacerbates the hemodynamic abnormalities of right ventricular myocardial infarction, so β-blocker therapy is contraindicated in this patient.

Nitroglycerin is contraindicated in patients with right ventricular myocardial infarction because of the potential for venodilation and hypotension.

> **KEY POINT**
> - Volume expansion is the primary supportive treatment for the hemodynamic abnormalities of a right ventricular myocardial infarction.

Bibliography
Antman EM, Anbe DT, Armstrong PW, et al. ACC/AHA guidelines for the management of patients with ST-elevation myocardial infarction: a report of the American College of Cardiology/American Heart Association Task Force on Practice Guidelines (Committee to Revise the 1999 Guidelines for the Management of Patients with Acute Myocardial Infarction) [erratum in Circulation. 2005;111(15):2013-4 and Circulation. 2007;115(15):e411.]. Circulation. 2004;110(9):e82-292. [PMID: 15339869]

Item 2   Answer: A
Educational Objective: Treat multivessel coronary artery disease.

This patient has several indications for coronary artery bypass graft surgery. He has stenosis of the left main coronary artery and multivessel coronary artery disease with mildly reduced left ventricular systolic function. Coronary artery bypass grafting is indicated in patients with left main coronary artery disease, severe three-vessel disease with reduced left ventricular systolic function, and severe three-vessel disease with involvement of the proximal left anterior descending artery. In addition, patients with diabetes mellitus and multivessel disease also derive benefit from coronary artery bypass graft surgery. In this setting, surgery would not only relieve angina and improve quality of life, but it would also prolong life expectancy. Patients achieve a significant clinical benefit when the left internal mamillary artery graft is used as the bypass conduit for lesions within the left anterior descending artery system.

Enhanced external counterpulsation (EECP) is an acceptable treatment for patients with medically refractory angina who are not candidates for revascularization. However, the patient presented is a candidate for coronary artery bypass graft surgery, and this should be performed prior to considering alternative options such as EECP.

Although percutaneous coronary intervention may occasionally be used for patients with multivessel coronary artery disease who are not appropriate candidates for surgery, it would not be the best choice for this patient. This patient is young and active, and he does not have any clear contraindications for surgery.

Ranolazine can be useful in patients with chronic stable angina on maximal medical therapy. However, this patient has severe obstructive coronary artery disease that requires revascularization. In patients who have failed to benefit from revascularization and remain symptomatic on maximal medical therapy, ranolazine can be considered.

KEY POINT

- Coronary artery bypass graft surgery is recommended for patients with diabetes mellitus and multivessel disease.

Bibliography

Elsässer A, Möllmann H, Nef HM, Hamm CW. How to revascularize patients with diabetes mellitus: bypass or stents and drugs? Clin Res Cardiol. 2006;95(4):195-203. [PMID: 16598587]

Item 3   Answer: C

Educational Objective: Manage symptomatic mitral stenosis.

This patient has symptomatic mitral stenosis with pulmonary hypertension, and intervention is now necessary. Given that moderate regurgitation is present in this patient, valve replacement surgery, rather than balloon valvuloplasty, is indicated. Clinical markers consistent with severe mitral stenosis are transmitral pressure gradients greater than 10 mm Hg, enlargement of the left atrium, mitral valve area less than 1.5 cm², and pulmonary pressures greater than 50 mm Hg. Clinical outcome in asymptomatic or minimally symptomatic patients with mitral stenosis is excellent (>80% survival at 10 years), but once patients are symptomatic, 10-year survival is less than 15%. Morbidity associated with untreated mitral stenosis includes pulmonary hypertension, right-sided heart failure, systemic embolism from atrial fibrillation, and valve infection.

In symptomatic patients, percutaneous valvuloplasty is the preferred intervention if valve anatomy is amenable. Valvuloplasty is less invasive than surgical intervention and avoids the need for lifelong anticoagulation. Major complications of percutaneous valvuloplasty include severe mitral regurgitation (1%-8%), systemic embolization (1%-3%), and tamponade (1%-2%). Procedural mortality rate is 1%. Valve characteristics that favor successful valvuloplasty include pliable mitral valve leaflets, minimal commissural fusion, and minimal valvular/subvalvular calcification, as evaluated by echocardiography. However, percutaneous valvuloplasty should not be performed if there is moderate or severe mitral regurgitation, as the procedure would likely worsen any mitral regurgitation already present. In patients under consideration for valvuloplasty, transesophageal echocardiography is necessary to definitively exclude a left atrial thrombus because of the risk of thrombus dislodgement and embolization during the procedure.

This patient has symptomatic mitral stenosis. Medical therapy with an angiotensin-converting enzyme inhibitor will not relieve the obstruction. Because of poor long-term outcome in untreated symptomatic patients with mitral stenosis, follow-up in 1 year with no intervention is incorrect.

KEY POINT

- Valvuloplasty or valve replacement is indicated once mitral stenosis becomes symptomatic.

Bibliography

Bonow RO, Carabello BA, Kanu C, et al. ACC/AHA 2006 guidelines for the management of patients with valvular heart disease: a report of the American College of Cardiology/American Heart Association Task Force on Practice Guidelines (writing committee to revise the 1998 Guidelines for the Management of Patients With Valvular Heart Disease): developed in collaboration with the Society of Cardiovascular Anesthesiologists: endorsed by the Society for Cardiovascular Angiography and Interventions and the Society of Thoracic Surgeons [erratum in Circulation. 2007;115(15):e409.]. Circulation. 2006;114(5):e84-231. [PMID: 16880336]

Item 4   Answer: D

Educational Objective: Diagnose peripartum cardiomyopathy.

Peripartum cardiomyopathy is defined as heart failure with a left ventricular ejection fraction less than 45% that is diagnosed between 3 months before and 6 months after delivery in the absence of an identifiable cause. It is usually diagnosed during the first month postpartum. This patient presents with clinical features consistent with peripartum cardiomyopathy, including timing of onset, evidence of left ventricular dilation (displaced and diffuse apical impulse), and typical signs of heart failure. Risk factors for peripartum cardiomyopathy in this patient include her age (>30 years at the time of the pregnancy), race (black, African, Haitian), and the presence of gestational hypertension. With a maternal mortality rate of approximately 10%, peripartum cardiomyopathy is the major cause of pregnancy-related death in North America.

In women suspected of having peripartum cardiomyopathy, urgent confirmation of global ventricular systolic dysfunction by transthoracic echocardiography and institution of treatment with standard heart failure therapy are critical. Improvement in left ventricular function occurs in about 50% of women with peripartum cardiomyopathy within 6 months after delivery. Intravenous immune globulin and pentoxifylline have been shown to improve outcomes in some studies. Anticoagulation is recommended for thromboembolic prophylaxis when left ventricular ejection fraction is less than 35%.

Acute myocardial infarction is a recognized cause of cardiovascular deterioration during pregnancy and in the postpartum period. It may be related to atherosclerotic coronary artery disease or coronary artery dissection, vasculitis, coronary embolism from a prosthetic valve, and atrial thrombus, and carries a high risk of maternal mortality and morbidity. Diagnosis of myocardial infarction is identical to that in the nonpregnant patient. This patient's presentation, however, does not suggest an acute coronary syndrome, given the absence of chest pain or electrocardiographic changes. If the echocardiogram were to demonstrate regional wall motion abnormalities, an assessment of coronary status might be warranted.

Aortic dissection may occur in the peripartum or postpartum period and is a particular concern in patients with aortopathy related to Marfan syndrome, familial thoracic aortic aneurysmal disease, or bicuspid aortic valve–related aortopathy. However, the current presentation does not suggest aortic dissection given the absence of chest pain, the presence of equal and normal blood pressures in the upper extremities, and the presence of normal lower extremity pulses. Aortic dissection cannot explain the patient's findings of a dilated left ventricle and signs of heart failure.

Coarctation of the aorta may rarely present initially as hypertension during pregnancy. However, the patient's current physical examination findings of easily palpable lower extremity pulses without delay and the absence of hypertension argue against coarctation. In addition, rib notching is not reported on the chest radiograph.

KEY POINT

- Peripartum cardiomyopathy is defined as heart failure with a left ventricular ejection fraction less than 45% that is diagnosed between 3 months before and 6 months after delivery in the absence of an identifiable cause.

Bibliography

Elkayam U, Tummala P, Rao K, et al. Maternal and fetal outcomes of subsequent pregnancies in women with peripartum cardiomyopathy [erratum in N Engl J Med. 2001;345(7):552.]. N Engl J Med. 2001;344(21):1567-1571. [PMID: 11372007]

Item 5   Answer: B

Educational Objective: Manage worsening heart failure in a patient with ischemic cardiomyopathy.

This patient has worsening heart failure symptoms (New York Heart Association [NYHA] class III) despite a good heart failure medication regimen. In addition, he has an increased risk of sudden death due to ischemic cardiomyopathy. Implantation of a biventricular pacemaker-defibrillator may afford him both symptomatic benefit and a reduced risk of death. The indications for biventricular pacemaker-defibrillator placement include NYHA class III or IV heart failure, an ejection fraction less than or equal to 35%, and a QRS width greater than 120 msec. Approximately 70% of patients who undergo biventricular device placement obtain a symptomatic benefit, thought to result from mechanical "resynchronization" of the timing of right and left ventricular contraction. These devices have been shown to improve ejection fraction, quality of life, and functional status, as well as to decrease heart failure hospitalizations and mortality.

Amiodarone does not improve symptoms of heart failure or decrease mortality and therefore would not be of use in this patient.

This patient is a candidate for an implantable defibrillator for prevention of sudden death. However, a single-lead primary prevention device will not provide amelioration of his symptoms. A dual-chamber (atrioventricular) pacemaker-defibrillator would provide additional protection

from sinus bradycardia by atrial pacing, while the defibrillator portion would reduce his risk of sudden death. Although a conventional dual-chamber pacemaker may allow increases of β-blocker dosage, there is no evidence that such a strategy results in improved cardiovascular outcome in patients treated for heart failure and it will not by itself provide symptomatic benefit or protect the patient from ventricular arrhythmia and sudden death. Additionally, some dual-chamber defibrillators oblige right ventricular pacing, which can cause worsening of heart failure symptoms and increase hospitalization for heart failure.

KEY POINT

- A biventricular pacemaker-defibrillator may provide symptomatic and mortality benefit in patients with ejection fraction less than or equal to 35%, QRS width greater than 120-130 msec, and New York Heart Association class III or IV heart failure.

Bibliography

Epstein AE, DiMarco JP, Ellenbogen KA, et al. ACC/AHA/HRS 2008 Guidelines for Device-Based Therapy of Cardiac Rhythm Abnormalities: A Report of the American College of Cardiology/American Heart Association Task Force on Practice Guidelines (Writing Committee to Revise the ACC/AHA/NASPE 2002 Guideline Update for Implantation of Cardiac Pacemakers and Antiarrhythmia Devices) Developed in Collaboration With the American Association for Thoracic Surgery and Society of Thoracic Surgeons [erratum in J Am Coll Cardiol. 2009;53(1):147.]. J Am Coll Cardiol. 2008;51(21):e1-62. [PMID: 18498951]

Item 6   Answer: D

Educational Objective: Diagnose pulmonary valve stenosis.

The patient has characteristic physical examination findings, electrocardiogram, and chest radiograph consistent with pulmonary valve stenosis. The jugular venous pulse contour demonstrates a prominent a wave. A right ventricular lift and systolic thrill are present. An ejection click is noted and is close to the S_1, suggesting severe pulmonary valve stenosis. This sound decreases in intensity during inspiration (the only right-sided sound that decreases during inspiration). An early systolic murmur is noted over the pulmonary area. The electrocardiogram demonstrates right ventricular hypertrophy and right axis deviation. The chest radiograph demonstrates pulmonary artery dilatation. The diagnosis can be confirmed by echocardiography.

A bicuspid aortic valve is a more common cause of an ejection click than is congenital pulmonary valve disease, and it is associated with the development of aortic stenosis. The classic symptoms of aortic stenosis include dyspnea, angina, and exertional syncope. Aortic stenosis is characterized by small and late carotid pulsations, a late-peaking systolic murmur loudest in the second right intercostal space, absent splitting of S_2, and a sustained apical impulse. The murmur characteristically radiates to one or both carotid arteries. Findings suggesting right ventricular hypertrophy would not be expected on physical examination or on the electrocardiogram.

The characteristic physical examination finding in atrial septal defect is fixed splitting of the S_2. Equal *a* and *v* waves may be noted on jugular venous assessment. A right ventricular impulse is present. An ejection click may be audible if the pulmonary artery is enlarged but is less common than in patients with pulmonary stenosis. A pulmonary midsystolic murmur and a tricuspid diastolic flow rumble may be heard owing to increased flow through the valves from the left-to-right shunt. A systolic thrill, loud systolic murmur, and post-stenotic dilation of the pulmonary artery would not be expected in a patient with an isolated atrial septal defect.

Chronic mitral valve regurgitation is characterized by a holosystolic murmur at the apex that radiates to the axilla without respiratory variation. Mitral valve regurgitation may cause secondary pulmonary hypertension, but an ejection click and a loud early systolic murmur would not be expected with mitral valve regurgitation, even in the presence of pulmonary hypertension.

Tricuspid valve regurgitation causes a holosystolic murmur noted at the left sternal border. This characteristically increases with inspiration, but marked right ventricular hypertrophy and right axis deviation would not be expected on the electrocardiogram with this valvular lesion. The jugular venous pulse contour demonstrates a prominent *v* wave with tricuspid regurgitation, rather than a prominent *a* wave.

KEY POINT

- Characteristic features of pulmonary valve stenosis include a prominent *a* wave in the jugular venous pulse contour, a parasternal impulse, an ejection click, a systolic thrill, and an early systolic murmur that increases with inspiration.

Bibliography

Warnes CA, Williams RG, Bashore TM, et al. ACC/AHA 2008 Guidelines for the Management of Adults with Congenital Heart Disease: a report of the American College of Cardiology/American Heart Association Task Force on Practice Guidelines (writing committee to develop guidelines on the management of adults with congenital heart disease). Circulation. 2008;118(23):e714-833. [PMID: 18997169]

Item 7   Answer: C

Educational Objective: Manage moderate mitral regurgitation with exertional dyspnea.

This patient has limited exercise tolerance and exertional dyspnea. The clinical examination and echocardiogram demonstrate mitral valve prolapse with moderate regurgitation and no evidence of adverse hemodynamic effect (left ventricular size, function, and pulmonary pressures are normal). Cardiopulmonary symptoms with less than severe valvular regurgitation and in the absence of adverse hemodynamic effects usually indicate other disease processes, such as coronary artery disease, physical deconditioning, or pulmonary disease. This patient's pulmonary examination indicates an increased expiratory phase. With his history of smoking, a primary pulmonary process as the etiology of dyspnea should be suspected. Pulmonary function testing is indicated.

The origin of this patient's symptoms is not yet clear. His exercise tolerance is limited and his exertional dyspnea is out of proportion to his mitral valve disease. During exercise, his pulmonary systolic pressure only increased from 30 mm Hg to 45 mm Hg, a normal physiologic response to exercise (normal increase with exercise between 10 and 25 mm Hg), suggesting that mitral regurgitation is not the etiology of his dyspnea. Proceeding directly to mitral valve annuloplasty repair is not indicated. Additional diagnostic testing is necessary.

Right heart catheterization allows for direct evaluation of intrapulmonary pressure, central venous pressure, and cardiac output, but will not aid in determining whether the etiology of exertional dyspnea is a consequence of a primary pulmonary process, coronary artery disease, or valve dysfunction. The echocardiogram demonstrates normal left ventricular function with normal resting pulmonary pressures. Right heart catheterization would add little to this patient's diagnostic evaluation.

In a patient with an anatomically normal mitral valve but with ventricular dilation and volume overload (for example, in dilated cardiomyopathy), mitral annular dilation and leaflet tethering cause poor coaptation, leading to "functional" mitral regurgitation. In this setting, afterload reduction benefits the poorly functioning ventricle and decreases ventricular volume and annular dilation, thus reducing regurgitation severity. In a patient with a primary valve dysfunction, such as mitral valve prolapse, the underlying hemodynamic state is not one of volume overload, however, and pharmacologic afterload therapy would not be of benefit.

KEY POINT

- Cardiopulmonary symptoms in patients with less than severe valvular regurgitation usually indicate other disease processes.

Bibliography

Bonow RO, Carabello BA, Kanu C, et al. ACC/AHA 2006 guidelines for the management of patients with valvular heart disease: a report of the American College of Cardiology/American Heart Association Task Force on Practice Guidelines (writing committee to revise the 1998 Guidelines for the Management of Patients With Valvular Heart Disease): developed in collaboration with the Society of Cardiovascular Anesthesiologists: endorsed by the Society for Cardiovascular Angiography and Interventions and the Society of Thoracic

Surgeons [erratum in Circulation. 2007;115(15):e409.]. Circulation. 2006;114(5):e84-231. [PMID: 16880336]

Item 8   Answer: D

Educational Objective: Treat a patient with hypertrophic cardiomyopathy and heart failure refractory to medications.

This young man presents with progressively worsening dyspnea and New York Heart Association (NYHA) functional class III symptoms. Biventricular heart failure is evident by symptoms (dyspnea, fatigue, weight gain) and signs (jugular venous distention, S_3 gallop, crackles, peripheral edema). Echocardiography confirms a hypertrophic obstructive cardiomyopathy (HOCM) with diastolic dysfunction, marked septal hypertrophy, and a severe outflow tract obstruction. The patient's heart failure has been refractory to aggressive medical therapy, including negative inotropic and chronotropic agents and diuretics. Surgical septal myectomy should be considered in patients with outflow obstruction who are NYHA functional class III or IV and whose symptoms are refractory to medical therapy. Septal myectomy has been beneficial in improving symptoms of heart failure and may lead to a better prognosis. Thus, this patient who is refractory to medical therapy with no significant comorbidities should undergo surgical septal myectomy.

An implantable cardioverter-defibrillator is not indicated in this patient with no significant predictors of sudden cardiac death.

Negative inotropic agents, particularly β-blockers, are important medications in the treatment of heart failure in HOCM. However, this patient has achieved maximal β-blockade with metoprolol on the basis of heart rate and blood pressure response. No further β-blockade with carvedilol is indicated. Carvedilol has vasodilator properties that could further lower blood pressure as well as potentially exacerbate outflow gradient. In addition, this patient is being treated with disopyramide as a negative inotropic agent.

Ventricular pacing reduces the vigor of left ventricular septal contraction by causing an asynchronous or disorganized pattern of contraction. This reduces left ventricular outflow tract obstruction in HOCM. However, permanent pacing has not shown long-term benefit in improving heart failure in patients with HOCM. Thus, this approach is not the best treatment choice.

KEY POINT

- Surgical septal myectomy is the treatment of choice in patients with hypertrophic obstructive cardiomyopathy who have New York Heart Association functional class III or IV symptoms and are refractory to medical therapy.

Bibliography

Smedira NG, Lytle BW, Lever HM, et al. Current effectiveness and risks of isolated septal myectomy for hypertrophic obstructive cardiomyopathy. Ann Thorac Surg. 2008;85(1):127-33. [PMID: 18154797].

Item 9   Answer: A

Educational Objective: Treat high-risk unstable angina.

This patient has progressive chest pain, an elevated serum troponin level, and an electrocardiogram that shows ST-segment depression. These features indicate a non–ST-elevation myocardial infarction (NSTEMI). The TIMI risk score can be used in patients with unstable angina and NSTEMI to further assess their short-term risk. The TIMI risk score consists of the sum of four historical and three presentation characteristics. This patient's age, elevated troponin, ST-segment deviation, recent history of angina, recent use of aspirin, and presence of three traditional cardiovascular risk factors (family history, diabetes mellitus, hypertension) give him a TIMI risk score of 6, which places him at high risk of death or nonfatal myocardial infarction over the next 14 days. Patients with high TIMI risk scores benefit from aggressive medical therapy and referral for early coronary angiography (early invasive approach).

Although an elevated B-type natriuretic peptide (BNP) level in the setting of a NSTEMI predicts a worse clinical outcome, it does not assist in the early management of patients with unstable angina or NSTEMI. BNP measurement is useful in patients presenting to the emergency department with shortness of breach and can assist in differentiating a cardiac from a noncardiac cause.

In the setting of this patient's acute event, stress testing, including pharmacologic stress testing, is contraindicated. A stress test could potentially extend the infarction. Following initial medical therapy and in the absence of recurrent chest pain, a stress test could be performed after 48 hours if a conservative treatment approach is pursued.

Thrombolytic therapy is not indicated for a NSTEMI, as previous studies found no clinical benefit and excessive bleeding complications. In contrast, patients presenting with an ST-elevation myocardial infarction benefit from either primary percutaneous coronary intervention or thrombolytic therapy.

KEY POINT

- Patients with unstable angina or a non–ST-elevation myocardial infarction and a high TIMI risk score benefit from aggressive medical therapy and referral for early coronary angiography.

Bibliography

Antman EM, Cohen M, Bernink PJ, et al. The TIMI risk score for unstable angina/non-ST elevation MI: a method for prognostication and therapeutic decision making. JAMA. 2000;284(7):835-842. [PMID: 10938172]

Item 10   Answer: C

Educational Objective: Diagnose coronary artery disease in a cardiac transplant patient.

Coronary artery disease (transplant vasculopathy) increases in frequency with time after cardiac transplantation and is present in almost half of all patients by 5 years after transplantation. As in this patient, coronary artery disease in a cardiac transplant patient often presents atypically and may manifest with new-onset heart failure symptoms, decreased exercise tolerance, syncope (usually due to arrhythmias or conduction defects), or cardiac arrest. Because transplant-related coronary artery disease is frequently asymptomatic or manifests with very atypical symptoms, regular screening with coronary angiography and/or noninvasive stress testing is generally performed, with specific testing schedules varying by center preferences. Traditional risk factors (hypertension, diabetes mellitus, dyslipidemia, smoking) and immunologic factors contribute to the development and progression of transplant-related coronary artery disease. Because the pathophysiology is a diffuse intimal thickening, standard revascularization methods are frequently not feasible. There is evidence that statins help prevent and retard progression of transplant vasculopathy. Prognosis is poor once significant transplant vasculopathy becomes symptomatic, and in appropriate candidates, another cardiac transplantation is a possible treatment option.

Cardiac transplant rejection most frequently occurs in the first 1 to 2 years after transplantation. It is frequently asymptomatic, but suspicion should be raised with the occurrence of new-onset heart failure symptoms or new-onset atrial arrhythmias. Currently, cardiac transplant rejection can only be diagnosed by endomyocardial biopsy. In this patient, who is 10 years post-transplant, rejection is not the most likely diagnosis.

Posttransplant lymphoproliferative disease is a known complication of chronic immunosuppression after transplantation. Typically, the malignancy is a B-cell lymphoma, with variable presentation (abdominal or central nervous system mass, nonspecific flu-like illness). It would be unusual for a central nervous system mass to present with syncope, as in this patient, rather than with focal neurologic deficits. In general, the treatment for posttransplant malignancy includes decreasing the intensity of immunosuppression.

Side effects for cyclosporine include hypertension, nephrotoxicity, hypertriglyceridemia, hirsutism, gingival hyperplasia, and tremor. High levels of cyclosporine can cause seizures, but syncope is not an established side effect.

KEY POINT

- Presentation of coronary artery disease in a cardiac transplant patient is frequently atypical, and may manifest with new-onset heart failure symptoms, decreased exercise tolerance, syncope (usually due to arrhythmias or conduction defects), or cardiac arrest.

Bibliography

Schmauss D, Weis M. Cardiac allograft vasculopathy: recent developments. Circulation. 2008;117(16):2131-41. [PMID: 18427143]

Item 11   Answer: D

Educational Objective: Manage risk of sudden death in a patient with ischemic cardiomyopathy.

This patient has New York Heart Association (NYHA) class II heart failure, ischemic cardiomyopathy, and an ejection fraction below 35%. Despite advances in medical therapy, sudden cardiac death remains a major cause of death for patients with heart failure. Implantable cardioverter-defibrillators (ICDs) have repeatedly been shown to reduce the risk of death due to arrhythmia and overall mortality in certain populations of heart failure patients. ICD implantation is indicated for primary prevention of sudden death in patients with NYHA class II or III heart failure and either ischemic or nonischemic cardiomyopathy with an ejection fraction of 35% or less.

The SCD-HeFT trial, which included patients with ejection fractions below 35% and either an ischemic or a nonischemic cause of cardiomyopathy, found a 23% reduction in the risk of death over a 5-year period in patients who received an ICD compared with treatment with amiodarone or placebo. In addition, a plethora of side effects and organ system toxicities limits the use of amiodarone.

Furosemide would be a reasonable treatment if this patient had volume overload; however, this does not appear to be the case, and as furosemide does not provide mortality benefit, there is no indication for its use in this patient.

If patients continue to have NYHA class III or IV symptoms despite therapy with angiotensin-converting enzyme inhibitors and β-blockers, low-dose spironolactone results in a further 35% reduction in mortality. However, based on this patient's symptoms (NYHA class II), low-dose spironolactone is not indicated.

KEY POINT

- Implantable cardioverter-defibrillators reduce the risk of death in patients with New York Heart Association class II or III heart failure and either ischemic or nonischemic cardiomyopathy and an ejection fraction of 35% or less.

Bibliography

Epstein AE, DiMarco JP, Ellenbogen KA, et al. ACC/AHA/HRS 2008 Guidelines for Device-Based Therapy of Cardiac Rhythm Abnormalities: A Report of the American College of Cardiology/

American Heart Association Task Force on Practice Guidelines (Writing Committee to Revise the ACC/AHA/NASPE 2002 Guideline Update for Implantation of Cardiac Pacemakers and Antiarrhythmia Devices) Developed in Collaboration With the American Association for Thoracic Surgery and Society of Thoracic Surgeons [erratum in J Am Coll Cardiol. 2009;53(1):147.]. J Am Coll Cardiol. 2008;51(21):e1-62. [PMID: 18498951]

Item 12   Answer: B

Educational Objective: Treat New York Heart Association class I and II systolic heart failure.

Angiotensin-converting enzyme (ACE) inhibitor and β-blocker therapy is indicated for all patients with systolic heart failure regardless of symptoms or functional status, including asymptomatic or very functional patients. The combination of these two classes of medications has additive benefits with regard to morbidity and mortality in systolic heart failure. The patient, who has New York Heart Association (NYHA) functional class II heart failure, is already taking an ACE inhibitor, so a β-blocker such as carvedilol should be added. Potential contraindications to β-blocker therapy include bronchospastic lung disease, low baseline blood pressure, and poor hemodynamic status. β-Blocker therapy rarely exacerbates chronic lung disease, particularly if there is not a bronchospastic component to the lung disease. Even in patients with reactive airways disease, the risk of exacerbation is low for most patients. This patient's blood pressure is not too low to start a β-blocker. With systolic heart failure, particularly with a lower ejection fraction, the blood pressure is expected to be lower than the usual normal ranges owing to the lower cardiac output generated. Trials of β-blocker therapy in systolic heart failure have used systolic blood pressure cutoffs as low as 85 mm Hg for study entry. Finally, the patient appears euvolemic. β-Blockers should not be initiated or increased during decompensated states, such as volume overload or hypotension, because of the transient decline in cardiac output, which may worsen a decompensated state.

Amlodipine is the only calcium channel blocker demonstrated to have a neutral (rather than detrimental) effect on morbidity and mortality in heart failure in a large randomized controlled trial (PRAISE). Thus, it is an acceptable agent to use for angina or hypertension that is not adequately controlled with ACE inhibitors or β-blockers. However, this patient has neither angina nor hypertension, and amlodipine is not indicated.

There are currently no robust data to support addition of an angiotensin receptor blocker (ARB), such as losartan, to ACE-inhibitor therapy for treatment of systolic heart failure. No definitive improvement in survival has been demonstrated using the combination of these two agents, although some trials do suggest reduced hospitalizations. ARBs are currently recommended only for patients who are intolerant of ACE inhibitors, primarily owing to ACE inhibitor–induced cough. The incidence of hyperkalemia, renal failure, and hypotension is similar to that with ACE inhibitors. There have been reports of angioedema occurring with ARB use among patients who developed angioedema with ACE inhibitor treatment, so caution should be exercised in this setting.

Digoxin is indicated for moderately to severely symptomatic heart failure patients (NYHA class III-IV) or for rate control in patients with atrial fibrillation. Digoxin improves symptoms and reduces hospitalizations, but does not affect survival. Spironolactone is indicated only for treatment of moderate to severe (NYHA class III-IV) heart failure; in this setting, its use is associated with a 30% reduction in mortality. This patient, however, is only minimally symptomatic (NYHA class II), and treatment with either medication is not indicated.

KEY POINT

- **Angiotensin-converting enzyme inhibitor and β-blocker therapy is indicated for all patients with systolic heart failure regardless of symptoms or functional status, including asymptomatic or very functional patients.**

Bibliography

Hunt SA; American College of Cardiology; American Heart Association Task Force on Practice Guidelines (Writing Committee to Update the 2001 Guidelines for the Evaluation and Management of Heart Failure). ACC/AHA 2005 guideline update for the diagnosis and management of chronic heart failure in the adult [erratum in J Am Coll Cardiol. 2006;47(7):1503-1505.]. J Am Coll Cardiol. 2005;46(6):e1-82. [PMID: 16168273]

Item 13   Answer: E

Educational Objective: Treat heart failure during pregnancy.

It has been reported that the ejection fraction decreases during a subsequent pregnancy in patients with a prior episode of peripartum cardiomyopathy with persistent reduction in systolic function. β-Blockers and angiotensin-converting enzyme inhibitors are generally recommended for patients with asymptomatic left ventricular systolic dysfunction. However, angiotensin-converting enzyme inhibitors are contraindicated during pregnancy because of recognized teratogenicity. Thus, it would be appropriate to start a β-blocker in this pregnant patient with asymptomatic left ventricular dysfunction.

All available β-blockers cross the placenta and are present in human breast milk, resulting in significant levels in the fetus or newborn. Therefore, when used during pregnancy, fetal and newborn heart rate and blood glucose monitoring are indicated. Adverse fetal effects, such as low birth weight, early delivery, and small size for gestational age, have been associated with the use of atenolol, especially when initiated early in the pregnancy. The World Health Organization considers atenolol (U.S. Food and Drug Administration [FDA] pregnancy risk category D) unsafe during breastfeeding as it concentrates in breast milk, resulting in a significant dose to the breast-fed infant with associated risks for hypoglycemia and bradycardia. Metoprolol (pregnancy risk category C) should be considered as an alternative.

Digoxin is a FDA pregnancy risk category C drug. Although it readily passes to the fetal circulation, no teratogenic effect has been reported in humans. Digoxin is often used as a maintenance medication in patients with heart failure or atrial arrhythmias during pregnancy. The indications for digoxin are identical to those for nonpregnant patients with heart failure. It is recommended for patients with New York Heart Association class III heart failure to improve symptoms and reduce hospitalization. It is not indicated in this asymptomatic patient.

No single diuretic is clearly contraindicated during pregnancy. Experience is greatest with thiazide diuretics and furosemide. Diuretics impair uterine blood flow and placental perfusion. Continuation of diuretic therapy initiated before conception does not seem to have unfavorable effects. Maternal use of furosemide during pregnancy has not been associated with toxic or teratogenic effects, although metabolic complications have been observed. Neonatal hyponatremia and fetal hyperuricemia have been reported. Use of diuretics should be limited to the treatment of symptomatic heart failure with clear evidence of elevated central venous pressure. Furosemide (pregnancy risk category C) is not indicated for this patient at this time because she is has no manifestations of volume overload.

Hydralazine (pregnancy risk category C) can be used during pregnancy. Although it crosses the placenta, hydralazine is the most widely used drug in the acute treatment of hypertensive emergencies in pregnancy. Hydralazine could be added during pregnancy if the patient develops symptoms while on β-blocker therapy; however, she is currently asymptomatic and hydralazine is not indicated at this time. Hydralazine can be safely used during lactation.

The use of angiotensin-converting enzyme (ACE) inhibitors and angiotensin II–receptor blockers is contraindicated during pregnancy. Maternal-fetal transfer has been documented, and there is a recognized increased risk of congenital cardiovascular or central nervous system malformations in the fetus with exposure to ACE inhibitors during the first trimester. In addition, there is a 30% risk of fetal morbidity when ACE inhibitors are used during the second trimester, with increased risk of early delivery, low birth weight, oligohydramnios, or neonatal anuria and renal failure. These agents can be safely used during lactation.

KEY POINT

- **The use of angiotensin-converting enzyme inhibitors and angiotensin II–receptor blockers is contraindicated during pregnancy.**

Bibliography

Cooper WO, Hernandez-Diaz S, Arbogast PG, et al. Major congenital malformations after first-trimester exposure to ACE inhibitors. N Engl J Med. 2006;354(23):2443-2451. [PMID: 16760444]

Item 14   Answer: A

Educational Objective: Treat supraventricular arrhythmia in pregnancy.

Maternal arrhythmias during pregnancy may jeopardize the health of both mother and fetus. The correct identification of the arrhythmia is critical. Treatment is indicated for arrhythmias that are hemodynamically unstable or cause debilitating symptoms. Few drugs are approved specifically for use during pregnancy. When medications are necessary, the physician should use as few drugs as possible at the lowest effective dose and choose drugs with a history of safe use in pregnancy.

The electrocardiogram demonstrates a narrow-complex tachycardia. The patient has symptoms but is hemodynamically stable; therefore, medical therapy is recommended initially. Adenosine is the drug of choice for narrow-complex tachycardia presenting during pregnancy. Adenosine is classified as a U.S. Food and Drug Administration (FDA) pregnancy risk category C drug, and animal reproduction studies have shown adverse fetal effects. In making the decision to administer this drug during pregnancy, the potential risks to the fetus must be weighed against the potential benefits to the mother.

Intravenous amiodarone can be used in patients with atrial or ventricular arrhythmias during pregnancy that are not controlled by other medications. Amiodarone is classified as an FDA pregnancy risk category D drug. Amiodarone crosses the placenta, affecting fetal heart rate and causing fetal hypothyroidism or goiter. Amiodarone is only used when absolutely mandatory during pregnancy. It would not be appropriate to use amiodarone in this patient while safer medication options exist.

Digoxin is classified as a pregnancy risk category C drug. Digoxin readily passes to the fetal circulation; however, no teratogenic effect has been reported in humans. Digoxin is often used as a maintenance medication in patients with atrial arrhythmias or other cardiac disorders during pregnancy and is generally well tolerated. It has also been used to treat fetal arrhythmias. However, it is unlikely that intravenous digoxin would convert a supraventricular tachycardia.

Diltiazem is classified as a pregnancy risk category C drug. Use of diltiazem in pregnancy should be restricted to patients in whom therapeutic benefits outweigh the potential risk to the fetus. Diltiazem is effective in slowing ventricular response to atrial fibrillation or atrial flutter. It is also used for atrioventricular reentrant tachycardia. However, diltiazem decreases blood pressure and may cause maternal hypotension, particularly when administered as an intravenous infusion. Diltiazem thus would not be the drug of choice in this pregnant patient.

Metoprolol is classified as a pregnancy risk category C drug. Metoprolol is often used in patients with supraventricular tachycardia during pregnancy, but would be less likely to convert this narrow-complex tachycardia than adenosine. In addition, it would further decrease the patient's blood pressure. Metoprolol is considered safe to use during pregnancy, but may cause intrauterine growth retardation, fetal bradycardia, polycythemia, hyperbilirubinemia, and prolonged labor. However, oral β-blockers and calcium-channel blockers are often used for chronic therapy of recurrent supraventricular arrhythmias during pregnancy.

> **KEY POINT**
>
> - Adenosine is the treatment of choice for a hemodynamically stable supraventricular tachycardia that occurs during pregnancy.

Bibliography

Elkayam U, Goodwin TM. Adenosine therapy for supraventricular tachycardia during pregnancy. Am J Cardiol. 1995;75(7):521-523. [PMID: 7864004]

Item 15   Answer: C

Educational Objective: Manage asymptomatic abdominal aortic aneurysm found on routine screening.

Abdominal aortic aneurysms are an important and treatable cause of mortality, and risk factors such as male sex, smoking history, and aging have been well established. This patient has an asymptomatic small infrarenal aortic aneurysm found on appropriate screening for a man older than 65 years who had previously smoked. Larger aneurysms expand more rapidly, and the rate of growth is important in clinical decision-making regarding intervention. Therefore, the larger the aneurysm is at index detection, the sooner follow-up surveillance should be performed. Two large prospective studies have documented the safety of semi-annual surveillance in patients with aneurysms from 4.0 to 5.4 cm in diameter. Data from the UK Small Aneurysm Trial suggest that a surveillance interval of 24 months may be more appropriate for aneurysms smaller than 4 cm.

An abdominal CT scan with intravenous contrast would clearly demonstrate the aneurysm; however, it would not affect current treatment for this patient and would expose him to unnecessary radiation and the risks of an iodinated contrast agent.

There is no indication for antithrombotic therapy in the treatment of this patient's aneurysm. However, antiplatelet therapy should be considered for cardiovascular primary prevention. Data from several large trials, taken together, suggest benefit of aspirin in middle-aged men for prevention of a first myocardial infarction.

In asymptomatic patients, repair is indicated for aneurysms with a transverse diameter of 5.5 cm or larger, or those demonstrating an expansion rate of more than 0.5 cm/year. In this patient with a 4-cm aneurysm, there is no indication for either surgical or endovascular repair

at this time, and the focus should be on surveillance and medical therapy.

This patient has hyperlipidemia and hypertension, and treatment for these conditions is indicated regardless of the aneurysm. Evidence from small randomized trials suggests that statins may inhibit aneurysm expansion. Observational human data suggest that angiotensin-converting enzyme (ACE) polymorphisms may predispose to risk of aneurysm formation, making ACE inhibitors potentially attractive for treatment of hypertension in patients with risk factors for aortic aneurysm. Animal studies with ACE inhibitors and angiotensin receptor blockers have shown a decrease in the rate of aneurysm expansion, but this has not been demonstrated in humans.

> **KEY POINT**
>
> - For asymptomatic abdominal aortic aneurysms 4.0 to 5.4 cm in diameter, an ultrasound surveillance interval of 6 months has been shown to be safe.

Bibliography

Baxter BT, Terrin MC, Dalman RL. Medical management of small abdominal aortic aneurysms. Circulation. 2008;117(14):1883-1889. [PMID: 18391122]

Item 16   Answer: D

Educational Objective: Treat a patient with non–ST-elevation myocardial infarction experiencing ongoing pain despite standard medical therapy.

This patient's elevated troponin value and ST-segment depression and T-wave inversions on electrocardiogram are indicative of a non–ST-elevation myocardial infarction (NSTEMI). After the initiation of aggressive medical therapy, she experiences recurrent symptoms. This is an appropriate indication to add a glycoprotein IIb/IIIa inhibitor to standard medical therapy. Patients undergoing early coronary angiography in this setting also derive benefit from a glycoprotein IIb/IIIa inhibitor. Glycoprotein IIb/IIIa inhibitors may also be considered in patients with dynamic electrocardiographic changes, diabetes mellitus, or heart failure. This patient has a TIMI risk score of 3. While patients with an elevated TIMI risk score derive benefit from glycoprotein IIb/IIIa inhibitors, these agents should not be withheld for patients with ongoing anginal symptoms and a low TIMI risk score. The main side effect of these agents is increased bleeding events.

Both β-blockers and calcium channel blockers are effective anti-anginal medications. β-Blockers are first-line therapy for unstable angina and NSTEMI unless contraindications are present. With ongoing angina, a calcium channel blocker can be added to a β-blocker. However, there is no benefit in substituting a calcium channel blocker for a β-blocker in the absence of significant side effects.

The decision to use low-molecular-weight heparin versus unfractionated heparin is multifactorial and related to the presence of renal insufficiency (low-molecular-weight heparin is contraindicated if creatinine clearance is less than 30 mL/min) and the timing of coronary angiography. However, for patients initially started on low-molecular-weight heparin, there would be no indication and no benefit to changing to unfractionated heparin.

Recent studies have suggested the possibility that angiotensin-converting enzyme inhibitors may be effective in reducing exercise-induced ischemia. The studies are small and the data are conflicting, however, and in any event, do not apply to a patient with ongoing chest pain due to an acute coronary syndrome.

KEY POINT

- Glycoprotein IIb/IIIa inhibitors should be added to standard anti-anginal and antithrombotic therapy in patients with unstable angina or non–ST-elevation myocardial infarction with ongoing anginal symptoms.

Bibliography

Anderson JL, Adams CD, Antman EM, et al. ACC/AHA 2007 guidelines for the management of patients with unstable angina/non-ST-Elevation myocardial infarction: a report of the American College of Cardiology/American Heart Association Task Force on Practice Guidelines (Writing Committee to Revise the 2002 Guidelines for the Management of Patients With Unstable Angina/Non-ST-Elevation Myocardial Infarction) developed in collaboration with the American College of Emergency Physicians, the Society for Cardiovascular Angiography and Interventions, and the Society of Thoracic Surgeons endorsed by the American Association of Cardiovascular and Pulmonary Rehabilitation and the Society for Academic Emergency Medicine [erratum in J Am Coll Cardiol. 2008;51(9):974.]. J Am Coll Cardiol. 2007;50(7):e1-e157. [PMID: 17692738]

Item 17   Answer: B

Educational Objective: Manage anticoagulation therapy in a patient with a non–ST-elevation myocardial infarction.

This patient's electrocardiographic findings and elevated troponin levels indicate that she is having a non–ST-elevation myocardial infarction (NSTEMI). Medical management for NSTEMI includes aspirin, β-blockers, nitrates, and anticoagulants. Recent randomized trials have shown that full-dose low-molecular-weight heparin is more effective than full-dose unfractionated heparin without an increase in bleeding events. The advantages of low-molecular-weight heparin include ease of dosing (subcutaneous route) and achievement of predictable levels of anticoagulation without the need for monitoring. However, low-molecular-weight heparin is renally excreted, and if estimated glomerular filtration rate is below 30 mL/min/1.73 m^2, the level of anti–factor Xa activity is increased, resulting in increased bleeding events. Full-dose unfractionated heparin is, therefore, preferable to full-dose low-molecular-weight heparin in patients with renal insufficiency.

Low-dose unfractionated heparin and low-dose low-molecular-weight heparin do not achieve sufficient systemic levels and therefore do not provide a benefit for patients with NSTEMI.

KEY POINT

- Low-molecular-weight heparin is contraindicated in patients with renal insufficiency and estimated glomerular filtration rate below 30 mL/min/1.73 m^2.

Bibliography

Lim W, Dentali F, Eikelboom JW, Crowther MA. Meta-analysis: low-molecular-weight heparin and bleeding in patients with severe renal insufficiency. Ann Intern Med. 2006;144(9):673-684. [PMID: 16670137]

Item 18   Answer: A

Educational Objective: Treat left atrial myxoma.

This patient has evidence of a systemic embolism to the left kidney causing flank pain and hematuria. No evidence of renal calculi is present. The history of fever, night sweats, and weight loss is consistent with a systemic illness. Echocardiography shows a left atrial mass with features consistent with a tumor, as evidenced by attachment to the atrial septum, echogenic texture, mobility, and protrusion into the mitral valve orifice obstructing inflow. This mass is most likely a left atrial myxoma, the most common tumor type of the left atrium. A left atrial myxoma does not metastasize to other organs, but it has significant associated morbidity. Left atrial myxoma causes fever, night sweats, and weight loss, and may embolize to the brain or other organs such as the kidney, as seen in this patient. Cardiac surgery to remove the left atrial mass is the best treatment and would be curative if the mass is a benign tumor. A primary malignant tumor is also a possibility, but surgical removal would also be the correct approach.

Echocardiography in this patient shows severe transmitral valve obstruction with a mean gradient of 15 mm Hg. Rheumatic mitral stenosis on auscultation can cause an early high-pitched diastolic sound (an opening snap) and a diastolic decrescendo murmur, similar to the findings in this patient. However, the opening sound in this patient is a low-pitched sound associated with a left atrial myxoma, a so-called "tumor plop." Furthermore, the patient's echocardiogram is inconsistent with primary mitral valve disease. The diastolic murmur in this patient is secondary to obstruction of the mitral valve orifice by the tumor, effectively a functional mitral stenosis. Thus, the appropriate cardiac surgery is removal of the left atrial mass rather than mitral valve replacement.

The left atrial mass is highly unlikely to be a thrombus given the presence of sinus rhythm and not atrial fibrillation. Systemic anticoagulation with heparin is not indicated.

The presentation of fever, night sweats, and weight loss is typical of endocarditis, and thus this diagnosis should be considered. However, blood cultures failed to confirm bacteremia, and echocardiography showed no vegetations. Empiric antibiotic therapy with vancomycin and tobramycin for presumed endocarditis in this patient who is hemodynamically stable and has an alternative explanation for her symptoms is not warranted.

Bibliography

D'Alfonso A, Catania S, Pierri MD, et al. Atrial myxoma: a 25-year single-institutional follow-up study. J Cardiovasc Med (Hagerstown). 2008;9(2):178-181. [PMID: 18192811]

Item 19 Answer: C
Educational Objective: Treat a patient presenting late with an ST-elevation myocardial infarction.

This patient is presenting late (>12 hours from onset of symptoms) with an ST-elevation myocardial infarction (STEMI). Reperfusion strategies for STEMI patients include either thrombolytic therapy or primary percutaneous coronary intervention (PCI). Most STEMI patients in the United States present to hospitals without on-site PCI capabilities; thrombolytic therapy is thus the main form of reperfusion used. However, thrombolytic therapy has not shown a clear benefit for patients presenting more than 12 hours from symptom onset. In this patient, therefore, coronary angiography and primary PCI are indicated as the treatment of choice for a patient presenting with ongoing chest pain more than 12 hours after onset of symptoms. Primary PCI is also useful for STEMI patients with contraindications to thrombolytic therapy, such as prior intracerebral hemorrhage, ischemic stroke within 3 months, suspected aortic dissection, or active bleeding.

An echocardiogram is occasionally useful in the management of patients presenting with chest pain and a nondiagnostic electrocardiogram (ECG). A focal wall motion abnormality suggests a cardiac basis to the symptoms. In this patient presenting with a late STEMI and a markedly abnormal ECG with ST-segment elevation, however, echocardiography would not add to the management.

A chest CT can be a useful diagnostic tool in patients being evaluated for chest pain if there is a high clinical suspicion for an aortic dissection. This patient described "crushing" chest pain that is not radiating to the back, blood pressures are normal and symmetric bilaterally, and the electrocardiogram shows ST-segment elevation. Given these factors, the possibility of an acute aortic dissection is extremely low, and further imaging with a chest CT would likely not add to the management and would further delay treatment for the STEMI.

Bibliography

Antman EM, Hand M, Armstrong PW, et al. 2007 Focused Update of the ACC/AHA 2004 Guidelines for the Management of Patients With ST-Elevation Myocardial Infarction: a report of the American College of Cardiology/American Heart Association Task Force on Practice Guidelines: developed in collaboration with the Canadian Cardiovascular Society endorsed by the American Academy of Family Physicians: 2007 Writing Group to Review New Evidence and Update the ACC/AHA 2004 Guidelines for the Management of Patients With ST-Elevation Myocardial Infarction, Writing on Behalf of the 2004 Writing Committee [erratum in Circulation. 2008;117(6):e162.]. Circulation. 2008;117(2):296-329. [PMID: 18071078]

Item 20 Answer: A
Educational Objective: Manage infective endocarditis with paravalvular extension.

This patient has aortic valve endocarditis. There is echocardiographic evidence of paravalvular extension with abscess (echolucency) and color Doppler evidence of an aorto-cavitary fistula from the aortic root to the right ventricle. Emergent surgery for endocarditis is indicated when there is hemodynamic instability, valvular destruction, or paravalvular extension, and should not be delayed while the acute infection is cleared. Additional factors favoring earlier surgical intervention include significant heart failure, resistant infections, vegetations greater than 1 cm in diameter (which pose an embolic risk), and recurrent distal emboli. This patient has paravalvular extension and manifestations of heart failure and therefore meets the criteria for emergent surgery. Paravalvular extension complicates up to 40% of native valve endocarditis, and most often occurs at the weakest portion of the valve annulus, near the membranous interventricular septum. In some patients, conduction abnormalities can occur if there is involvement of the atrioventricular node.

Broadening antibiotic coverage for this patient is not indicated. The culprit organism, *Staphylococcus aureus*, is covered by the antibiotics currently prescribed, and antibiotic treatment alone will not be adequate to fully clear the infection for endocarditis complicated by paravalvular abscess. Following surgery, however, antibiotics should be continued for at least 4 to 6 weeks to ensure clearance of the infection.

The use of aspirin to prevent embolization is of no benefit in patients with infective endocarditis. In one randomized trial, aspirin did not reduce the incidence of embolic events, but there was a trend toward excess bleeding.

An intra-aortic balloon pump for hemodynamic support is contraindicated in the settings of aortic regurgitation or aortic fistulous communication with the right ventricle because diastolic inflation of the balloon pump would exacerbate regurgitation severity. This patient requires surgery to repair the fistula, debride the paravalvular abscess, and replace the native valve.

Although preoperative coronary angiography would normally be ideal to exclude coronary artery disease prior to cardiac surgery, it would portend prohibitive risk in this patient. Placement of angiography catheters in the vicinity of the aortic root abnormalities already present would increase the risk of additional rupture or damage. The patient is young and has few clinical atherosclerotic risk factors, making the yield of coronary angiography low and the risk unnecessary.

> **KEY POINT**
>
> - Surgery for infective endocarditis is indicated if there is significant hemodynamic instability or paravalvular extension and should be considered if there is heart failure, resistant infections, or large mobile vegetations.

Bibliography

Chan KL, Tam J, Dumesnil JG, et al. Effect of long-term aspirin use on embolic events in infective endocarditis. Clin Infect Dis. 2008;46(1):37-41. [PMID: 18171211]

Item 21   Answer: D

Educational Objective: Treat elevated LDL cholesterol in the presence of other cardiovascular risk factors.

This patient has multiple risk factors for coronary artery disease (CAD), including diabetes mellitus, hypertension, and hypercholesterolemia. Given his age and risk factors, he is at high risk (20%) of having a CAD event within the next 10 years. The goal LDL cholesterol level for a patient with two or more risk factors for CAD is dependent on the 10-year risk for a CAD event based upon the Framingham risk equation. In patients with two or more risk factors and with an intermediate (10%-20%) 10-year risk, the goal LDL cholesterol level is below 130 mg/dL (3.4 mmol/L). However, in patients with two or more risk factors and a high risk (>20%) of a CAD event, the goal LDL cholesterol level is below 100 mg/dL (2.6 mmol/L). A statin is the first-line treatment for cholesterol reduction. Given the degree of LDL cholesterol reduction required to achieve this goal level in this patient (a 30% reduction), a 40-mg daily dose of simvastatin would likely be required for this reduction.

Colestipol interrupts bile acid reabsorption and reduces LDL cholesterol levels by 10% to 15%. It is often used as a second-line drug with statins because it acts synergistically to induce LDL receptors. However, it can interfere with the absorption of this patient's other medications, and for these reasons, is not the best initial management of his hyperlipidemia.

Although ezetimibe reduces LDL cholesterol levels by reducing cholesterol absorption from the intestine, there are presently no clinical trial results showing that this medication reduces cardiovascular disease events, in contrast to statins, such as simvastatin. Therefore, ezetimibe should be reserved as an adjunct to other cholesterol-lowering medications if goal level is not achieved or for patients intolerant or allergic to other proven medications.

Niacin is an effective medication for lowering LDL cholesterol and increasing HDL levels but is often not tolerated because of its side effects (nausea and flushing), particularly at the dosage needed to achieve adequate reduction of LDL cholesterol. Niacin would be a poor choice for this patient because it can cause glucose intolerance, potentially worsening his glucose control.

> **KEY POINT**
>
> - The indication to initiate cholesterol-lowering medication as well as the goal level for treatment are dependent on the absolute level of LDL cholesterol and the estimated 10-year risk for a coronary artery disease event.

Bibliography

Grundy SM, Cleeman JI, Merz CN, et al; National Heart, Lung, and Blood Institute; American College of Cardiology Foundation; American Heart Association. Implications of recent clinical trials for the National Cholesterol Education Program Adult Treatment Panel III guidelines [erratum in Circulation. 2004;110(6):763.]. Circulation. 2004;110(2):227-239. [PMID: 15249516]

Item 22   Answer: C

Educational Objective: Evaluate a patient with chest pain, a normal electrocardiogram, and normal cardiac enzymes.

Patients presenting with chest pain require careful assessment. The first step in the diagnosis of coronary artery disease (CAD) is to estimate the pretest probability of disease. The Diamond and Forrester approach to assessing pretest probability is based on the age and sex of the patient and the character of the symptoms. Noninvasive stress tests for detecting CAD perform best in patients with an intermediate pretest probability of disease. In patients with a high pretest probability of disease, a negative test result is most likely to be falsely negative. In that setting, coronary angiography may be required. In patients with a low pretest probability, a positive stress test result is likely to be falsely positive.

The patient presented has several cardiac risk factors and his description of chest pain is most consistent with atypical angina, placing him at intermediate pretest probability of having CAD. In this setting, it is appropriate to begin antianginal therapy and schedule an exercise stress test to confirm the diagnosis of CAD. Admission to the hospital is not required, as the probability of adverse cardiovascular events (death or nonfatal myocardial infarction) is low. Coronary angiography is not indicated at this point because the pretest probability of CAD is not high enough to warrant an invasive procedure.

For patients with multiple cardiac risk factors and chest pain, a cardiac evaluation should be performed prior to proceeding with other diagnostic testing. Although a trial with a proton pump inhibitor may be required at a later date to diagnose gastroesophageal reflux disease (GERD) causing chest symptoms, ruling out a cardiac basis for the current symptoms should be done first. In the absence of alarm features, esophagogastroduodenoscopy is not the first test of choice to evaluate possible GERD or dyspepsia symptoms.

> **KEY POINT**
>
> - Noninvasive stress tests for detecting coronary artery disease perform best in patients with an intermediate pretest probability of disease.

Bibliography

Anderson JL, Adams CD, Antman EM, et al. ACC/AHA 2007 guidelines for the management of patients with unstable angina/non-ST-Elevation myocardial infarction: a report of the American College of Cardiology/American Heart Association Task Force on Practice Guidelines (Writing Committee to Revise the 2002 Guidelines for the Management of Patients With Unstable Angina/Non-ST-Elevation Myocardial Infarction) developed in collaboration with the American College of Emergency Physicians, the Society for Cardiovascular Angiography and Interventions, and the Society of Thoracic Surgeons endorsed by the American Association of Cardiovascular and Pulmonary Rehabilitation and the Society for Academic Emergency Medicine [erratum in J Am Coll Cardiol. 2008;51(9):974.]. J Am Coll Cardiol. 2007;50(7):e1-e157. [PMID: 17692738]

Item 23   Answer: C

Educational Objective: Treat restrictive cardiomyopathy caused by acquired hemochromatosis.

This patient has signs and symptoms of heart failure, particularly of the right side of the heart (peripheral edema, jugular venous distention, and Kussmaul sign or inspiratory increase in jugular venous distention). Disproportionate involvement of the right side of the heart should always raise the suspicion for restrictive cardiomyopathy, particularly in a patient at risk for iron overload. This patient's iron studies confirm an acquired iron-overload state, or acquired hemochromatosis.

Hemochromatosis is the only cause of restrictive cardiomyopathy that is potentially reversible by medication therapy that induces regression of symptoms. Because the body lacks an intrinsic method of increasing elimination of excessive iron, therapeutic methods are needed. Restrictive cardiomyopathy from iron overload may improve with removal of iron by chelation therapy in iron-overload states, such as lifelong transfusion-dependent anemias. Iron chelation therapy is indicated only in patients who cannot tolerate phlebotomy therapy, such as those with significant anemia. Iron chelation therapy would be the most appropriate treatment in this patient.

Iron overload secondary to multiple blood transfusions in the treatment of sickle cell anemia is a recognized cause of acquired hemochromatosis. Other causes of acquired iron overload include parenteral iron supplementation and hematologic disorders with ineffective erythropoiesis or increased erythrocyte turnover, such as thalassemia major, sideroblastic anemia, and hereditary spherocytosis.

Echocardiographic findings in this patient are consistent with restrictive cardiomyopathy, as evidenced by restrictive left ventricular filling without respiratory variation in peak filling velocity, biatrial enlargement, and preserved ventricular systolic function. Infiltration of the myocardium by iron would account for the cardiomyopathy. Endomyocardial biopsy is positive for iron deposition in this patient, but this biopsy finding is not invariably present because iron deposition is often predominantly in the epicardial layer. Thus, a negative endomyocardial biopsy would not exclude myocardial iron infiltration.

Heart transplant has been used with variable results for treatment of refractory cases of restrictive cardiomyopathy due to hereditary hemochromatosis. Heart transplant has not been studied and is not of proven benefit in restrictive cardiomyopathy from acquired hemochromatosis. In addition, in this setting the ongoing need for blood transfusions would subject the transplanted heart to iron deposition.

Diuretic therapy plays a major role in the symptomatic treatment of patients with restrictive cardiomyopathy. Importantly, because of these patients' pathophysiologic dependence on maintaining higher atrial pressures (preload) to achieve adequate ventricular filling, excessive diuresis often results in orthostatic hypotension by lowering atrial pressures. This patient has evidence of orthostatic hypotension that is probably related to his diuretic therapy. Thus, increasing furosemide (a loop diuretic) would not be the best treatment for this patient.

Hereditary hemochromatosis is a storage disease from iron overload due to increased intestinal absorption. Excessive deposition into organs such as the heart results in the disease manifestations. In hereditary forms of hemochromatosis, iron overload is appropriately treated by phlebotomy. Phlebotomy effectively removes excess iron and circumvents the need for chelation therapy. However, phlebotomy would not be appropriate for this patient with acquired hemochromatosis and sickle cell anemia. Phlebotomy would exacerbate anemia in patients with sickle cell anemia, and thus is not a feasible treatment option.

> **KEY POINT**
>
> - Iron chelation therapy can be effective in the treatment of restrictive cardiomyopathy from acquired hemochromatosis in patients who cannot tolerate phlebotomy therapy.

Bibliography

Madani TA, Bormanis J. Reversible severe hereditary hemochromatotic cardiomyopathy. Can J Cardiol. 1997;13(4):391-4. [PMID: 9141972]

Item 24   Answer: E
Educational Objective: Manage an asymptomatic murmur.

This patient has a benign midsystolic murmur that is grade 2/6 in intensity. Midsystolic murmurs grade 2/6 or less are considered innocent murmurs, especially when they are short in duration, associated with a physiologically split (normal) S_2, and are not accompanied by any other abnormal cardiac sounds or murmurs. The most common etiology of this type of murmur in persons older than 65 years is minor valvular abnormalities due to aortic sclerosis. Aortic sclerosis is characterized by focal areas of valve thickening leading to mild valvular turbulence, producing the auscultated murmur. A hyperdynamic circulation (for example, from severe anemia, thyrotoxicosis, or pregnancy) also may produce an innocent midsystolic pulmonary or aortic flow murmur. A physiologically split S_2 (no delay in the aortic component of S_2) excludes severe aortic stenosis as a diagnosis.

This patient is physically active, and her only symptoms are consistent with premature ventricular contractions not increasing in intensity or frequency. Further diagnostic testing is not warranted. Transthoracic echocardiography is indicated when a grade 3/6 or greater systolic murmur is heard on examination, in the presence of any diastolic or continuous murmur, or if a new murmur is diagnosed in the interval since a normal prior physical examination; none of these criteria are met by this patient. A screening cardiac stress test is not warranted because she has no symptoms indicative of angina or risk factors for coronary artery disease. In a patient with a low pretest probability of coronary artery disease, an exercise stress test would carry a high false-positive rate.

Endocarditis prophylaxis is not indicated. According to current American Heart Association guidelines, the only patients who should receive endocarditis prophylaxis are those with prosthetic cardiac valves, those with a known history of prior infective endocarditis, those with unrepaired cyanotic congenital heart disease, those with complex congenital heart disease with residual abnormalities, and cardiac transplant recipients with valve abnormalities.

Continuous 24-hour ambulatory electrocardiographic monitoring is useful to identify a cardiac arrhythmia during symptoms of palpitations, syncope, or presyncope during a 24-hour period of time, and can diagnose arrhythmias such as atrial fibrillation, supraventricular arrhythmias, or ventricular ectopy. However, this patient describes rare (approximately every 6 months) "single skipped beats" most consistent with premature ventricular contractions. It is unlikely that this rare event would occur during the 24-hour monitoring period. Regardless, in the absence of other cardiopulmonary symptoms, her isolated beats are most likely a benign condition and do not warrant further diagnostic testing.

KEY POINT
- **Short, soft, midsystolic murmurs in the elderly are usually benign and due to minor, age-related changes of the aortic valve (aortic sclerosis).**

Bibliography
Douglas PS, Khandheria B, Stainback RF, et al. ACCF/ASE/ACEP/ASNC/SCAI/SCCT/SCMR 2007 appropriateness criteria for transthoracic and transesophageal echocardiography: a report of the American College of Cardiology Foundation Quality Strategic Directions Committee Appropriateness Criteria Working Group, American Society of Echocardiography, American College of Emergency Physicians, American Society of Nuclear Cardiology, Society for Cardiovascular Angiography and Interventions, Society of Cardiovascular Computed Tomography, and the Society for Cardiovascular Magnetic Resonance endorsed by the American College of Chest Physicians and the Society of Critical Care Medicine. J Am Coll Cardiol. 2007;50(2):187-204. [PMID: 17616306]

Item 25   Answer: B
Educational Objective: Diagnose acute viral pericarditis.

Specific history and, occasionally, physical examination findings are essential in guiding the diagnostic evaluation of patients who present with severe chest pain, which may signify potentially life-threatening illnesses. Acute viral pericarditis is the most likely diagnosis in this patient who presents with constitutional symptoms (myalgias, malaise), pleuritic chest pain, low-grade fever, pericardial friction rub, lymphocytosis, and ST-segment elevation. Although unusual, the serum troponin level or the MB fraction of creatine kinase may be modestly elevated, indicative of epicardial inflammation.

An acute myocardial infarction is a possible diagnosis in a patient with chest pain, ST-segment elevation, and risk factors for coronary artery disease that include diabetes mellitus, hypertension, tobacco use, and illicit drug use. However, ST-segment elevation in acute myocardial infarction is typically concave downward and not upward, as in this patient. In addition, myocardial infarction would not explain this patient's constitutional symptoms, pericardial friction rub, and lymphocytosis.

Costochondritis is a classic cause of pleuritic chest pain. It is associated with reproducible pain with palpation of the upper costal cartilages at the costochondral or costosternal junctions. However, this diagnosis is unlikely in this patient given the lack of palpable chest wall tenderness and the presence of ST-segment elevation, constitutional symptoms, friction rub, elevated troponin level, and febrile illness.

A viral pleuritis could account for many of this patient's symptoms, such as pleuritic chest pain, low-grade fever, constitutional symptoms, and lymphocytosis. However, it would not explain a pericardial friction rub, elevated troponin level, or ST-segment elevation.

Pulmonary embolism may cause pleuritic chest pain and should be considered in this patient. However, the constitutional symptoms prior to the onset of chest pain would not be explained by this etiology. In addition, ST-segment elevation, pericardial friction rub, and an elevated troponin level would not be expected on the basis of pulmonary embolism.

- Acute viral pericarditis is typically characterized by pleuritic chest pain, fever, pericardial friction rub, lymphocytosis, and ST-segment elevation.

Bibliography

Tingle LE, Molina D, Calvert CW. Acute pericarditis. Am Fam Physician. 2007;76(10):1509-1514. [PMID: 18052017]

Item 26   Answer: D

Educational Objective: Manage a post–myocardial infarction patient with reduced left ventricular ejection fraction.

Results from the DINAMIT trial showed no benefit from cardioverter-defibrillator implantation early after myocardial infarction. For this reason, patients with reduced ejection fraction are not candidates for device placement within 40 days after acute myocardial infarction or immediately after percutaneous or surgical revascularization. This patient underwent primary percutaneous coronary intervention for treatment of acute myocardial infarction; he should be treated medically and reevaluated with a repeat echocardiogram to reassess his ejection fraction and determine his risk for sudden death. In addition, although his ejection fraction is reduced immediately after the myocardial infarction, this finding is likely related to myocardial stunning. He may have substantial improvement in his ejection fraction over the next few months, particularly with angiotensin-converting enzyme (ACE) inhibitor therapy.

In patients with acute myocardial infarction with reduced left ventricular function (ejection fraction ≤40%) and clinical heart failure or diabetes mellitus, and who were on therapeutic doses of a β-blocker and an ACE inhibitor, the addition of eplerenone reduced total mortality and cardiovascular mortality. (Patients with serum creatinine levels of ≥2.5 mg/dL [190.8 μmol/L] or baseline serum potassium levels >5.0 meq/L [5.0 mmol/L] were excluded from the trial.) Since this patient has neither clinical heart failure nor diabetes, treatment with eplerenone is not indicated.

Like ACE inhibitors, angiotensin-receptor blockers can improve clinical outcomes in patients with acute myocardial infarction complicated by clinical heart failure, systolic dysfunction, or both. It is reasonable to initiate therapy with valsartan after myocardial infraction as an alternative to an ACE inhibitor in patients with clinical heart failure and/or a left ventricular ejection fraction less than or equal to 35% who are intolerant of an ACE inhibitor. Clinical studies have not demonstrated that the combination of captopril and valsartan improves survival, and the combination is associated with an increased incidence of side effects.

- Post–myocardial infarction patients with reduced ejection fraction are not candidates for implantable cardioverter-defibrillator placement until 40 days after infarction.

Bibliography

Hohnloser SH, Kuck KH, Dorian P, et al; DINAMIT Investigators. Prophylactic use of an implantable cardioverter-defibrillator after acute myocardial infarction. N Engl J Med. 2004;351(24):2481-2488. [PMID: 15590950]

Item 27   Answer: E

Educational Objective: Diagnose atypical chest pain in a patient with an intermediate risk of coronary artery disease.

This 59-year-old man with atypical chest pain and coronary artery disease (CAD) risk factors of hypertension and hypercholesterolemia has an intermediate risk of a coronary event (a 10%-20% 10-year risk based on the Framingham risk score). His electrocardiogram and cardiac enzyme results are not consistent with an acute coronary syndrome, so the most appropriate next step in management is a stress test to evaluate for the presence and severity of CAD. However, owing to his knee injury, a pharmacologic stress test, rather than an exercise stress test, is required. A "negative" exercise stress study result is not useful for diagnosis unless the patient works at a level of at least 85% of the maximum predicted heart rate because ischemia will be missed at lower workloads. Thus, a pharmacologic stress test with imaging is most appropriate in this patient—either a nuclear perfusion imaging stress test or an echocardiographic stress test.

Adenosine positron emission tomography (PET) stress testing is more sensitive (91%) and specific (92%) than thallium single photon emission computed tomography (SPECT) nuclear perfusion imaging (87% sensitivity and 77% specificity). PET stress testing is particularly valuable in overweight and obese patients because of better image quality in larger patients. However, this patient has a normal BMI, so a standard nuclear perfusion stress test is appropriate. Currently, PET stress testing is not widely available.

Cardiac catheterization and angiography would be appropriate as the initial diagnostic approach in the setting of an acute coronary syndrome defined by ST-segment elevation on electrocardiography and elevated cardiac enzyme levels. Patients who present with ischemic chest pain but without diagnostic ST-segment elevation are categorized as having unstable angina or non–ST-elevation myocardial infarction (NSTEMI). These two conditions are closely related and have similar pathophysiology and clinical presentations, but they differ in the severity of the myocardial ischemia. Patients with either condition typically present with angina at rest; some patients describe a pattern of new-onset or increasing angina. In NSTEMI, ischemia is severe and results in a detectable release of biomarkers of myocardial injury within hours. In unstable angina, there is no detectable increase in these enzymes. However, because unstable angina and NSTEMI may be indistinguishable at the time of the initial presentation, principles of risk stratification and management apply to both entities and may include coronary angiography. This patient does not have either condition, so coronary angiography is not indicated.

Current guidelines indicate that coronary artery calcium (CAC) scores are reasonable in asymptomatic patients at intermediate risk of coronary artery disease in order to refine the risk stratification to determine the appropriate intensity of risk factor reduction. However, CAC scores are not a functional study of coronary ischemia and are not a substitute for noninvasive testing to determine if chest pain is caused by CAD.

CT coronary angiography can provide detailed images of the proximal coronary anatomy, and the role of CT coronary angiography in the emergency department is under study, particularly because of its utility in ruling out CAD, aortic dissection, and pulmonary embolism with a single test. However, this patient has symptoms that would best be evaluated by a functional study instead of CT coronary angiography. In addition, CT coronary angiography requires a high resolution scan, intravenous contrast, and significant radiation exposure and is not an appropriate test for a patient with low or intermediate probability of coronary artery disease.

KEY POINT

- **Exercise stress testing is only diagnostic at an adequate workload, defined as achieving 85% of the maximum predicted heart rate.**

Bibliography

Breen DP. Stress tests: how to make a calculated choice. J Fam Pract. 2007;56(4):287-93. [PMID: 17403327]

Item 28   Answer: C

Educational Objective: Treat medically refractory angina.

This patient is best classified as having medically refractory angina. He is on maximal medical therapy and is not a candidate for either percutaneous or surgical revascularization. Therapeutic options include external enhanced counterpulsation (EECP) and spinal cord stimulation. Of the options provided, EECP is the best choice for managing this patient's angina. EECP uses three sets of pneumatic cuffs wrapped around the lower extremities to achieve a hemodynamic effect that is similar to an intra-aortic balloon pump and is associated with an improvement in angina and exercise capacity. Contraindications to EECP include severe aortic regurgitation and severe peripheral vascular disease.

Spinal cord stimulation involves placement of an electro-catheter within the epidural space that is connected to a pulse generator and stimulates the spinal cord region receiving the cardiac nerve fibers. In a placebo-controlled trial, spinal cord stimulation was shown to reduce angina and improve functional status. Spinal cord stimulation would also be a reasonable option for this patient with medically refractory angina.

Clopidogrel is a reasonable alternative to aspirin in the treatment of chronic stable angina, although it is significantly more expensive and increases the risk of bleeding. Among high-risk subjects, clopidogrel resulted in a greater reduction in the risk for major cardiovascular events than aspirin, although the incremental benefit was small. Ticlopidine has not been shown to reduce coronary events or improve symptoms.

Calcium-channel blockers are second-line agents for stable angina. They are used in addition to β-blockers if symptoms persist or instead of β-blockers if unacceptable side effects supervene. Short-acting nifedipine is not recommended because of the increased risk of adverse cardiovascular events. Additionally, the use of two calcium-blocking agents is not more effective than appropriate doses of a single agent.

β-Blockers are first-line agents in patients with stable angina. However, symptomatic bradycardia, pre-existing second- or third-degree atrioventricular block, sick sinus syndrome, and symptomatic left ventricular failure are absolute contraindications. Severe asthma, severe depression, and severe peripheral vascular disease are relative contraindications. All β-blockers appear equally effective in treating angina, but their use is limited by the development of hypotension or bradycardia. With the patient's heart rate at 48/min, additional β-blockade is not indicated.

KEY POINT

- **Alternative therapies for patients with medically refractory angina, such as external enhanced counterpulsation, are appropriate after medical therapy is optimized and complete percutaneous and/or surgical coronary revascularization has been achieved.**

Bibliography

Michaels AD, Linnemeier G, Soran O, Kelsey SF, Kennard ED. Two-year outcomes after enhanced external counterpulsation for stable angina pectoris (from the International EECP Patient Registry [IEPR]). Am J Cardiol. 2004;93(4):461-464. [PMID: 14969624]

Item 29   Answer: D

Educational Objective: Treat symptomatic recurrent atrial flutter.

This patient has recurrent atrial flutter (AFL) that is symptomatic despite reasonable rate control at rest. "Typical" AFL is a macroreentrant circuit that rotates counter-clockwise around the tricuspid valve. The atrial cycle length is 250 to

300 msec, and negative "saw-tooth" deflections are seen in the inferior leads. The dyspnea on exertion may be due to AFL or to inadequate rate control with exercise. It is notoriously difficult to achieve rate control with AFL. Often, as in this patient, the doses of atrioventricular (AV) nodal blocking medications required for adequate rate control in AFL cause symptomatic bradycardia during sinus rhythm. Antiarrhythmic medications, such as flecainide or amiodarone, are an option, but their efficacy is limited. Radiofrequency ablation of typical AFL has a long-term success rate of greater than 90% and a risk of complications of 1% to 2%, and is the most appropriate treatment for this patient.

The addition of digoxin would further slow conduction during flutter and sinus rhythm at rest, but would not provide enhanced rate control during activity because of its vagotonic mechanism of action. Digoxin has no antiarrhythmic benefit over other AV nodal blocking agents.

Flecainide should not be used as a single agent in patients with AFL. It can enhance AV nodal conduction, which may cause 1:1 transmission of AFL waves and result in ventricular fibrillation. Flecainide may be used in conjunction with AV nodal blocking agents, such as a β-blocker or a nondihydropyridine calcium channel blocker. The actual efficacy rate of flecainide in the long-term maintenance of sinus rhythm in patients with atrial flutter, however, is unclear. In atrial fibrillation, the recurrence rate is approximately 30% per year.

Amiodarone is a more effective antiarrhythmic agent than class I agents such as flecainide or other class III agents. However, in comparison with radiofrequency ablation, the high risk of thyroid, lung, and liver toxicity presents an adverse risk/benefit ratio in this setting. A small prospective, randomized trial revealed improved efficacy and reduced complications with radiofrequency ablation compared with amiodarone in the treatment of AFL. Notably, in both groups, there was a substantial rate of incident atrial fibrillation.

KEY POINT

- **Radiofrequency ablation of recurrent atrial flutter is highly successful with a low risk of complications and recurrence.**

Bibliography

Da Costa A, Thévenin J, Roche F, et al. Results from the Loire-Ardèche-Drôme-Isère-Puy-de-Dôme (LADIP) trial on atrial flutter, a multicentric prospective randomized trial comparing amiodarone and radiofrequency ablation after the first episode of symptomatic atrial flutter. Circulation. 2006;114(16):1676–1681. [PMID: 17030680]

Item 30   Answer: B

Educational Objective: Treat acute aortic intramural hematoma.

The abrupt onset of severe chest pain is consistent with acute aortic disease. The CT scan findings for this patient are characteristic of an acute distal (type B) intramural hematoma. Analgesia is imperative in the treatment of acute aortic syndromes, as pain control is integral in management of blood pressure and heart rate. Medical management, consisting of control of heart rate with intravenous β-blockade, followed by intravenous administration of a rapidly titratable parenteral arterial vasodilator (such as sodium nitroprusside, fenoldopam, or enalaprilat) is the preferred therapy. Heart rate should be reduced to 60 to 80/min with the use of a parenteral β-blocking agent, such as esmolol, labetalol, or metoprolol. Blood pressure should be lowered to a systolic pressure of 100 to 120 mm Hg, mean arterial pressure of 60 to 75 mm Hg, or the lowest blood pressure commensurate with vital end-organ perfusion.

Certain findings on physical examination, including unequal upper extremity blood pressures and a pulse deficit, increase the likelihood of acute aortic disease (including dissection and intramural hematoma); however, the absence of these findings, as in this patient, should not influence the decision to pursue further diagnostic testing.

Surgical therapy together with medical hemodynamic control would be appropriate for an ascending aortic (type A) hematoma. Whereas endovascular repair has been used for treatment of aortic dissection, there is no current role for endovascular treatment of isolated acute intramural hematoma. Surgical therapy of type B aortic syndromes is associated with significant morbidity and mortality. Endovascular repair or surgical intervention should be considered when distal intramural hematoma arises in association with a deep (≥10 mm) and wide (≥20 mm) penetrating atherosclerotic ulcer.

Aortic hematoma is caused by acute bleeding, possibly from rupture of the vasa vasorum, contained within the media of the aorta. There is no role for anticoagulation as part of management.

With treatment, patients with type B acute intramural hematomas fare as well as, or better than, patients with type B aortic dissection. Over time, intramural hematomas may follow one of three courses: resorption and normalization, aneurysmal dilation, or conversion to typical dissection. Because of this, follow-up surveillance by CT is reasonable.

KEY POINT

- **Medical management of pain, heart rate, and blood pressure is the preferred treatment for type B (distal) acute intramural hematoma.**

Bibliography

Evangelista A, Mukherjee D, Mehta RH, et al; International Registry of Aortic Dissection (IRAD) Investigators. Acute intramural hematoma of the aorta: a mystery in evolution. Circulation. 2005;111(8):1063-1070. [PMID: 15710757]

Item 31　　Answer:　C

Educational Objective: Evaluate recurrent syncope in a patient with a structurally normal heart.

Syncope remains a difficult diagnostic dilemma, particularly in the setting of a structurally normal heart. Syncopal events are common; up to 40% of persons will experience a loss-of-consciousness event in their lifetime, and such events account for 1% to 3% of emergency department visits. Common causes include neurocardiogenic (vasovagal) syncope, bradyarrhythmia, tachyarrhythmia, outflow tract obstruction, and seizures. In patients with underlying heart disease, cardiovascular causes of syncope have been associated with an increased mortality rate. This patient has a structurally normal heart by echocardiogram, no ischemia on exercise testing, and no evidence of an underlying inherited ion channel–associated disorder (long QT, Wolff-Parkinson-White, or Brugada syndrome) on the electrocardiogram. The goal of diagnosis of syncope is, therefore, to prevent injury to the patient from subsequent events and improve quality of life.

The next step in the evaluation of this patient is monitoring for an arrhythmia. The gold standard for diagnosis of an arrhythmic cause of syncope is documentation of a rhythm disturbance at the time of symptom occurrence. The choice of monitoring test should be related to the frequency of the symptoms. This patient has had recurrent, infrequent events; therefore, an implantable loop recorder would be the most likely test to result in a useful finding (either positive or negative). An implanted loop recorder records patient-activated events and automatically records bradycardic and tachycardic events; it is, therefore, significantly less prone to acquisition errors than an event monitor. Implantable loop recorder batteries now last approximately 2 years. The implantable loop recorder has repeatedly been shown to be cost effective and highly likely to result in a useful finding compared with a 24-hour ambulatory monitor or an event monitor. External event monitors are of two types: loop monitors, which are worn and record continuously but only save when the patient activates the monitor, and hand-held event monitors, which must be held to the chest to record. Loop monitors are useful for syncope because patient activation saves data from a short period of time (programmable and varying by company) before the monitor is activated by the patient. Hand-held event monitors are not useful for syncope, since the patient cannot activate the monitor when consciousness is lost.

This patient has had three syncopal events in 3 years. Neither a 24-hour ambulatory monitor nor an event monitor would be a good choice because of the infrequency of the patient's symptoms. He is highly unlikely to have an event during the standard 24 hours of ambulatory monitoring or the standard event monitor duration of 30 days. In addition, event monitors are complex enough in their use that patient acquisition errors can occur, rendering the results less reliable. Some newer event monitor systems do have the capability of automatic recording, and this has been shown to increase diagnostic yield. However, this capability is not likely to improve the diagnostic yield in a patient being monitored for infrequent syncopal episodes.

Electrophysiology study is incorrect because the diagnostic yield for syncope with an otherwise normal evaluation is extremely low.

KEY POINT

- **The implantable loop recorder has been shown to have the greatest diagnostic yield and cost-effectiveness for the evaluation of infrequent syncope in the setting of a structurally normal heart.**

Bibliography

Strickberger SA, Benson DW, Biaggioni I, et al. AHA/ACCF scientific statement on the evaluation of syncope: from the American Heart Association Councils on Clinical Cardiology, Cardiovascular Nursing, Cardiovascular Disease in the Young, and Stroke, and the Quality of Care and Outcomes Research Interdisciplinary Working Group; and the American College of Cardiology Foundation In Collaboration With the Heart Rhythm Society. J Am Coll Cardiol. 2006;47(2):473-484. [PMID: 16412888]

Item 32　　Answer:　B

Educational Objective: Manage a patient with a non–ST-elevation myocardial infarction after diagnostic angiography.

The patient has had a non–ST-elevation myocardial infarction (NSTEMI). The electrocardiogram and results of angiography and left ventriculography are congruent with a small apical infarction that is not amenable to percutaneous coronary intervention (PCI). Further medical therapy, in addition to continuation of the statin, aspirin, and β-blocker, is indicated. The CURE trial demonstrated a significant reduction in the composite endpoint of death, nonfatal myocardial infarction, and stroke in patients with NSTEMI treated with both aspirin and clopidogrel even if they did not undergo PCI. Based on these results, this patient should receive clopidogrel in addition to aspirin, and the clopidogrel should be continued for up to 1 year from the time of discharge. Aspirin should ideally be continued for life in this patient who has had a documented myocardial infarction.

In a patient with NSTEMI who has ongoing or frequently recurrent ischemia and a contraindication to β-blockade, the use of a non-dihydropyridine calcium channel blocker should be considered. Contraindications to the use of a β-blocker, such as shock or atrioventricular block greater than first-degree block, would also be contraindications to the use of verapamil. In patients with active, uncontrolled reactive airways disease, which this patient does not have, verapamil could be considered as second-tier therapy.

The aldosterone antagonist eplerenone has been shown to be effective in reducing all-cause and cardiovascular mortality after myocardial infarction in patients with a left ventricular ejection fraction of 40% or less. Given the lack of heart failure signs or symptoms and the preserved ejection fraction, there is no current indication for the addition of an aldosterone antagonist in this patient.

The combined use of 'mini-dose' warfarin in conjunction with aspirin versus aspirin alone was evaluated in the CHAMP trial. In post–myocardial infarction patients, warfarin therapy (at a mean INR of 1.8) combined with low-dose aspirin did not provide a clinical benefit beyond that achievable with aspirin monotherapy.

KEY POINT

- **Patients who have sustained a non–ST-elevation myocardial infarction benefit from the addition of clopidogrel to aspirin regardless of whether percutaneous coronary intervention was performed.**

Bibliography

Yusuf S, Zhao F, Mehta SR, Chrolavicius S, Tognoni G, Fox KK; Clopidogrel in Unstable Angina to Prevent Recurrent Events Trial Investigators. Effects of clopidogrel in addition to aspirin in patients with acute coronary syndromes without ST-segment elevation [erratum in N Engl J Med. 2001;345(23):1716. and N Engl J Med. 2001;345(20):1506.]. N Engl J Med. 2001;345(7):494-502. [PMID: 11519503]

Item 33   Answer: B

Educational Objective: Treat symptomatic mitral stenosis in a pregnant woman.

This patient recently emigrated from a region where rheumatic fever is prevalent. Her clinical history and physical examination are consistent with rheumatic mitral valve stenosis. Mitral stenosis is usually due to rheumatic valve disease. In the United States, clinical presentation tends to be in the fifth decade, or 20 to 30 years after the initial episode of rheumatic fever, and most cases are in women. Patients with mitral stenosis may be asymptomatic for some time, but become symptomatic with additional hemodynamic stress, such as the increased volume load of pregnancy. This hemodynamic stress may precipitate an arrhythmia, such as atrial fibrillation, that can further exacerbate heart failure symptoms. This patient has atrial fibrillation with increased heart rate. This relative decrease in diastolic filling time contributes to heart failure symptoms. Intravascular volume management with diuretics is essential and will greatly relieve symptoms. A β-blocker should be administered to slow the heart rate, and can be given safely in pregnancy as long as the fetal heart rate is concurrently monitored. Because the patient's underlying ventricular function is normal, she will tolerate β-blockade well. In order to prevent systemic embolization, intravenous unfractionated heparin or therapeutic subcutaneous low-molecular-weight heparin can be used until the infant is delivered, and then warfarin can be initiated and heparin discontinued.

Direct-current cardioversion can be performed during pregnancy without adverse effects to the fetus. If cardioversion were to be performed, transesophageal echocardiography would need to be performed first to exclude a left atrial thrombus to reduce the risk of an embolic stroke. The indication for immediate cardioversion would be hemodynamic instability. In this hemodynamically stable patient, adequate acute diuresis will relieve her symptoms, and long-term maintenance of normal volume status will decrease the risk of respiratory distress during delivery and greatly increase the propensity to remain in sinus rhythm. Therefore, cardioversion is not needed.

In the setting of decompensated rheumatic mitral valve disease, optimization of medical management is preferred over urgent percutaneous mitral balloon valvuloplasty. A transthoracic echocardiogram aids in evaluating the severity of mitral stenosis, pulmonary pressures, involvement of other cardiac valves, and the presence of concurrent mitral regurgitation. If the patient can be treated medically and the pregnancy carried to term, valvuloplasty can be delayed until after delivery to reduce radiation exposure to the fetus and provide an opportunity to reassess the patient. With the decrease in volume load, a previously symptomatic pregnant patient may improve following delivery, delaying or eliminating the need for valvuloplasty. If despite aggressive medical therapy, the pregnant patient remains severely symptomatic, however, percutaneous balloon valvuloplasty may be performed (preferred gestational age >8 weeks) if significant mitral regurgitation is absent and a left atrial thrombus is excluded by transesophageal echocardiography.

Pregnancy induction and delivery should not be undertaken as the initial step in this acutely decompensated patient, but could be considered if symptoms persist following aggressive diuretic and medical therapy.

KEY POINT

- **In acutely decompensated patients with mitral stenosis, medical therapy optimization should be provided initially before contemplating valvuloplasty.**

Bibliography

Esteves CA, Munoz JS, Braga S, et al. Immediate and long-term follow-up of percutaneous balloon mitral valvuloplasty in pregnant patients with rheumatic mitral stenosis. Am J Cardiol. 2006; 98(6):812-816. [PMID: 16950192]

Item 34   Answer: A

Educational Objective: Treat recurrent pericarditis.

This young patient has a history of acute viral pericarditis and presents with pleuritic chest pain and a pericardial friction rub. The likely diagnosis is recurrent pericarditis. The ST-segment elevation on the electrocardiogram is concave upward and PR-segment depression is present, further supporting the diagnosis. Prior treatment of acute viral pericarditis with prednisone predisposes to recurrent pericarditis. Because of its efficacy, colchicine has emerged as the treatment of choice for acute bouts of recurrent pericarditis and can be useful in the prevention of recurrences. Treatment duration is 6 months. Treatment of pericarditis with colchicine is an off-label use. Colchicine is contraindicated in patients with chronic kidney disease. However, this patient has no signs of chronic kidney disease.

High-dose aspirin and NSAIDs are first-line agents for the treatment of an initial episode of viral or idiopathic pericarditis. However, high-dose aspirin therapy is less effective in the treatment of recurrent pericarditis and is complicated by gastrointestinal adverse effects with long-term use. High-dose NSAIDs, such as ibuprofen, are useful adjuncts to colchicine therapy in the treatment of recurrent pericarditis, but are less effective as first-line agents in the treatment of recurrent bouts of pericarditis.

The use of systemic corticosteroids early in the course of acute pericarditis is associated with an increased frequency of relapse, as was seen in this patient. Corticosteroids are considered third-line agents for refractory cases of recurrent pericarditis.

KEY POINT

- **Colchicine is the treatment of choice for acute bouts of recurrent pericarditis.**

Bibliography

Imazio M, Bobbio M, Cecchi E, et al. Colchicine as first-choice therapy for recurrent pericarditis: results of the CORE (COlchicine for Recurrent pericarditis) trial. Arch Intern Med. 2005;165(17):1987-1991. [PMID: 16186468]

Item 35   Answer: D

Educational Objective: Treat chest pain after recent cocaine use.

Cocaine is one of the most commonly used illicit drugs. Cocaine was responsible for nearly half a million visits to emergency departments in the United States in 2005, and chest discomfort is reported in approximately 40% of these patients after cocaine use. Cocaine is a potent vasoconstrictor that can result in acute coronary syndrome, and these symptoms may occur several days after drug use. In addition, cocaine use has been associated with aortic dissection, which should be considered in the differential diagnosis of chest pain after recent cocaine use.

Because of the relatively common use of cocaine, all patients presenting with symptoms of unstable angina or an acute coronary syndrome should be asked about any use of these drugs. Vasodilator therapy is the mainstay of treatment of chest pain related to cocaine use. Administration of nitroglycerin or calcium channel antagonists is strongly recommended. In addition, unlike patients with acute coronary syndrome unrelated to cocaine, patients with chest pain after cocaine use should be treated with benzodiazepines.

Coronary angiography is not recommended in the evaluation of cocaine-associated chest pain unless ongoing chest pain is not relieved by vasodilator therapy or the electrocardiogram or cardiac enzyme levels are consistent with myocardial ischemia or infarction. In the absence of these findings, patients who experience chest pain after cocaine use should be observed and medically managed for 9 to 12 hours and then may be discharged, as the incidence of myocardial infarction is only 0.7% to 6% in patients with cocaine-associated chest pain.

Intravenous heparin is not indicated as a first-line treatment of cocaine-induced chest pain in the absence of vasodilator therapy. Antithrombotic and antiplatelet therapy should be used in patients with evidence of myocardial ischemia unresponsive to vasodilator therapy or infarction.

Treatment with metoprolol and other β-blockers is controversial due to possible unopposed α-receptor agonism of cocaine with β-receptor antagonism, resulting in coronary artery spasm. Although treatment with cardioselective $β_1$-receptor antagonists (such as metoprolol) or combined α- and β-antagonists (such as labetalol or carvedilol) has a theoretical benefit over nonselective β-blockers, there is no conclusive evidence of clinical benefit or safety of these agents in patients with cocaine-induced chest pain. Therefore, these agents should be used very cautiously in such patients.

KEY POINT

- **Vasodilator therapy is the primary treatment of cocaine-induced chest pain.**

Bibliography

McCord J, Jneid H, Hollander JE, et al. Management of cocaine-associated chest pain and myocardial infarction: a scientific statement from the American Heart Association Acute Cardiac Care Committee of the Council on Clinical Cardiology. Circulation. 2008;117(14):1897-1907. [PMID: 18347214]

Item 36   Answer: B

Educational Objective: Recognize complications and residua related to coarctation of the aorta.

A bicuspid aortic valve is present in more than 50% of patients with aortic coarctation. Other associations include ventricular septal defect, patent ductus arteriosus, aortic stenosis (valvular, subvalvular, or supravalvular), and mitral stenosis. This patient has physical findings consistent with severe aortic valve regurgitation, including a wide pulse pressure, rapidly collapsing pulse, pulsating nailbeds, a brief systolic and long diastolic murmur, and features of left ventricular enlargement. The displaced apical impulse suggests left ventricular dilation and the presence of chronic aortic regurgitation.

Patients with coarctation of the aorta are prone to aneurysm formation. This can affect the ascending aorta, region of coarctation repair, descending thoracic aorta, and also the intracranial vessels. There are no physical findings that would suggest an aortic aneurysm in this patient, such as hoarseness due to left vagus or left recurrent laryngeal nerve compression, dysphagia due to esophageal compression, recurrent pneumonia due to bronchial compression, or superior vena cava syndrome. Furthermore, the presence of an aortic systolic murmur argues against aortic aneurysm as a cause of aortic annular dilation causing valvular regurgitation. Nevertheless, routine imaging is recommended to exclude these complications.

Mitral valve prolapse is not generally associated with coarctation of the aorta. Occasionally, coarctation is part of the Shone complex, a syndrome of multiple congenital abnormalities on the left side of the heart, including one or more of the following: supravalvular mitral ring and mitral inflow obstruction, a "parachute" mitral valve, subaortic stenosis, bicuspid aortic valve, and coarctation of the aorta. However, this patient's finding of a diastolic murmur is not compatible with the systolic cardiac findings associated with mitral valve prolapse and mitral regurgitation.

The patient has a history of coarctation repair, and systemic hypertension is a common problem even after successful coarctation repair, occurring in more than 50% of patients. The presence of hypertension, therefore, does not indicate recoarctation; however, this should be excluded prior to operative intervention for the aortic regurgitation, and the hypertension should be aggressively treated. The large pulse pressure and absence of pulse lag between the radial and femoral arteries argue against recurrent coarctation.

KEY POINT

- **Bicuspid aortic valve occurs in more than 50% of patients with aortic coarctation, and these patients should be monitored for aortic stenosis and aortic valve regurgitation.**

Bibliography

Aboulhosn J, Child JS. Left ventricular outflow obstruction: subaortic stenosis, bicuspid aortic valve, supravalvar aortic stenosis, and coarctation of the aorta. Circulation. 2006;114(22):2412-2422. [PMID: 17130357]

Item 37   Answer: B

Educational Objective: Treat chronic stable angina with worsening symptoms.

Medical therapy for chronic stable coronary artery disease (CAD) includes both antianginal and vascular-protective agents. Antianginal therapy includes β-blockers, calcium channel blockers, and nitrates. Vascular-protective therapy includes aspirin, angiotensin-converting enzyme (ACE) inhibitors, and statins. This patient is already on a β-blocker, aspirin, a statin, and an ACE inhibitor. Switching to a long-acting nitrate will help relieve his angina symptoms. However, his resting heart rate of 85/min suggests a suboptimal dose of β-blocker, and the patient's dosage of metoprolol should be increased. The β-blocker dose should

be titrated to achieve a resting heart rate of approximately 55 to 60/min and approximately 75% of the heart rate that produces angina with exertion. The patient should be re-evaluated in a few weeks to assess the response to therapy.

Ranolazine is a novel antianginal agent that is approved for the treatment of chronic stable angina. It should only be used, however, in additional to baseline therapy with a β-blocker, a calcium channel blocker, and a long-acting nitrate. Given that this patient was on suboptimal doses of metoprolol and is just being started on a long-acting nitrate, the addition of ranolazine would be premature.

Coronary angiography would not be indicated at this time because the patient is not receiving maximal medical therapy. In the setting of continued angina despite maximal medical therapy, coronary angiography could be considered.

Exercise treadmill stress testing would not provide useful information in this setting. It would only confirm the high pretest probability that this patient has underlying CAD as a cause for the current symptoms. In selected patients with chronic stable angina, exercise stress testing may be useful to assess the response to medical therapy (the effectiveness of current antianginal therapy) and to objectively evaluate the severity of angina (the level of activity at which angina occurs). Given that this patient is not on maximal medical therapy, exercise treadmill stress testing would not provide additional useful information.

KEY POINT

- **Maximal medical therapy for chronic stable angina includes aspirin, an angiotensin-converting enzyme inhibitor, a β-blocker, a long-acting nitrate, and a statin.**

Bibliography

Fraker TD Jr, Fihn SD, Gibbons RJ, et al. 2007 chronic angina focused update of the ACC/AHA 2002 guidelines for the management of patients with chronic stable angina: a report of the American College of Cardiology/American Heart Association Task Force on Practice Guidelines Writing Group to Develop the Focused Update of the 2002 guidelines for the management of patients with chronic stable angina [erratum in Circulation. 2007;116(23):e558.]. Circulation. 2007;116(23):2762-2772. [PMID: 17998462]

Item 38   Answer: B

Educational Objective: Manage relative anemia in a patient with cyanotic congenital heart disease.

This patient has features of cyanotic congenital heart disease with Eisenmenger syndrome. Eisenmenger syndrome is a form of cyanotic congenital heart disease characterized by irreversible pulmonary vascular disease due to the presence of a long-standing cardiac shunt. Patients with Eisenmenger syndrome typically have a hemoglobin level of 18 to 20 g/dL (180 to 200 g/L) and a hematocrit greater than 65%. The hemoglobin level and hematocrit in this patient are markedly reduced for a patient with cyanotic congenital heart disease. A decrease in hemoglobin and hematocrit, such as that associated with menorrhagia in this patient, often causes fatigue and exertional dyspnea owing to the reduced oxygen-carrying capacity in the cyanotic patient. The treatment of choice, unless the patient is acutely volume depleted, would be low-dose iron therapy (325 mg/d) for 1 week to 10 days followed by assessment of the hemoglobin and hematocrit. Therapy should be discontinued at this point if the hemoglobin level and hematocrit have begun to increase.

Blood transfusion is occasionally required in patients with Eisenmenger syndrome around the time of surgery or in the presence of excessive bleeding. A transfusion is usually recommended if the hemoglobin level drops to 10 g/dL (100 g/L) or if the patient has severe symptoms related to the anemia.

Patients with Eisenmenger syndrome often do well for many years. Treatment options for symptomatic patients with Eisenmenger syndrome include pulmonary vasodilator therapy and lung transplantation with intracardiac repair or heart-lung transplantation. Pulmonary vasodilators have been demonstrated to improve symptoms in patients with Eisenmenger syndrome, but this therapy would not be indicated in this patient until the hemoglobin level has been corrected. If symptoms persist after correction of the anemia, then the patient may benefit from pulmonary vasodilator therapy.

Observation and follow-up would not be appropriate at this time. The patient has symptomatic anemia that requires intervention. She may also require additional short courses of iron therapy.

KEY POINT

- **The treatment of choice for a patient with Eisenmenger syndrome with anemia is low-dose iron therapy with reassessment of the hemoglobin and hematocrit after 7 to 10 days.**

Bibliography

Warnes CA, Williams RG, Bashore TM, et al. ACC/AHA 2008 Guidelines for the Management of Adults with Congenital Heart Disease: a report of the American College of Cardiology/American Heart Association Task Force on Practice Guidelines (writing committee to develop guidelines on the management of adults with congenital heart disease). Circulation. 2008;118(23):e714-833. [PMID: 18997169]

Item 39   Answer: C

Educational Objective: Differentiate spinal stenosis from peripheral arterial disease.

In this patient, the normal ankle-brachial index, the lack of secondary skin or hair changes, the lack of a bruit, and the clinical history all suggest a diagnosis other than peripheral arterial disease. Her symptoms are more typical of lumbosacral spinal stenosis, also termed *pseudoclaudication*. The discomfort of spinal stenosis may be very similar to that of peripheral arterial disease. However, whereas the pain of peripheral arterial disease is precipitated by a predictable degree of exertion and relieved by rest and is unaffected by lumbar flexion or extension, that of spinal stenosis is provoked by prolonged standing and is relieved by sitting, lying down, or flexing at the waist. In addition, the pain of spinal stenosis may occur with walking, especially downhill (lumbar extension). Deep tendon reflexes are reduced at the ankle in about half of patients with spinal stenosis; reduced reflexes at the knee are less common. MRI of the lumbosacral spine would be the most useful first test in confirming the clinical suspicion of spinal stenosis.

Measuring the ankle-brachial index during exercise can be useful in diagnosing peripheral arterial disease when the resting ankle-brachial index is normal and there is a high clinical suspicion of peripheral arterial disease. A decrease of the ankle-brachial index by 20% after exercise suggests significant peripheral arterial disease.

Lower-extremity CT angiography could be used to help plan an interventional approach in a patient with documented peripheral arterial disease, but should not be used for the diagnosis of peripheral arterial disease. Segmental limb plethysmography is useful in better localizing the point of arterial compromise in a patient with symptoms of peripheral arterial disease and an abnormal ankle-brachial index.

KEY POINT

- **Unlike the pain of peripheral arterial disease, the pain of spinal stenosis is aggravated by prolonged standing and is relieved with sitting or lumbar flexion.**

Bibliography

Watters WC 3rd, Baisden J, Gilbert TJ, et al; North American Spine Society. Degenerative lumbar spinal stenosis: an evidence-based clinical guideline for the diagnosis and treatment of degenerative lumbar spinal stenosis. Spine J. 2008;8(2):305-310. [PMID: 18082461]

Item 40   Answer: C

Educational Objective: Treat hemodynamically significant ventricular arrhythmia in a patient with systolic heart failure.

This patient's syncopal event is strongly suggestive of syncope induced by ventricular arrhythmia, with a sudden onset, no prodromal symptoms, and no evidence for other causes of syncope. Syncope in the setting of systolic heart failure and in the absence of obvious reversible causes is very likely related to ventricular arrhythmia and indicates a high risk for sudden death. A patient with left ventricular dysfunction and a hemodynamically significant ventricular arrhythmia (that is, causing syncope, near syncope, or cardiac arrest) should receive an implantable cardioverter-defibrillator (ICD).

Amiodarone can be used to treat patients with heart failure who have ventricular arrhythmias and contraindications to ICD placement or those who have recurrent ventricular arrhythmias causing repeated ICD shocks. The first-line therapy for prevention of sudden death in patients with heart failure, however, is ICD implantation.

In the setting of a high enough clinical suspicion for syncope caused by ventricular arrhythmia, it is not necessary to formally document the arrhythmia with an event monitor before proceeding with ICD implantation, given the extremely high risk for sudden death in this setting. If this patient's ejection fraction remained low after optimal medical therapy, she would also qualify for ICD implantation for a primary prophylaxis indication.

Midodrine is an α-sympathomimetic drug used to treat orthostatic hypotension. This patient does not demonstrate evidence for orthostatic hypotension on examination, and the description of the event also is not consistent with orthostatic hypotension—it occurred while seated rather than when arising to an upright position, and there was no typical presyncopal prodrome. In addition, midodrine would counteract the vasodilating effects of the patient's enalapril and carvedilol. If symptomatic hypotension were a problem, the appropriate intervention would be to decrease either agent rather than to add a vasoconstricting agent.

A pacemaker is indicated for treatment of bradyarrhythmias, such as type 2 second-degree (Mobitz) atrioventricular block or complete heart block, or chronotropic incompetence. The patient does not have evidence for heart block on electrocardiogram, and her reasonable exercise tolerance argues against chronotropic incompetence. She would not meet criteria for a biventricular pacemaker given her good functional status (New York Heart Association functional class I) and her narrow QRS complex (94 msec).

KEY POINT

- **Placement of an implantable cardioverter-defibrillator is indicated in a patient with left ventricular dysfunction and a hemodynamically significant ventricular arrhythmia.**

Bibliography
Bardy GH, Lee KL, Mark DB, et al; Sudden Cardiac Death in Heart Failure Trial (SCD-HeFT) Investigators. Amiodarone or an implantable cardioverter-defibrillator for congestive heart failure [erratum in N Engl J Med. 2005;352(20):2146.]. N Engl J Med. 2005;352(3):225-237. [PMID: 15659722]

Item 41   Answer: E
Educational Objective: **Evaluate aortic stenosis.**

This patient has severe aortic stenosis based on clinical and echocardiographic examination findings. An absent aortic component of S_2, a long and late-peaking systolic murmur, and a sustained apical impulse are all associated with severe aortic stenosis with likelihood ratios between 4.1 and 4.5. The primary indication for valve replacement in aortic stenosis is the presence of cardiopulmonary symptoms (angina, syncope, exertional dyspnea, heart failure). Aortic valve replacement is indicated in any symptomatic patient, regardless of age, because of the substantial improvements in long-term survival and quality of life. Aortic valve replacement is not performed in asymptomatic patients because of the increased surgical risk incurred, with potential complications including thromboembolism, bleeding from anticoagulation, prosthetic valve dysfunction, and endocarditis. This patient is asymptomatic, without angina complaints, and further diagnostic testing, including cardiac stress testing and coronary angiography, is not indicated. However, if aortic valve replacement is eventually recommended, preoperative coronary angiography is usually performed so that bypass surgery can be done at the time of valve surgery if needed.

The role of cardiac CT angiography in routine diagnostic evaluation of valvular anatomy is not established. Cardiac CT angiography would provide little additional diagnostic information to transthoracic echocardiography for aortic stenosis due to shadowing and artifact from the calcified aortic valve. Cardiac CT angiography is most useful for coronary disease evaluation when images from standard coronary angiography are suboptimal or for evaluation of congenital or acquired coronary anomalies and aortic pathology.

Exercise treadmill stress testing would allow for an objective evaluation of exercise tolerance and symptom provocation. This patient would not be able to perform an exercise treadmill stress test, as she walks with the aid of a cane. Exercise testing for valvular heart disease is contraindicated in patients with unstable angina, congestive heart failure symptoms, or exertional syncope. Pharmacologic stress testing with dobutamine echocardiography is occasionally used for patients with aortic stenosis and systolic dysfunction. If the valve area increases with augmentation of cardiac output during dobutamine infusion, then the "obstruction" was due to the inability of the left ventricle to fully open the valve (pseudostenosis). If the valve area does not increase, the obstruction is fixed and true aortic stenosis is the culprit. This patient's systolic function is normal, however, and pharmacologic stress testing is not indicated.

Transesophageal echocardiography is semi-invasive and requires conscious sedation. Anatomy and hemodynamics of the aortic valve are generally well evaluated by transthoracic echocardiographic imaging, and additional transesophageal imaging is rarely needed. The physical examination and echocardiogram in this patient are diagnostic for aortic stenosis.

KEY POINT

- **Aortic valve replacement should be recommended in any symptomatic patient with aortic stenosis, regardless of age, owing to the improvement in long-term survival and quality of life.**

Bibliography

Freeman RV, Otto CM. Spectrum of calcific aortic valve disease: pathogenesis, disease progression, and treatment strategies. Circulation. 2005;111(24):3316-3326. [PMID: 15967862]

Item 42   Answer: D

Educational Objective: Manage a patient with inappropriate shocks from an implanted cardioverter-defibrillator.

Inappropriate implantable cardioverter-defibrillator (ICD) shocks can be caused by mechanical lead dysfunction; supraventricular tachycardias, including atrial fibrillation with rapid ventricular response; sinus tachycardia at rates higher than the ICD detection rate; and electromagnetic interference. The incidence of inappropriate ICD shocks is approximately 9% to 20%. This patient has experienced multiple ICD firings in the absence of tachycardia, and the device should be disabled by immediate magnet application. This allows the patient to wait comfortably for assessment by ICD interrogation with a programmer. Magnet application will suspend the ability of the ICD to detect arrhythmia, and therefore stop ICD firing. Magnet application to an ICD does not change the pacing modality, unlike in pacemakers, where a magnet will cause temporary reversion of the pacemaker programming to an asynchronous mode. The patient should be in a telemetry-monitored setting when the ICD is disabled by a magnet or programmed to "off."

ICD shocks for both appropriate and inappropriate reasons are common. In the absence of symptoms, a single isolated shock does not require emergent evaluation. However, patients experiencing cardiac symptoms or multiple shocks should be referred to the emergency department. ICD shocks are usually painful and frightening, and anxiolytics can be helpful in the treatment of both appropriate and inappropriate shocks.

Amiodarone has been shown to reduce the incidence of appropriate and inappropriate shocks due to supraventricular tachycardias. Because the ICD firings in this patient are unrelated to a tachycardia, however, amiodarone would not provide clinical benefit. Similarly, substituting atenolol for metoprolol or starting verapamil is unlikely to be helpful in a patient with inappropriate shocks in the absence of tachycardia.

KEY POINT

- **An implanted cardioverter-defibrillator giving inappropriate shocks should be disabled pending further evaluation.**

Bibliography

Gehi AK, Mehta D, Gomes JA. Evaluation and management of patients after implantable cardioverter-defibrillator shock. JAMA. 2006;296(23):2839-2847. [PMID: 17179461]

Item 43   Answer: C

Educational Objective: Treat acute pericarditis complicated by cardiac tamponade.

This patient has examination findings that indicate cardiac tamponade. Physical examination reveals tachycardia, reduced blood pressure, distended jugular veins, elevated pulsus paradoxus (>10 mm Hg), and an unremarkable lung examination. This constellation of signs should always raise the possibility of cardiac tamponade but is not pathognomonic. Other acute conditions, such as pulmonary embolism or myocardial infarction, could account for these findings. However, cardiac tamponade is confirmed by echocardiography, specifically by a pericardial effusion with associated right atrial and ventricular free wall diastolic collapse. In addition, this patient presents with symptoms consistent with an infectious illness. A viral pericarditis is the most likely source. The definitive treatment for this patient's hemodynamic derangement is pericardiocentesis, which is typically performed via a percutaneous route but may be performed surgically if indicated.

Cardiac tamponade is typically caused by a circumferential pericardial effusion, but a loculated pericardial effusion also can cause tamponade, particularly in patients with prior cardiac surgery. The rapidity of fluid accumulation, rather than the absolute size of an effusion, is the major determinant of developing tamponade. Thus, a small but rapidly developing effusion may cause tamponade, whereas a large but slowly accumulating effusion may not.

Vasoactive medications can be used as temporizing measures to improve hemodynamic alterations from cardiac tamponade while awaiting definitive treatment. Vasopressors such as dopamine or norepinephrine may have a role. However, dobutamine acts primarily as an inotropic agent. In this setting, with dynamic left ventricular function documented by echocardiography, it would be unlikely to improve the hemodynamic compromise of cardiac tamponade. In addition, dobutamine can be detrimental by exacerbating hypotension via inducing dynamic left ventricular intracavitary obstruction, or systemic vasodilation. Rapid intravascular volume infusion (typically 250 to 500 mL of normal saline over 10 to 20 minutes) is an important temporizing measure to maintain systemic blood pressure in patients with cardiac tamponade and hypotension, as was given in this patient, until the definitive treatment, pericardiocentesis, can be performed.

Sepsis from bacteremia should always be a consideration in a patient who presents with hypotension. Empiric broad-spectrum antibiotic therapy may be warranted in such situations. However, the specific findings of cardiac tamponade (jugular venous distention and pulsus paradoxus) would not be directly explained by sepsis. Treatment with levofloxacin and tobramycin is unlikely to immediately improve potentially life-threatening hypotension in this patient.

Constrictive pericarditis is characterized by thickened, fibrotic, and adherent pericardium that restrains ventricular diastolic expansion, leading to impaired filling. The visceral and parietal pericardium are typically fused and a pericardial effusion is most commonly absent. Calcification occurs in the chronic phase, contributing to pericardial stiffening. Constrictive pericarditis typically presents with either signs of fluid overload or symptoms of fatigue and dyspnea. Pericardiectomy is useful for treatment of constrictive pericarditis, but is not a specific treatment for cardiac tamponade from a pericardial effusion.

KEY POINT

- Pericardiocentesis is the appropriate immediate treatment for cardiac tamponade.

Bibliography

Meltser H, Kalaria VG. Cardiac tamponade. Catheter Cardiovasc Interv. 2005;64(2):245-255. [PMID: 15678459]

Item 44   Answer: A

Educational Objective: Evaluate a patient with new-onset heart failure.

This patient has typical angina (substernal chest pain precipitated by exertion and relieved by rest) and new-onset heart failure, as evidenced by symptoms (exertional dyspnea and orthopnea), examination findings (elevated jugular venous pressure and pulmonary crackles), and echocardiogram with a subnormal ejection fraction. Definitive testing for coronary artery disease (CAD) by cardiac catheterization is warranted. The primary aim of an evaluation for CAD is to identify possible targets for revascularization (percutaneous or surgical) with the goals of reducing angina, improving systolic function, reducing the risk of heart failure progression, and improving survival.

Cardiac MRI is useful for evaluating for infiltrative cardiomyopathies or for viable myocardium after myocardial infarction. In this patient, the history of exertional chest pain does not suggest infiltrative cardiomyopathy. While the echocardiogram does show increased left ventricular wall thickness, it is mild and likely related to the patient's hypertension; typically, left ventricular wall thickness is markedly increased with infiltrative cardiomyopathies. There is no evidence that the patient has had a myocardial infarction: the electrocardiogram (ECG) and troponin level are normal, and the echocardiogram does not show focal akinesis or scar. In any case, a diagnosis of coronary disease and ischemic cardiomyopathy would have to be established first before performing a viability evaluation using cardiac MRI.

A radionuclide ventriculogram can be useful in confirming the ejection fraction if clarification is needed. In this patient, however, the ejection fraction value is not in dispute. Furthermore, a radionuclide ventriculogram would not assist in determining the cause of the new-onset heart failure.

For patients with an intermediate likelihood of CAD who have no features of unstable angina, stress testing is the preferred approach when assessing for CAD. An exercise stress test is recommended for assessing for CAD in a patient with an intermediate probability of disease and a normal resting ECG. A nuclear medicine stress test is helpful if the resting ECG is abnormal. In this patient, however, the pretest probability for CAD is high based on his age, sex, and the presence of typical anginal symptoms. Because a negative result on stress testing in a patient with a high pretest probability of coronary artery disease would have a high likelihood of being a false negative, catheterization would still be needed for a definitive diagnosis.

KEY POINT

- Patients with new-onset heart failure and angina should be evaluated with cardiac catheterization if they are possible candidates for revascularization.

Bibliography

Hunt SA; American College of Cardiology; American Heart Association Task Force on Practice Guidelines (Writing Committee to Update the 2001 Guidelines for the Evaluation and Management of Heart Failure). ACC/AHA 2005 guideline update for the diagnosis and management of chronic heart failure in the adult [erratum in J Am Coll Cardiol. 2006;47(7):1503-1505.]. J Am Coll Cardiol 2005;46(6):e1-82. [PMID: 16168273]

Item 45   Answer: D

Educational Objective: Diagnose patent foramen ovale.

Decompression sickness can result in air embolism through a patent foramen ovale (PFO). A PFO can also permit paradoxical embolization from other causes of air embolism. Testing for PFO should be considered in patients with a cerebral ischemic event of uncertain origin. In addition, a PFO is associated with up to a 5-fold increase in the odds ratio for developing serious decompression sickness. The patient presented has a history of severe decompression sickness that involved confusion and seizure in addition to new-onset atrial arrhythmia, raising the possibility of air embolism through a PFO. The diagnostic test of choice for a PFO is a transesophageal echocardiogram with agitated saline contrast injection. It is highly sensitive and relatively noninvasive. Some experts recommend beginning with transthoracic echocardiography and if negative, proceeding to transesophageal echocardiography. If a PFO is found in a patient who wants to continue diving, closure is recommended to reduce the likelihood of recurrent decompression illness and air embolism.

Cardiac catheterization may confirm the presence of a PFO, but because of the invasive nature of the procedure, it is not the diagnostic test of choice.

Cardiac magnetic resonance (CMR) imaging is not the diagnostic procedure of choice to determine the presence or absence of a PFO. When directly compared with transesophageal echocardiography as a diagnostic modality, CMR imaging has shown reduced sensitivity for PFO detection both before and after device closure.

Intracardiac echocardiography is used primarily during procedures performed in the catheterization laboratory. Intracardiac echocardiography can readily demonstrate a PFO but requires venous access and passage of the catheter into the right heart to adequately image the atrial septum and is therefore unnecessarily invasive.

KEY POINT

- **Transesophageal echocardiography is the test of choice to detect a patent foramen ovale.**

Bibliography

Messé SR, Silverman IE, Kizer JR, et al. Practice parameter: recurrent stroke with patent foramen ovale and atrial septal aneurysm: report of the Quality Standards Subcommittee of the American Academy of Neurology. Neurology. 2004;62(7):1042-1050. [PMID: 15078999]

Item 46   Answer: D

Educational Objective: Manage ST-elevation myocardial infarction.

This patient with chest pain, tachycardia, crackles, and a left bundle branch block of unknown duration has ongoing discomfort despite therapy. Regardless of her equivocal troponin level, her condition should be treated as an ST-elevation myocardial infarction (STEMI). For the patient who presents with STEMI and symptoms of less than 12 hours in duration, reperfusion therapy must be considered in order to salvage myocardium. The ISIS-2 study demonstrated efficacy of thrombolysis for STEMI for up to 12 hours from the onset of symptoms. However, the greatest benefit of thrombolytic therapy is seen when it can be administered very early in the course of infarction (especially <1 hour). Current guidelines suggest that after 3 hours, PCI is preferable.

In this particular patient, PCI is not immediately available. Since the degree of myocardial salvage is directly related to the time from symptom onset to the time of reperfusion of the infarct-related artery, a decision must be made quickly whether to administer thrombolytic therapy or transfer the patient to another facility for PCI. For the purpose of investigating treatment outcomes in STEMI with respect to thrombolysis versus PCI, several terms have been defined. "Medical contact–to-balloon time" is the elapsed time from the first contact of the patient with the medical system to the time an angioplasty balloon is inflated in the infarct-related artery. This includes the inter-facility transfer time if the patient first arrives at a hospital without PCI capability. "Door-to-balloon time" is the elapsed time from arrival to PCI in a facility with this capability. "Door-to-needle time" is the elapsed time from arrival to delivery of thrombolytic therapy. When the medical contact–to-balloon time is less than 90 minutes, or the door-to-balloon time minus the door-to-needle time is less than 60 minutes, an invasive strategy is preferred.

Outcomes are worse when there are delays in achieving patency of the infarct-related artery, and a national initiative has targeted a door-to-balloon time of less than 90 minutes as a goal. For this patient, transfer to a catheterization laboratory with PCI capability can be performed in 45 minutes, and this is preferred. Additionally, since there is some doubt regarding the diagnosis (left bundle branch block and equivocal biomarker value), angiography may provide a better risk/benefit ratio, as it can establish the correct diagnosis.

A glycoprotein IIb/IIIa inhibitor is not indicated as part of the routine treatment of a STEMI unless it is being delivered as upstream therapy in preparation for urgent PCI. Waiting for additional cardiac enzyme results would allow further myocardial necrosis, and definitive therapy should not be delayed unnecessarily.

KEY POINT

- **Primary percutaneous coronary intervention is favored over thrombolytic therapy for ST-elevation myocardial infarction if it is available in fewer than 90 minutes; it is also favored in patients with late presentation, shock, contraindications to thrombolysis, or if the diagnosis is unclear.**

Bibliography

Antman EM, Hand M, Armstrong PW, et al. 2007 Focused Update of the ACC/AHA 2004 Guidelines for the Management of Patients With ST-Elevation Myocardial Infarction: a report of the American College of Cardiology/American Heart Association Task Force on Practice Guidelines: developed in collaboration With the Canadian Cardiovascular Society endorsed by the American Academy of Family Physicians: 2007 Writing Group to Review New Evidence and Update the ACC/AHA 2004 Guidelines for the Management of Patients With ST-Elevation Myocardial Infarction, Writing on Behalf of the 2004 Writing Committee [erratum in Circulation. 2008;117(6):e162.]. Circulation. 2008;117(2):296-329. [PMID: 18071078]

Item 47   Answer: D

Educational Objective: Manage acute severe mitral regurgitation.

Although this patient does not have a known history of coronary artery disease, the electrocardiogram suggests an inferior wall myocardial infarction, with Q waves in leads II, III, and aVF. Clinical presentation is consistent with cardiogenic shock, with posteromedial papillary muscle rupture causing acute severe mitral regurgitation. The echocardiogram demonstrates hypokinesis of the inferior wall and significant mitral regurgitation. Acute, severe mitral regurgitation is associated with high mortality and is a surgical emergency. In the SHOCK Trial Registry, although patients with cardiogenic shock who underwent urgent mitral valve surgery had significant in-hospital mortality (40%), those who did not receive surgery fared worse, with mortality above 70%.

Clinical presentation for papillary muscle rupture is generally several days after the infarct event (in this case, 1 week later), once infarcted tissue has had time to necrose. Posteromedial papillary muscle rupture is more common than anteromedial papillary muscle rupture because of its single coronary artery supply, as opposed to the dual coronary supply of the anteromedial papillary muscle. As a consequence, acute severe mitral regurgitation complicating an acute myocardial infarct is more common with inferior versus anterior infarcts and should be suspected in patients with pulmonary edema and respiratory distress in that setting. The murmur of mitral regurgitation may not be prominent because of the acutely elevated left atrial pressure and relatively lower transmitral systolic pressure gradient. Echocardiography is diagnostic, and early clinical recognition with aggressive support (intra-aortic balloon pump and/or afterload reduction if blood pressure allows) is essential. This condition is often misdiagnosed as respiratory decompensation due to pneumonia, acute respiratory distress syndrome, or endocarditis.

CT of the chest aids in assessment of the aorta and great vessels to assess for aortic aneurysm and/or dissection, and allows for evaluation of the lung parenchyma. Chest CT is not indicated in this patient, however, as echocardiography was diagnostic for severe mitral regurgitation as the etiology of his respiratory distress.

This patient should undergo emergent diagnostic coronary angiography to identify targets for bypass grafting to be performed at the time of mitral valve replacement. Although percutaneous intervention would address any residual intracoronary lesions identified at angiography, papillary muscle rupture with severe mitral regurgitation can only be treated surgically.

Compared with transthoracic imaging, transesophageal imaging may provide improved visualization of cardiac anatomy and function, particularly of posterior cardiac structures such as the mitral valve. However, in this patient, the regional wall motion abnormalities, mitral regurgitation, and ruptured papillary muscle were adequately identified by transthoracic echocardiography, and the more invasive transesophageal imaging is not necessary.

KEY POINT

- **The treatment for acute ischemic mitral regurgitation and cardiogenic shock is mitral valve replacement.**

Bibliography

Thompson CR, Buller CE, Sleeper LA, et al. Cardiogenic shock due to acute severe mitral regurgitation complicating acute myocardial infarction: A report from the SHOCK Trial Registry. SHould we use emergently revascularize Occluded Coronaries in cardiogenic shocK? J Am Coll Cardiol. 2000;36(3 Suppl A):1104-1109. [PMID: 10985712]

Item 48   Answer: A

Educational Objective: **Manage fever in a patient with a pacemaker.**

The most appropriate next step in the management of this patient is to obtain blood and urine cultures. In patients with implanted cardiac devices, fever raises concerns of infection. This patient has had a recent urinary tract infection, which is a risk factor for bloodstream infection with gram-negative bacteria, subsequent secondary infection of the device, and possible right-sided endocarditis. A systemic infection is suggested by the presence of positive blood cultures in the absence of an obviously infected pocket or eroded device. Negative blood cultures do not, however, exclude systemic infection, particularly in the setting of previous antibiotic therapy.

The two categories of infection associated with implanted devices are pocket infection and systemic infection. Pocket infection refers to infection of the subcutaneous pocket containing the device and the subcutaneous segment of the leads. A pocket infection is characterized by local swelling, erythema, pain, and, occasionally, wound drainage or erosion of the device through the skin. As the intravascular leads are connected to the generator within the pocket, even pocket infections are seldom entirely localized. Systemic infection refers to infection of the portion of the lead within the venous system and/or endovascular infection. Systemic infection is usually associated with bacteremia. Systemic infection can occur alone (50% of patients) or in combination with right-sided endocarditis. Systemic infections from other causes are risk factors for secondary infection of implanted cardiac devices. Other risk factors for device infection include older age, diabetes mellitus, and the use of an indwelling vascular catheter. Antibiotic treatment of device infections, even for prolonged periods of time, rarely results in eradication of infection unless the device is removed; therefore, complete device system removal is usually indicated.

In stable patients without localizing signs, empiric antibiotic therapy is typically withheld until the source of the infection can be verified. Antibiotic therapy without obtaining blood and urine cultures is not correct because the source and nature of the fever are unknown, and this information should guide appropriate therapy. Besides pacemaker system infection, a likely source of infection includes relapsed urinary tract infection.

Pocket aspiration should rarely be performed because of the high risk of infecting a sterile device pocket or damaging the leads. In this patient, the pocket itself is benign. Even if the pocket is obviously infected, there is no indication for aspiration, since the device system will require explantation as part of therapy.

Transthoracic echocardiography is noninvasive and is the initial diagnostic test of choice for patients with a moderate or high probability of infective endocarditis but has a sensitivity of only 50% to 80% for detection of vegetations on valves or leads. However, the finding of normal valves on transthoracic echocardiography substantially reduces the probability of infective endocarditis. Transesophageal echocardiography increases both the sensitivity and specificity to detect vegetations to approximately 95% but is invasive and requires conscious sedation. In a patient with a low probability of infective endocarditis, both transthoracic and transesophageal echocardiography are associated with low diagnostic yield and should not be performed. Because a bloodstream infection has not yet been documented, neither a transthoracic nor transesophageal echocardiogram is indicated for this patient.

KEY POINT

- **In patients with an implanted cardiac device, pocket aspiration should rarely be performed because of the high risk of infecting a sterile device pocket or damaging the leads.**

Bibliography

Uslan DZ, Sohail MR, St Sauver JL, et al. Permanent pacemaker and implantable cardioverter defibrillator infection: a population-based study. Arch Intern Med. 2007;167(7):669-675. [PMID: 17420425]

Item 49   Answer: D

Educational Objective: Diagnose anthracycline cardiotoxicity.

This patient has a history of anthracycline exposure in the treatment of her childhood leukemia together with other clinical risk factors for the development of anthracycline cardiotoxicity (female sex, black race, young age at administration, hypertension). She presents with bilateral lower extremity edema and elevated estimated central venous pressure, consistent with a cardiogenic etiology. Anthracycline cardiotoxicity may occur any time after administration, from immediate acute toxicity to long-term (even decades). Chronic and long-term cardiotoxicities are dose-dependent, and approximately 20% of survivors who received 300 mg/m^2 of anthracycline have been found to have evidence of ventricular systolic dysfunction over the long term. Transthoracic echocardiography is indicated in this patient to assess ventricular function.

Although left ventricular dysfunction may be asymptomatic, patients who develop cardiotoxicity are at higher risk of cardiovascular events, and thus may benefit from appropriate pharmacologic therapy. Given the high cure rate of childhood cancer in the current era, awareness and monitoring for possible long-term adverse effects of chemotherapy may improve outcomes for these survivors.

An adenosine nuclear perfusion imaging study is not the first choice of a diagnostic test because the patient has a low pretest probability of coronary artery disease based upon her age and absence of ischemic or angina equivalent symptoms.

Lower extremity venous duplex ultrasound is incorrect because bilateral deep venous thrombosis is unlikely, particularly in light of the elevated central venous pressure.

Additional diuretic therapy would be inappropriate, as this offers only symptomatic improvement of her lower extremity edema, without diagnosis of the underlying cause and treatment with possible proven therapies for left ventricular dysfunction.

KEY POINT

- **Risk of anthracycline cardiotoxicity is related to cumulative dosage and may occur many years after administration.**

Bibliography

Shankar SM, Marina N, Hudson MM, et al. Monitoring for cardiovascular disease in survivors of childhood cancer: report from the Cardiovascular Disease Task Force of the Children's Oncology Group. Pediatrics. 2008;121(2):e387-396. [PMID: 18187811]

Item 50   Answer: B

Educational Objective: Diagnose irradiation-induced constrictive pericarditis.

This patient has symptoms and signs of heart failure. The physical examination is notable for findings of right heart failure (jugular venous distention, peripheral edema) in the absence of left heart failure (clear lung fields, absence of gallop). The most important physical examination findings are a Kussmaul sign (accentuated jugular venous pressure during inspiration) and an early diastolic sound (pericardial knock). These findings help to confirm constrictive pericarditis as the most likely diagnosis.

Constrictive pericarditis is characterized by thickened, fibrotic, and adherent pericardium that restrains ventricular diastolic expansion, leading to impaired filling. Orthostatic hypotension may occur as an adverse effect from excessive diuresis in patients with constrictive pericarditis, as seen in this patient, who was being treated with a high dosage of furosemide. Constrictive pericarditis is a well-known complication of chest irradiation therapy and may occur 10 to 15 years after exposure. Mediastinal radiation therapy results in approximately a three-fold increase in the risk of cardiac death. Most deaths are due to myocardial infarction, and the remainder are due to heart failure, constrictive pericarditis, cardiomyopathy, or valvular heart disease.

Cirrhosis with portal hypertension could account for this patient's peripheral edema and ascites. However, it would not explain the elevated right heart pressures, orthostatic hypotension, pericardial knock, or Kussmaul sign. In addition, the patient does not have any cutaneous findings of chronic liver disease such as gynecomastia, spider angioma, or palmar erythema. The elevated aminotransferase levels reflect passive hepatic congestion and are a feature of constrictive pericarditis.

Nephrotic syndrome is a reasonable consideration in a patient with diabetes mellitus, hypercholesterolemia, hypoalbuminemia, and peripheral edema. However, the absence of proteinuria excludes this diagnosis. In addition, nephrotic syndrome would not explain the jugular venous distention, pericardial knock, or orthostatic hypotension.

Systolic heart failure can explain many of the patient's findings, including dyspnea on exertion, elevated central venous pressure, and peripheral edema. However, systolic failure is also associated with crackles on pulmonary auscultation and an S_3, which are absent in this patient. Furthermore, murmurs characteristic of mitral regurgitation and tricuspid regurgitation are frequently associated with systolic failure but are absent in this patient. Systolic failure cannot explain the pericardial knock or Kussmaul sign.

KEY POINT

- **The most important physical examination findings of constrictive pericarditis are a Kussmaul sign (accentuated jugular venous pressure during inspiration) and an early diastolic sound (pericardial knock).**

Bibliography

Gaya AM, Ashford RF. Cardiac complications of radiation therapy. Clin Oncol (R Coll Radiol). 2005;17(3):153-159. [PMID: 15900998]

Item 51   Answer: E

Educational Objective: Recognize long-term cardiovascular complications of radiotherapy.

The patient has symptoms of left upper extremity claudication precipitated by exertion involving the left arm. Examination findings suggestive of left subclavian artery stenosis include the low blood pressure in the left arm compared with the right, the diminished left radial and brachial pulses, and the systolic murmur in the left clavicular region. Another possible symptom is syncope or near-syncope due to subclavian steal syndrome, which occurs in the setting of significant stenosis of the subclavian artery and retrograde flow in the ipsilateral vertebral artery during upper extremity exertion.

Patients with Hodgkin lymphoma who were previously treated with radiation therapy are at an increased risk of long-term cardiovascular complications. In a single-center cohort study of 415 patients with Hodgkin lymphoma treated with radiation therapy, 16% of patients developed coronary artery disease (CAD), peripheral arterial disease, or clinically important valvular disease (particularly aortic stenosis) by 20 years after radiation therapy. Although CAD was the most common cardiovascular complication found, all patients with CAD had at least one cardiovascular risk factor, and the observed-to-expected ratio for any coronary revascularization procedure was 1.63. In contrast, the observed-to-expected ratio for valve surgery was 8.42. For peripheral arterial disease, which occurred in 7.4% of the cohort at a median of 17 years after radiotherapy, the only treatment or

patient-related covariates for carotid or subclavian artery disease were hypertension and diabetes mellitus.

Although pericardial disease is a known complication of radiation therapy involving the chest, it would be unusual for cardiac tamponade due to a pericardial effusion to occur so late after radiotherapy, and this could not account for the patient's signs and symptoms. Rather, at this point in time, constrictive pericarditis presenting as signs of right heart failure (edema, ascites) would be more likely.

CAD is incorrect because the patient has no history of angina and has had symptoms only in the setting of left arm exertion and an abnormal peripheral vascular examination.

Radiation therapy may result in left ventricular systolic or diastolic (restrictive cardiomyopathy) dysfunction owing to its effect on the myocardium, but this patient does not have symptoms or signs of heart failure.

This patient has no examination findings consistent with severe aortic stenosis (no radiation of the murmur to the right clavicle or carotid regions; no late-peaking murmur; no decrease in the S_2; no decrease or delay in carotid upstrokes), and aortic stenosis cannot account for the differences in the arm pulses or blood pressures.

KEY POINT

- **The long-term risks of radiotherapy include pericardial disease, cardiomyopathy, peripheral arterial disease, coronary artery disease, and valvular heart disease.**

Bibliography

Hull MC, Morris CG, Pepine CJ, Mendenhall NP. Valvular dysfunction and carotid, subclavian, and coronary artery disease in survivors of Hodgkin lymphoma treated with radiation therapy. JAMA. 2003;290(21):2831-2837. [PMID: 14657067]

Item 52   Answer: D

Educational Objective: Manage idiopathic uncomplicated pericardial effusion.

Pericardiocentesis is warranted if an effusion persists for longer than 3 months and may be curative in approximately 50% of patients with idiopathic effusions. In addition, pericardiocentesis prevents the development of cardiac tamponade. Pericardiocentesis is the best management option in this patient. An expectant strategy of delaying pericardiocentesis in such patients is dependent on clinical findings that show no evidence of systemic disease or concern for malignancy, as was the initial approach adopted in this patient.

In patients who present with pericardial effusion, management should be based on the etiology and hemodynamic significance of the effusion. In the absence of cardiac tamponade, pericardiocentesis may be indicated if clinical suspicion exists for bacterial, tubercular, or systemic inflammatory causes of pericarditis. In this patient, none of these entities would be suspected. In patients with an isolated pericardial effusion, if clinical assessment fails to reveal a likely obvious cause, it is unlikely that extensive laboratory testing will yield a diagnosis. In such circumstances, it is reasonable to test serum electrolytes, blood urea nitrogen, serum creatinine (to exclude renal insufficiency), thyroid-stimulating hormone, complete blood count, and antinuclear antibodies; and perform a chest radiograph, as was done in this patient. An idiopathic pericardial effusion lasting less than 3 months in a stable patient requires no specific therapy, but serial echocardiography based on clinical status, as was done in this patient, is advisable.

This patient has no findings that suggest pericarditis, such as pleuritic chest pain, fever, a pericardial friction rub, or ST-segment elevation. Anti-inflammatory agents such as colchicine, indomethacin, or prednisone are not indicated without further evidence of pericarditis.

Pericardiectomy is an appropriate treatment in constrictive pericarditis, but is not appropriate in the management of patients with asymptomatic pericardial effusion.

KEY POINT

- Pericardiocentesis should be performed when an idiopathic pericardial effusion persists longer than 3 months.

Bibliography

Little WC, Freeman GL. Pericardial disease [erratum in Circulation. 2007;115(15):e406.]. Circulation. 2006;113(12):1622-1632. [PMID: 16567581]

Item 53   Answer: B

Educational Objective: Select an imaging modality in a patient with an implanted cardiac device.

CT arthrography of the shoulder is the indicated test in this patient. Conventional arthrography is also an acceptable choice, as is shoulder ultrasonography, although the availability of shoulder ultrasonography is quite limited in the United States. Plain-film radiography is typically the first imaging modality for shoulder pathology, particularly for the evaluation of acute shoulder trauma, calcific tendinitis, and arthritis.

The primary indication for CT arthrography is when MRI arthrography is contraindicated; for example, in a patient with a pacemaker, incompatible vascular clips, or claustrophobia. Rotator cuff pathology, as is highly likely in this patient, can be visualized, including tears of the supraspinatus and infraspinatus muscles, with similar accuracy as MRI arthrography.

The primary indication for CT of the shoulder is evaluation of fracture/fracture-dislocation or a prosthetic shoulder.

Although recent small studies in patients with implantable cardiac rhythm devices have provided data showing some safe use of MRI, current device labeling cautions against its use in this population. Strong magnetic fields have been shown to cause a variety of problems in patients with implanted devices, including heating at the lead tip interface, device reprogramming, induced arrhythmias (including ventricular fibrillation), reed switch malfunction, pacing threshold increases, and inhibition of therapy. Further studies must be completed before MRI is used routinely as a diagnostic tool in patients with pacemakers and implantable cardioverter-defibrillators.

Arthrography, CT arthrography, plain radiography, and ultrasonography all can be safely used in patients with implanted cardiac devices.

KEY POINT

- MRI is contraindicated in patients with pacemakers or implantable cardioverter-defibrillators.

Bibliography

Faris OP, Shein M. Food and Drug Administration perspective: magnetic resonance imaging of pacemaker and implantable cardioverter-defibrillator patients. Circulation. 2006;114(12):1232–1233. [PMID: 16982951]

Item 54   Answer: A

Educational Objective: Diagnose atrial septal defect in an adult.

The patient presents with physical examination findings consistent with an atrial septal defect, which include fixed splitting of the S_2, a parasternal impulse due to right-sided chamber enlargement, and tricuspid diastolic and pulmonary systolic murmurs related to the increased right heart volume from the left-to-right shunt. The right-sided murmurs increase with inspiration due to the increased systemic venous return. The chest radiograph demonstrates right heart and pulmonary artery enlargement, consistent with long-standing right-to-left shunt. The test of choice for confirming the diagnosis of atrial septal defect suspected on physical examination is transthoracic echocardiography.

Hypertrophic cardiomyopathy is generally associated with a dynamic systolic murmur that increases with Valsalva maneuver release. The apical impulse is often displaced and bifid. A parasternal impulse would not be expected, and the S_2 should be normal. The electrocardiogram in patients with hypertrophic cardiomyopathy demonstrates left ventricular hypertrophy.

Patients with a left atrial myxoma may have a diastolic sound known as a "tumor plop" noted on physical examination. The S_2 is normal, and a parasternal impulse would not be expected. A diastolic murmur related to an inflow gradient may be heard when the tumor obstructs mitral inflow. The electrocardiogram may be normal in patients with left atrial myxoma.

A patient with pulmonary arterial hypertension manifests a parasternal impulse and a loud pulmonic component of the S_2, which changes with respiration. The electrocardiogram in patients with pulmonary arterial hypertension demonstrates features of right axis deviation, right ventricular hypertrophy with tall R waves in the right precordial leads (V_1 and V_2) and deep S waves in the left precordial leads (V_5 and V_6), and, occasionally, a right ventricular strain pattern.

Patients with rheumatic mitral stenosis classically manifest a loud S_1, variable S_2, and an opening snap, followed by a low-pitched diastolic murmur. In the setting of concomitant pulmonary hypertension, the S_2 is loud and splits during inspiration but does not remain split during expiration. The electrocardiogram in patients with mitral stenosis demonstrates features of left atrial enlargement and hypertrophy. When pulmonary hypertension occurs, right ventricular hypertrophy is also demonstrated.

KEY POINT

- **The characteristic physical examination findings in atrial septal defect are a right ventricular impulse, fixed splitting of the S_2, a pulmonary mid-systolic murmur and a tricuspid diastolic flow rumble.**

Bibliography

Webb G, Gatzoulis MA. Atrial septal defects in the adult: recent progress and overview. Circulation. 2006;114(15):1645-1653. [PMID: 17030704]

Item 55   Answer: B

Educational Objective: Treat acute pericarditis after myocardial infarction.

The correct diagnosis in this middle-aged man is acute pericarditis associated with post–myocardial infarction syndrome, or Dressler syndrome. Post–myocardial infarction syndrome develops several weeks (rarely within a week) to months after an ST-elevation myocardial infarction and is characterized by pleuritic chest pain, pericardial friction rub, fever, leukocytosis, and, sometimes, pleural effusion or pulmonary infiltrates. This is distinguished from infarction pericarditis, which is characterized by a pericardial friction rub with or without chest pain and typically occurs within 1 to 2 days of the myocardial infarction. On electrocardiogram, acute pericarditis is characterized by diffuse ST-segment elevation that is characteristically concave upward (as opposed to downward, as in the case of a myocardial infarction) and PR-segment depression, which is nearly pathognomonic for pericarditis.

Anti-inflammatory therapy is the mainstay of treatment for pericarditis. Treatment with aspirin is preferred over NSAIDs if an acute myocardial infarction is the cause of acute pericarditis because its antiplatelet effects are beneficial and because of a prevailing concern that NSAIDs may promote ventricular rupture by impairing myocardial scar formation. Although animal data support this proposition, no definite proof for this concern exists in humans. However, expert opinion supports avoidance of these agents in this setting until further evidence is available. Thus, treatment of this patient's pericarditis with aspirin is the best option. Pharmacologic gastric protection (for example, a proton pump inhibitor) may be necessary in select patients to improve the gastric tolerability of aspirin.

Colchicine is an effective drug in the treatment of acute bouts of recurrent pericarditis. In addition, colchicine added to aspirin has been reported to be more effective than aspirin alone in the treatment of a first episode of idiopathic acute pericarditis. However, its efficacy in the treatment of acute pericarditis in the setting of myocardial infarction has not been firmly established. Colchicine therapy has no specific role in the treatment of patients after myocardial infarction. Thus, it would not be the best choice in this patient.

Corticosteroids such as prednisone may promote the development of recurrent pericarditis and should be avoided if possible in the treatment of acute pericarditis. They should be considered only in patients who are refractory to or have contraindications for the use of all alternative agents (aspirin, NSAIDs, and colchicine).

KEY POINT

- **Aspirin is preferred over NSAIDs to treat acute pericarditis that is caused by acute myocardial infarction.**

Bibliography

Imazio M, Bobbio M, Cecchi E, et al. Colchicine in addition to conventional therapy for acute pericarditis: results of the COlchicine for acute Pericarditis (COPE) trial. Circulation. 2005;112(13):2012-2016. [PMID: 16186437]

Item 56   Answer: B

Educational Objective: Manage a patient with an asymptomatic bicuspid aortic valve.

A bicuspid aortic valve is a common congenital abnormality. Because a bicuspid valve is subject to higher mechanical and shear stress than a tricuspid valve, the disease process of progressive calcification is accelerated, and clinical presentation tends to be earlier—in the fourth or fifth decades of life. This patient has a bicuspid aortic valve with moderate aortic regurgitation. Echocardiography demonstrates normal left ventricular size and systolic function. Pulmonary pressures are in the normal range, and there is no evidence of adverse hemodynamic effects of valve regurgitation on the ventricle (ventricular size and function are normal). No specific treatment is needed at this time. However, because worsening of aortic regurgitation can be insidious, routine clinical follow-up is indicated in at least yearly intervals, typically with repeat transthoracic echocardiography to monitor for disease progression. The presence of a bicuspid aortic valve is associated with ascending aorta dilation, and transthoracic echocardiography can also monitor for aortic enlargement. Most patients with bicuspid valves will eventually develop significant abnormalities—aortic stenosis, regurgitation, or aortic root dilation or dissection—that require surgery.

Many patients with bicuspid aortic valves have underlying disorders of vascular connective tissue with loss of elastic tissue, which leads to progressive dilation of the ascending aorta. Surgery is recommended when the aortic root or proximal ascending aorta exceeds 5 cm in diameter. If there is moderate dilatation (diameter 4.0-4.9 cm), serial imaging is recommended to monitor for progressive dilation and dysfunction.

Endocarditis prophylaxis is now recommended only in patients at the highest risk of developing endocarditis and in whom an adverse outcome would be most severe. This includes those with prosthetic cardiac valves, those with a known history of prior infective endocarditis, cardiac transplant recipients with valve abnormalities, those with unrepaired cyanotic congenital heart disease, and those with complex congenital heart disease with residual abnormalities. Antibiotic prophylaxis is no longer recommended in all other patient subsets. This patient, therefore, should not receive antibiotic prophylaxis prior to dental procedures.

Aortic valve replacement surgery is recommended in patients with severe aortic regurgitation and cardiopulmonary symptoms. In asymptomatic patients with severe regurgitation, surgery is recommended once there are signs of adverse hemodynamic effects on the left ventricle, left ventricular enlargement, or the ejection fraction falls below 55%. This patient has moderate aortic regurgitation. He is asymptomatic and his left ventricular size and function are normal. Valve replacement surgery is not indicated at this time.

Transthoracic echocardiography is generally adequate for visualization of the proximal 4 cm of the aortic root, but additional transesophageal echocardiography, cardiac MRI, or CT may aid in further imaging if inadequate visualization with transthoracic imaging is present. Transesophageal echocardiography is not indicated in this patient because adequate diagnostic information was obtained from the transthoracic echocardiography study.

> **KEY POINT**
>
> • Guidelines for prevention of infective endocarditis now recommend antibiotic prophylaxis only for persons with prosthetic valves, prior endocarditis, cardiac transplant recipients with valvulopathy, and complex congenital heart disease.

Bibliography

Wilson W, Taubert KA, Gewitz M, et al. Prevention of infective endocarditis: guidelines from the American Heart Association: a guideline from the American Heart Association Rheumatic Fever, Endocarditis, and Kawasaki Disease Committee, Council on Cardiovascular Disease in the Young, and the Council on Clinical Cardiology, Council on Cardiovascular Surgery and Anesthesia, and the Quality of Care and Outcomes Research Interdisciplinary Working Group [erratum in Circulation. 2007;116(15):e376-7.]. Circulation. 2007;116(15):1736-1754. [PMID: 17446442]

Item 57   Answer: D

Educational Objective: Choose a diagnostic test to evaluate a patient with cardiovascular symptoms.

The most appropriate test for this patient is a dobutamine echocardiographic stress test. This 65-year-old woman has atypical angina, and her pretest probability of coronary artery disease (CAD) is, therefore, intermediate. For patients with an intermediate likelihood of CAD who have no features of unstable angina, exercise stress testing is the preferred approach when assessing for CAD. For patients who cannot exercise because of pulmonary or mobility limitations, pharmacologic stress testing can be performed using agents that mimic the catecholamine increases of exercise, such as dobutamine, or agents that cause coronary artery vasodilation, such as adenosine or dipyridamole. The presence of severe degenerative arthritis of the knees would most likely limit the ability of this patient to achieve an adequate level of stress with exercise treadmill stress testing. Therefore, the diagnostic accuracy of treadmill stress testing would be too low in this setting to exclude CAD, and a noninvasive stress test with imaging (nuclear or echocardiography) is therefore needed.

Adenosine and dipyridamole are contraindicated in patients with hypotension, sick sinus syndrome, high-degree atrioventricular block, and bronchospastic disease. These agents may cause dyspnea and reduced FEV_1 in persons with chronic obstructive pulmonary disease. For these reasons, dobutamine is the preferred pharmacologic agent for stress testing in the presence of underlying bronchospastic lung disease.

Coronary angiography remains the gold standard to evaluate patients for CAD. However, this is an invasive test which carries a small, but inherent risk of vascular complications. For patients at intermediate risk for CAD, in the absence of a recent acute coronary syndrome, noninvasive stress testing is the recommended diagnostic approach.

A coronary artery calcium score allows quantification of coronary artery calcium, but in this patient would not confirm that the current symptoms were due to underlying CAD. Quantification of coronary artery calcium may be useful in asymptomatic patients at intermediate risk for CAD, and in this setting may further refine risk stratification. The patient presented is symptomatic, however, and assessment of coronary artery calcium would not provide functional information for coronary ischemia. In this setting, coronary artery calcium scanning would not be a substitute for noninvasive stress testing to determine if this patient's chest pain is caused by CAD.

> **KEY POINT**
>
> • Adenosine and dipyridamole stress testing are contraindicated in patients with severe bronchospastic disease.

Bibliography

Fletcher GF, Mills WC, Taylor WC. Update on exercise stress testing. Am Fam Physician. 2006;74(10):1749-1754. [PMID: 17137006]

Item 58   Answer: D

Educational Objective: Treat a heart failure patient who has angiotensin-converting enzyme inhibitor intolerance.

Angiotensin-converting enzyme (ACE) inhibitors improve the survival and quality of life in patients with heart failure. This patient has developed hyperkalemia and a rise in creatinine level (greater than 30% above baseline) related to ACE inhibitor treatment. For most patients, if the initial dose of an ACE inhibitor is poorly tolerated, lower doses should be used. However, this patient was started on the lowest dose of enalapril, and a dose reduction is not practical. Beginning ACE inhibitors at low doses and slowly titrating toward the maximum doses used in clinical trials increases the probability that the medication will be tolerated by most patients. For patients intolerant of ACE inhibitors due to hyperkalemia or renal insufficiency, the combination of hydralazine and a nitrate is a suitable alternative, with hemodynamic effects of vasodilation and afterload reduction. Treatment with this combination is also associated with a reduction in mortality, although to a lesser degree than is seen with ACE inhibitors, and this combination does not have the same positive impact on quality of life as an ACE inhibitor.

The incidence of drug-induced hyperkalemia and renal insufficiency is similar with ACE inhibitors and angiotensin receptor blockers (ARBs); therefore, switching to the ARB candesartan would not be appropriate in this patient. The primary reason to use an ARB rather than an ACE inhibitor is to avoid the side effect of cough.

Digoxin is indicated for symptom amelioration in heart failure, but this patient is asymptomatic, so digoxin is not indicated. The addition of digoxin does not impact survival but is associated with a risk of toxicity if drug levels are not carefully managed.

Eplerenone is a selective aldosterone blocker that is currently approved for treatment of hypertension and for left ventricular dysfunction after myocardial infarction. Eplerenone is a suitable alternative to spironolactone in treatment of severe heart failure (New York Heart Association class III or IV) if gynecomastia develops as a side effect of spironolactone treatment. This patient has New York Heart Association class I heart failure and does not meet the criteria for treatment with an aldosterone agonist. Furthermore, eplerenone would exacerbate hyperkalemia.

KEY POINT

- **For patients intolerant of angiotensin-converting enzyme inhibitors due to hyperkalemia or renal insufficiency, the combination of hydralazine and a nitrate is a suitable alternative.**

Bibliography

Hunt SA; American College of Cardiology; American Heart Association Task Force on Practice Guidelines (Writing Committee to Update the 2001 Guidelines for the Evaluation and Management of Heart Failure). ACC/AHA 2005 guideline update for the diagnosis and management of chronic heart failure in the adult [erratum in J Am Coll Cardiol. 2006;47(7):1503-1505.]. J Am Coll Cardiol. 2005;46(6):e1-82. [PMID: 16168273]

Item 59   Answer: B

Educational Objective: Manage a patient with ventricular fibrillation arrest in the setting of acute myocardial infarction.

The best option for the patient at this time is to continue medical management. Ventricular tachyarrhythmias are common in the setting of acute myocardial infarction, occurring in up to 20% of patients. Despite a 6-fold increase in in-hospital mortality, the overall mortality at 1 year is not increased in patients with ventricular fibrillation that occurs early in this setting. Therefore, unlike sudden cardiac death occurring in other settings, cardiac arrest occurring within the first 48 hours of transmural acute myocardial infarction does not require defibrillator placement. Primary ventricular fibrillation should be distinguished from ventricular fibrillation that occurs later in the course, usually as a result of heart failure. All patients, even those who have not suffered arrhythmia during myocardial infarction, should be re-evaluated after myocardial infarction by transthoracic echocardiogram to further stratify risk. If the ejection fraction is found to be reduced (<35%), the patient may be a candidate for defibrillator placement.

Amiodarone has not been shown to improve overall mortality following myocardial infarction, although some studies have shown a decrease in deaths due to arrhythmias. In the general population of cardiac arrest survivors, however, amiodarone does not improve mortality.

Implantable cardioverter-defibrillator placement is not indicated for patients who experience ventricular arrhythmias less than 48 hours after an acute ST-elevation myocardial infarction. Implantable cardioverter-defibrillators have demonstrated a mortality benefit for essentially all other groups of cardiac arrest survivors.

Electrophysiology study can be useful in the long-term management of myocardial infarction patients whose left ventricular ejection fractions are borderline (35%–45%) after the event, particularly if high-risk markers, such as nonsustained ventricular tachycardia on ambulatory monitoring, are seen. However, it is not indicated in the setting of an asymptomatic patient after myocardial infarction.

KEY POINT

- **Unlike sudden cardiac death occurring in other settings, cardiac arrest occurring within the first 48 hours of an acute, transmural myocardial infarction does not require secondary prevention therapy other than standard post–myocardial infarction care.**

Bibliography

Zipes DP, Camm AJ, Borggrefe M, et al. ACC/AHA/ESC 2006 Guidelines for Management of Patients With Ventricular Arrhythmias and the Prevention of Sudden Cardiac Death: a report of the American College of Cardiology/American Heart Association Task Force and the European Society of Cardiology Committee for Practice Guidelines (writing committee to develop Guidelines for Management of Patients With Ventricular Arrhythmias and the Prevention of Sudden Cardiac Death): developed in collaboration with the European Heart Rhythm Association and the Heart Rhythm Society. Circulation. 2006;114(10):e385-484. [PMID: 16935995]

Item 60   Answer: C

Educational Objective: Manage primary prophylaxis of sudden death in a patient with systolic heart failure.

The most common cause of sudden death in patients with heart failure is arrhythmia, including both ventricular tachyarrhythmia and bradyarrhythmia. Current guidelines recommend implantable cardioverter-defibrillator (ICD) placement in patients with ischemic or nonischemic cardiomyopathy and an ejection fraction of less than or equal to 35%. ICD placement is, therefore, indicated in this setting (primary prevention), regardless of symptoms or functional status. This patient's most recent left ventricular ejection fraction was 25%; ICD placement is the correct option.

This patient does not meet current criteria for implantation of a biventricular pacemaker in addition to ICD implantation. This patient is asymptomatic (New York Heart Association [NYHA] class I) and does not have a prolonged QRS complex on electrocardiogram. Current criteria for biventricular pacemaker implantation include left ventricular ejection fraction less than or equal to 35%, QRS duration greater than or equal to 120 msec, sinus rhythm, and NYHA class III or IV symptoms (that is, symptoms with mild activity or at rest) on optimal medical therapy for heart failure.

This patient has a very good functional capacity and no symptoms to suggest angina. He does not have other clinical evidence to suggest worsening coronary artery disease, such as worsening heart failure. The primary aim of stress testing or coronary angiography would be to evaluate for ischemia that might be treated with revascularization, which is not an issue in this patient.

The role of warfarin solely for treatment of a low ejection fraction is currently controversial; trials to study this issue are ongoing. Patients with heart failure often have concurrent conditions that do warrant treatment with warfarin, such as atrial fibrillation or ventricular thrombus, but this patient does not.

KEY POINT

- **Implantable cardioverter-defibrillator placement is indicated for patients with ischemic or nonischemic cardiomyopathy and an ejection fraction less than or equal to 35% for mortality reduction, regardless of symptoms or functional status.**

Bibliography

Epstein AE, DiMarco JP, Ellenbogen KA, et al. ACC/AHA/HRS 2008 Guidelines for Device-Based Therapy of Cardiac Rhythm Abnormalities: a report of the American College of Cardiology/American Heart Association Task Force on Practice Guidelines (Writing Committee to Revise the ACC/AHA/NASPE 2002 Guideline Update for Implantation of Cardiac Pacemakers and Antiarrhythmia Devices) developed in collaboration with the American Association for Thoracic Surgery and Society of Thoracic Surgeons. J Am Coll Cardiol. 2008;117(21):e350-408. [PMID: 18483207]

Item 61   Answer: B

Educational Objective: Manage severe pulmonary valve stenosis.

This patient has features of severe symptomatic pulmonary valve stenosis with right ventricular pressure overload. The jugular venous pulse contour in pulmonary stenosis demonstrates a prominent a wave. A right ventricular lift is frequently present. An early systolic click is common, and increased proximity of the click to the S_1 suggests increased severity of pulmonary stenosis. A systolic murmur with a delayed pulmonic component of the S_2 is noted. In patients with severe valvular pulmonary stenosis, the pulmonic component of the S_2 and ejection click disappear due to reduced pliability of the valve. Right ventricular hypertrophy and right axis deviation are noted on the electrocardiogram.

The diagnosis of pulmonary valve stenosis is confirmed by transthoracic echocardiography. Echocardiography with Doppler evaluation determines the severity of pulmonary stenosis and the degree of right ventricular hypertrophy. Intervention is recommended when the gradient is greater than 50 mm Hg or when right ventricular hypertrophy is present. Systolic doming of the pulmonary valve noted on two-dimensional echocardiography suggests that the valve is likely amenable to percutaneous intervention.

The treatment of choice for pulmonary valve stenosis is pulmonary balloon valvuloplasty. This treatment was developed in the mid 1980s and is now the treatment of choice for isolated pulmonary valve stenosis and provides a durable reduction in pulmonary valve gradient. However, repeat intervention is needed more often in patients treated with balloon valvuloplasty rather than surgical intervention.

Angiotensin-converting enzyme inhibitors are not recommended for patients with pulmonary valve stenosis alone. The patient presented has normal blood pressure and ventricular function; there is no indication to initiate this medication.

Surgical intervention for pulmonary valve stenosis was the standard treatment for many years. Since the advent of balloon intervention, however, this has become the procedure of choice. Patients are at increased risk of pulmonary valve regurgitation following surgical intervention for pulmonary stenosis. Pulmonary regurgitation may also occur late after pulmonary balloon valvuloplasty, but because percutaneous intervention is noninvasive, less expensive, and carries a lower risk of morbidity and mortality than operative intervention, this is the procedure of choice.

Clinical observation would not be appropriate for this patient with symptoms related to severe pulmonary valve stenosis. Progressive symptoms of dyspnea, fatigue, and eventually right-sided heart failure will occur without intervention. In addition, the degree of right ventricular pressure overload and hypertrophy suggests that intervention is recommended.

KEY POINT

- **Pulmonary balloon valvuloplasty is the treatment of choice for patients with isolated congenital pulmonary valve stenosis.**

Bibliography
Warnes CA, Williams RG, Bashore TM, et al. ACC/AHA 2008 Guidelines for the Management of Adults with Congenital Heart Disease: a report of the American College of Cardiology/American Heart Association Task Force on Practice Guidelines (writing committee to develop guidelines on the management of adults with congenital heart disease). Circulation. 2008;118(23):e714-833. [PMID: 18997169]

Item 62   Answer: A

Educational Objective: Evaluate angina in a patient with a chronic inflammatory condition.

The patient is a young woman with hypertension but no other traditional risk factors for coronary heart disease. However, she has a long history of systemic lupus erythematosus, which is an autoimmune inflammatory disease. Inflammation is a possible mechanism of vascular endothelial injury and may promote the development of atherosclerotic disease. Coronary artery disease is a major cause of premature death in patients with systemic lupus erythematosus, and atherosclerosis has been found to develop prematurely in this disease. In addition, persons with systemic lupus erythematosus may have other cardiac involvement including pericardial disease (acute or recurrent pericarditis, pericardial effusion and tamponade, constrictive pericarditis), myocarditis, cardiomyopathy, and valvular regurgitation due to noninfective endocarditis.

The patient's presenting symptoms are typical of unstable angina: the pain is new in onset, progressive, and occurs with minimal activity or at rest. In light of the severity of her symptoms, electrocardiographic abnormalities consistent with ischemia (probably in the distribution of the proximal left anterior descending coronary artery), and the indeterminate troponin T level, coronary angiography and possible revascularization are indicated. Exercise stress echocardiography should not be performed because of her unstable symptoms and her high pretest probability of coronary artery disease.

High-sensitivity C-reactive protein level, a nonspecific biomarker of inflammation, would likely be abnormally elevated in this patient with systemic lupus erythematosus and is not diagnostically useful in this setting. In fact, this test, which is often used to assess ongoing inflammation as a predictor of future risk of cardiovascular events, is not valid in the setting of recent infection or chronic inflammatory conditions.

Transthoracic echocardiography is not indicated for this patient. Although she has a history of pericarditis, her symptoms, examination findings, and electrocardiographic findings are not consistent with either recurrent pericarditis or constrictive pericarditis. Acute pericarditis is associated with sharp, pleuritic, positional chest pain and diffuse ST-segment and T-wave abnormalities not in a distribution consistent with a coronary artery territory.

KEY POINT

- **Chronic inflammatory conditions, such as systemic lupus erythematosus, may be associated with cardiac complications, including premature atherosclerotic coronary artery disease.**

Bibliography
Knockaert DC. Cardiac involvement in systemic inflammatory diseases. Eur Heart J. 2007;28(15):1797-1804. [PMID: 17562669]

Item 63   Answer: B

Educational Objective: Diagnose right ventricular infarction complicating an inferior wall ST-elevation myocardial infarction.

Right ventricular infarction occurs in approximately 20% of patients with an inferior wall ST-elevation myocardial infarction (STEMI). This diagnosis should be considered in patients with the clinical triad of hypotension, clear lung fields, and jugular venous distention. Sublingual nitroglycerin further limits filling of the right ventricle and therefore worsens hypotension. The diagnosis can be made using a right-sided electrocardiogram, on which ST-segment elevation in leads V_3R and V_4R will be seen. In the patient presented, subtle (0.5 mm) ST-segment elevation in lead V_1 suggests the diagnosis, as lead V_1 is adjacent to the right ventricle. Treatment for right ventricular infarction consists of rapid restoration of blood flow to the right ventricle with either thrombolytic therapy or primary percutaneous coronary intervention, aggressive volume loading to increase filling of the right ventricle, and dopamine or dobutamine if hypotension persists.

Pericardial tamponade from rupture of the left ventricular free wall usually leads to sudden hypotension and death. Free wall rupture is second only to heart failure as the most common cause of death for patients who die in hospitals after myocardial infarction. Ventricular free wall rupture typically occurs 1 to 4 days after acute myocardial infarction. It would be unlikely for pericardial tamponade to be present upon initial presentation unless the patient had chest pain for several days prior to the hospitalization.

Increased vagal tone can cause bradycardia and decreased right ventricular preload, resulting in hypotension early in the course of a myocardial infarction. Although increased vagal tone is commonly associated with inferior wall myocardial infarction, the patient's tachycardia and hypotension suggest an alternative diagnosis.

A ventricular septal defect manifests as a new systolic murmur, hypotension, and respiratory distress 1 to 3 days following the onset of a myocardial infarction. It would be exceedingly uncommon for a patient to present initially with a ventricular septal defect, unless symptoms of chest pain were present for several days.

> **KEY POINT**
> - In the setting of an inferior wall ST-elevation myocardial infarction, the clinical triad of hypotension, clear lung fields, and jugular venous distention suggests a right ventricular infarction.

Bibliography
Kinch JW, Ryan TJ. Right ventricular infarction. N Engl J Med. 1994;330(17):1211-1217. [PMID: 8139631]

Item 64   Answer: C
Educational Objective: Evaluate palpitations in a healthy young person.

Palpitation is one of the most frequent symptom complaints evaluated in general medicine practice. Most patients (60%-80%) are not ultimately diagnosed with a cardiac arrhythmia; however, continuous loop recorders have been shown to provide a higher efficacy in diagnosis, and are cost effective compared with other modalities.

Loop recorders, as opposed to hand-held event monitors, continuously record data but only save when the patient manually activates the monitor because of symptoms. Rhythm data are saved preceding and following activation, usually for a period of 1 to 2 minutes. The advantages of loop recorders include a longer period of monitoring time (up to 1 month) compared with 24-hour ambulatory monitoring and continuous monitoring in patients with transient loss of consciousness. Hand-held event monitors are not useful in patients with transient symptoms or loss of consciousness, and are often not successfully used by patients.

β-Blockers are a key therapy for supraventricular tachycardia, however, this patient's resting sinus bradycardia and athletic regimen place her at risk for symptomatic bradycardia and exercise intolerance. In addition, further evaluation is necessary for diagnosis of this patient's symptoms prior to treatment. If she is diagnosed with supraventricular tachycardia, she would be an excellent candidate for catheter ablation, because she is highly symptomatic and the success rate of the procedure is very high.

Ambulatory monitors, which continuously record and save data over a 24- to 48-hour period, are often unrevealing, unless the patient is experiencing symptoms several times a day. Ambulatory monitoring has been shown to have less diagnostic efficacy and is less cost effective than continuous loop recording.

Cardiovascular symptoms are common in panic disorder, with more than 25% of patients reporting palpitations or tachycardia. The diagnosis of panic attack requires four or more of the following symptoms that develop abruptly and peak within 10 minutes: palpitations, pounding heart, or accelerated heart rate; sweating; trembling or shaking; sensations of shortness of breath or smothering; feeling of choking; chest pain or discomfort; nausea or abdominal distress; feeling dizzy, unsteady, lightheaded, or faint; derealization (feelings of unreality) or depersonalization (being detached from oneself); fear of losing control or going crazy; fear of dying; paresthesias (numbness or tingling sensations); chills or hot flushes. Selective serotonin-reuptake inhibitors, such as sertraline, are the first-line treatment of choice for panic disorder. The patient does not meet the diagnostic criteria for panic disorder, however, and treatment with sertraline is not indicated.

This patient is highly likely to be experiencing recurrent supraventricular tachycardia, and should be further evaluated with rhythm monitoring. Features that suggest supraventricular tachycardia in this patient include termination with a Valsalva maneuver, sustained episodes, and the triggers of her episodes.

> **KEY POINT**
> - Continuous-loop monitoring is more effective in diagnosis of tachycardia than ambulatory monitoring.

Bibliography
Abbott AV. Diagnostic approach to palpitations. Am Fam Physician. 2005;71(4):743-750. [PMID: 15742913]

Item 65   Answer: C
Educational Objective: Manage heart failure following ST-elevation myocardial infarction.

This patient has developed heart failure following treatment of his ST-elevation myocardial infarction (STEMI). Early complications of a STEMI include failure of thrombolytic therapy, arrhythmias, heart failure, and bleeding. The optimal treatment for patients who develop heart failure early in the course of a STEMI includes afterload reduction with an angiotensin-converting enzyme inhibitor and preload reduction with nitroglycerin and diuretics. At high doses, nitroglycerin variably reduces afterload and increases stroke volume and cardiac output. Heart failure is more commonly seen in patients with larger infarcts, such as an anterior STEMI. The absence of a murmur in this patient and the timing of the patient's respiratory distress (within 24 hours from the initial diagnosis of STEMI) argue against other causes of respiratory distress in the setting of a large myocardial infarction, such as ischemic mitral regurgitation and a ventricular septal defect.

Dobutamine may be useful in patients who develop heart failure early in the course of a STEMI if there is hypotension and evidence of systemic hypoperfusion, such as reduced urine output. Dobutamine should be used cautiously in patients with myocardial infarction, however, as it may induce ventricular arrhythmias and has the potential to increase oxygen demand and therefore extend the infarction. In this patient with stable blood pressure and no evidence of hypoperfusion, dobutamine is not indicated.

In this patient with worsening heart failure with severe volume overload, increasing metoprolol would exacerbate the heart failure by further impairing cardiac output. The key treatment of this patient should be aggressive preload reduction with an intravenous diuretic.

Repeat administration of thrombolytic therapy is not indicated because this patient does not have thrombolytic therapy failure. Although resolution of ST-segment elevation is incomplete in most patients, improvement of ST-segment elevation greater than 50% an hour after the administration of thrombolytic therapy generally indicates successful reperfusion. This patient's ST-segment elevation has improved substantially on the repeat electrocardiogram, and his chest pain has resolved. Potential treatment options for thrombolytic therapy failure include rescue percutaneous coronary intervention (PCI), conservative management, or repeat administration of thrombolytic therapy. In a randomized trial of these three options in patients with failure of thrombolytic therapy, repeat administration of thrombolytic therapy did not improve clinical outcome. Rescue PCI did provide clinical benefit.

KEY POINT

- **Heart failure following treatment of an ST-elevation myocardial infarction includes afterload reduction with an angiotensin-converting enzyme inhibitor and preload reduction with nitroglycerin and diuretics.**

Bibliography

Gershlick AH, Stephens-Lloyd A, Hughes S, et al; REACT Trial Investigators. Rescue angioplasty after failed thrombolytic therapy for acute myocardial infarction. N Engl J Med. 2005;353(26):2758-2768. [PMID: 16382062]

Item 66   Answer: E

Educational Objective: Manage asymptomatic aortic stenosis in a patient undergoing noncardiac surgery.

The best perioperative management option for this patient is to proceed directly to hip replacement. Preoperative assessment of cardiovascular risk includes a careful physical examination, a thorough assessment for cardiopulmonary symptoms and exercise tolerance, as well as an evaluation of the type of surgery contemplated and indication (high versus low risk, elective versus nonelective). In the evaluation of patients prior to noncardiac surgery, cardiac murmurs are

commonly encountered. This patient has clinical and echocardiographic findings consistent with aortic stenosis (delayed distal pulses, a radiating systolic murmur, and a single S_2 due to delayed closure of the calcified aortic valve). Aortic stenosis is a slowly progressive disease process, and asymptomatic patients can remain event-free for prolonged time periods. As a consequence, prophylactic valve replacement is not performed in asymptomatic patients. In patients with significant aortic stenosis but with good preoperative exercise tolerance, surgical procedures are generally well tolerated. The patient in this question was asymptomatic and active prior to her fall. Most asymptomatic aortic stenosis patients who need noncardiac surgery can be managed conservatively with careful intraoperative attention to fluid balance. For patients with advanced cardiac disease, an anesthesiologist with additional cardiovascular training (cardiac anesthesiologist) may be preferred.

Percutaneous aortic balloon valvuloplasty is generally not performed for calcific aortic stenosis because serious complications, including aortic regurgitation and embolic stroke, occur in more than 10% of procedures, and restenosis occurs within a year in most patients. Rarely, valvuloplasty is considered in patients with severe, symptomatic aortic stenosis who require emergent noncardiac surgery and are not candidates for valve replacement. This is not an appropriate course of action in this patient.

In symptomatic patients, postponement of noncardiac surgery until after valve replacement should be considered, particularly if surgery is elective. This patient is asymptomatic and valve replacement is not indicated, and it would be unwise to postpone this patient's hip replacement surgery.

This patient is hemodynamically stable, and neither an intra-aortic balloon pump nor intravenous nitroprusside is indicated.

KEY POINT

- **Prophylactic aortic valve replacement is not performed in asymptomatic patients with aortic stenosis.**

Bibliography

Zahid M, Sonel AF, Saba S, Good CB. Perioperative risk of noncardiac surgery associated with aortic stenosis. Am J Cardiol. 2005;96(3):436-438. [PMID: 16054477]

Item 67   Answer: A

Educational Objective: Manage repaired tetralogy of Fallot over the long term.

The best option for this patient is to undergo cardiac magnetic resonance imaging. Although repaired tetralogy of Fallot is associated with a higher risk of cardiac arrhythmias, the slow onset and offset and persistent nature of this patient's symptoms, in conjunction with excess caffeine intake and stress, are most consistent with sinus tachycardia. Many young adults with congenital heart disease mistakenly believe they no longer need regular evaluation and, like this patient, present to a primary care physician with unrelated symptoms. However, the finding of a diastolic murmur consistent with pulmonic regurgitation and right ventricular enlargement requires further evaluation because these findings would not be present if the pulmonic valve was still competent after surgical repair. In adults with repaired tetralogy of Fallot, the most common long-term adverse outcome is severe pulmonic regurgitation leading to right ventricular dilation and systolic dysfunction.

Surgical repair for tetralogy of Fallot includes closure of the ventricular septal defect and relief of right ventricular outflow obstruction. Usually, outflow obstruction is relieved by surgically opening fused valve leaflets or by placement of a patch to enlarge the pulmonic annulus (transannular patch). This approach avoids placement of a prosthetic valve because a prosthesis will not grow with the child and is prone to rapid degeneration in children. However, this approach often results in pulmonic regurgitation, which is initially well tolerated, but eventually results in right ventricular volume overload and systolic dysfunction. Cardiac magnetic resonance imaging is the most accurate method for quantitation of right ventricular volumes and ejection fraction, and can also provide quantitative measures of pulmonic regurgitant severity. Repeat pulmonic valve surgery will eventually be needed in this patient to prevent progressive right heart dysfunction.

Chest CT is useful for evaluation of coronary anomalies and aortic dimensions, but these are not the primary concern in this patient. Mild aortic root dilation is typical of tetralogy of Fallot and is rarely associated with progressive dilation.

There is no reason to discourage pregnancy in this patient because she has no high-risk features—she is not cyanotic, her left ventricular function is normal, she does not have severe left-sided valve obstruction, and she has an excellent functional status.

Endocarditis prophylaxis is no longer recommended for native valve disease. In persons with congenital heart disease, endocarditis prophylaxis is recommended only with cyanotic disease or in the first 6 months after implantation of prosthetic material.

Reassurance alone is inappropriate for this patient. Although her presenting symptoms are likely benign, she needs further diagnostic evaluation of her structural heart disease and should also be referred to an established center for management of adult congenital heart disease.

KEY POINT

- Endocarditis prophylaxis is no longer needed in native valve disease or most cases of repaired congenital heart disease.

Bibliography

Oosterhof T, van Straten A, Vliegen HW, et al. Preoperative thresholds for pulmonary valve replacement in patients with corrected tetralogy of Fallot using cardiovascular magnetic resonance. Circulation. 2007;116(5):545-551. [PMID: 17620511]

Item 68   Answer: B

Educational Objective: Treat symptomatic premature ventricular complexes.

This patient presents with frequent symptomatic premature ventricular complexes. Premature ventricular complexes are spontaneous depolarizations originating from the ventricles. A premature complex can be single, in pairs (couplets), or alternating with sinus beats in a specific multiple, such as in bigeminy, in which premature ventricular complexes and sinus beats alternate in a 1:1 ratio. These beats are usually followed by a compensatory pause, and patients may feel as if their heart is stopping. In the absence of structural heart disease, the prognosis is benign, and treatment is based on ameliorating significant symptoms, which may include palpitations, fatigue, and lightheadedness. β-Blockers, such as metoprolol, are reasonably effective at suppressing premature ventricular complexes. This prognosis is in contrast to patients with heart failure, hypertension, or left ventricular hypertrophy; in all of these groups, ventricular ectopy has been described as a marker of increased risk of cardiovascular events.

The high incidence of side effects and organ system toxicity that occurs with amiodarone therapy proscribes its use as a first-line agent for suppression of premature ventricular complexes.

A pacemaker has no primary role in the treatment of symptomatic premature ventricular complexes. In some rare cases, a patient may require pacemaker placement in order to tolerate the bradyarrhythmic side effects of medical therapy.

Radiofrequency ablation is generally reserved for patients with severe symptoms that are refractory to drug therapy and those with more sustained ventricular arrhythmias, particularly those with ectopy originating from the right ventricular outflow tract. In the present case, the multifocal nature of the patient's ectopy, as documented by the varying morphologies of the premature ventricular complexes, would reduce the efficacy of the procedure.

KEY POINT

- Suppression of premature ventricular complexes is only indicated in patients with severe and disabling symptoms; in these patients, β-blockers are the safest initial choice.

Bibliography

Ng GA. Treating patients with ventricular ectopic beats. Heart. 2006;92(11):1707-1712. [PMID: 17041126]

Item 69   Answer: A

Educational Objective: Manage a black patient with New York Heart Association functional class III or IV systolic heart failure.

The addition of hydralazine and isosorbide dinitrate to standard medical therapy is indicated for treatment of black patients with systolic heart failure and New York Heart Association functional class III or IV symptoms. Hydralazine and nitrates together provide afterload reduction in patients with left ventricular dysfunction. Hydralazine and isosorbide dinitrate have been shown to reduce mortality by 40% in black patients when added to standard medical therapy (angiotensin-converting enzyme inhibitor, β-blocker). Although the patient's blood pressure is lower than the usual normal ranges, patients with systolic heart failure will typically demonstrate lower than normal blood pressures owing to lower cardiac output and generally tolerate vasodilator medication without significant hypotension, as cardiac output is increased.

Digoxin is indicated in patients with NYHA class II to IV heart failure and left ventricular systolic dysfunction (ejection fraction <40%) despite optimal medical treatment with an angiotensin-converting enzyme (ACE) inhibitor and a β-blocker. Digoxin has been shown to alleviate symptoms and decrease hospitalizations in patients with heart failure but does not improve survival. This patient's digoxin level is therapeutic, and increasing the dose is not indicated. Higher levels of digoxin have been associated with increased mortality in the setting of heart failure.

This patient has no evidence of volume overload either by history or examination, so increasing diuresis with a higher dosage of furosemide is not indicated and may be detrimental, leading to a reduction in preload and resulting in decreased cardiac output.

Clinical outcomes are improved by the use of β-blockers, and the mortality rate is decreased in all classes of heart failure when these agents are used. The therapeutic goal for a β-blocker in most patients is titration to the highest therapeutic dose tolerated as limited by bradycardia, hypotension, or side effects. Although too high a dose of β-blocker can cause fatigue and decreased exercise capacity, this patient does not demonstrate bradycardia, which would suggest that the dosage of β-blocker is too high. In addition, the fatigue associated with β-blocker initiation or increase is typically a self-limited period that may last up to several weeks. This patient has been on a stable dose of medication for at least the past year. Therefore, stopping metoprolol is not the best option at this time.

KEY POINT

- **The addition of hydralazine and isosorbide dinitrate to standard medical therapy is indicated for treatment of black patients with systolic heart failure and New York Heart Association functional class III or IV symptoms.**

Bibliography

Taylor AL, Ziesche S, Yancy C, et al; African-American Heart Failure Trial Investigators. Combination of isosorbide dinitrate and hydralazine in blacks with heart failure [erratum in N Engl J Med. 2005;352(12):1276.]. N Engl J Med. 2004;351(20):2049-2057. [PMID: 15533851]

Item 70   Answer: C

Educational Objective: Manage a patient with highly symptomatic paroxysmal atrial fibrillation.

This patient with paroxysmal atrial fibrillation is experiencing frequent symptomatic episodes. Symptoms can result from inadequate rate control while in atrial fibrillation or from the atrial fibrillation itself in the absence of a rapid ventricular response. Given the frequency of episodes in this patient, 24-hour ambulatory monitoring will best allow correlation of symptoms with atrial fibrillation and permit assessment of rate control during atrial fibrillation. Pinpointing the cause of symptoms will allow formation of a management plan for effective rate control versus institution of a rhythm control strategy. Randomized controlled trials have not shown a mortality benefit from rhythm control; however, this finding may reflect the inadequacy of current antiarrhythmic medications.

Amiodarone, although more efficacious than other antiarrhythmic drugs, is an unappealing first-line antiarrhythmic agent owing to its side effect profile. This is particularly true in a young patient who presumably will require long-term management.

Even if a rate control strategy is ultimately chosen, the addition of digoxin is unlikely to be helpful in this young, healthy patient, owing to its vagotonic mechanism of action. Because vagal tone is higher in young persons, digoxin is less effective as a rate control agent. Correspondingly, its effects are diminished with activity, because vagal input is withdrawn and sympathetic input is enhanced with action. Digoxin can therefore be a useful rate-control adjunct in elderly or inactive patients but is still usually second-line therapy, as it is not as effective as β-blockers or calcium-channel blockers.

The patient's symptoms are of sufficient frequency to allow for external ambulatory monitoring; an implanted loop recorder, with its additional inconvenience and expense, is therefore not indicated.

KEY POINT

- **In patients with atrial fibrillation, it is important to correlate symptoms with episodes of arrhythmia and assess rate control to determine whether symptoms are caused by rapid heart rate or by the atrial fibrillation itself.**

Bibliography

Fuster V, Rydén LE, Cannom DS, et al. ACC/AHA/ESC 2006 guidelines for the management of patients with atrial fibrillation: full text: a report of the American College of Cardiology/American Heart Association Task Force on practice guidelines and the European Society of Cardiology Committee for Practice Guidelines (Writing Committee to Revise the 2001 guidelines for the management of patients with atrial fibrillation) developed in collaboration with the European Heart Rhythm Association and the Heart Rhythm Society [erratum in Europace. 2007;9(9):856.]. Europace. 2006;8(9):651-745. [PMID: 16987906]

Item 71   Answer: C

Educational Objective: Diagnose aortic dissection.

Clinical suspicion of aortic dissection is based upon presenting symptoms, physical findings, and radiographic tests. In this patient, the abrupt onset of chest discomfort of maximal intensity is consistent with an acute aortic syndrome. Physical examination findings typical of acute aortic dissection include severe aortic pain, blood pressure or pulse differential between the arms, and a widened mediastinum on chest radiograph. The positive likelihood ratio of aortic dissection in a patient with one of these findings is 0.5, with two of these findings, 5.3; and with all three of these findings, 66.

The recent use of cocaine increases the risks for aortic dissection acutely around the time of use. A transesophageal echocardiogram is the appropriate test at this time because it could be performed rapidly and would allow inspection of the ascending and descending thoracic aorta for dissection or other acute aortic pathology, as well as characterize the location and extent of such findings. Additionally, transesophageal echocardiography would allow evaluation of the pericardial space, competence of the aortic valve, and left ventricular function and regional wall motion analysis, elements that would be integral to treatment, especially if a proximal (type A) dissection is present.

A ventilation-perfusion lung scan would be useful for evaluation of pulmonary embolism. Although acute pulmonary embolism should be considered in a patient with chest pain, the lack of dyspnea, hypoxemia, or underlying risk factors for venous thrombosis and a reasonable alternative diagnosis make pulmonary embolism less likely.

Acute myocardial infarction is possible as a cause of chest pain, despite the lack of specific ST-T segment changes on the electrocardiogram and the initial normal cardiac troponin level. However, the normal myoglobin level measured 90 minutes after the onset of continuous symptoms makes this diagnosis less likely. Nuclear myocardial perfusion imaging is useful as part of the diagnosis of an acute coronary syndrome when the electrocardiogram is nonspecific, initial cardiac enzyme tests are negative, and clinical suspicion is high.

Transesophageal echocardiography (TEE), contrast-enhanced CT, and MRI (without contrast) have similar sensitivity and diagnostic accuracy for the detection of acute aortic dissection. TEE has the benefit of being a portable test that can be performed at bedside, and it yields additional information regarding ventricular and valvular function. Contrast-enhanced chest CT would normally be an acceptable test for further investigation of a suspected acute aortic syndrome. However, the patient's abnormal renal function makes this choice less attractive because of the risks of dye-induced nephropathy. Contrast is not necessary with MRI for definition of an acute aortic dissection, but it may be useful in the evaluation of chronic dissection for defining flow in the false lumen. However, gadolinium contrast should be avoided in this patient because of the risk of nephrogenic fibrosing dermopathy.

KEY POINT

- **When aortic dissection is suspected, transesophageal echocardiography can be performed quickly to assess the aorta, pericardium, aortic valve, and left ventricular function.**

Bibliography

Sommer T, Fehske W, Holzknecht N, et al. Aortic dissection: a comparative study of diagnosis with spiral CT, multiplanar transesophageal echocardiography, and MR imaging. Radiology. 1996;199(2):347-352. [PMID: 8668776]

Item 72   Answer: C

Educational Objective: Treat atrial septal defect.

The most common form of atrial septal defect (ASD) is the ostium secundum defect, located in the midportion of the atrial septum. This usually occurs as an isolated abnormality. Treatment of ostium secundum ASDs depends on the size and hemodynamic impact of the defect. An ASD should be closed if there is evidence of a left-to-right shunt with a pulmonary flow to systemic flow ratio that is greater than or equal to 1.5:1.0, volume overload of right-sided cardiac chambers, or symptoms related to the defect. This patient with an ostium secundum ASD has a significant left-to-right shunt, manifested by right-sided cardiac chamber enlargement and reduced exercise capacity. ASD closure is performed in an effort to prevent right-sided heart failure, arrhythmias, and paradoxical embolism, and is indicated in this patient. Studies have demonstrated improvement in survival and symptoms even when closure is performed in adulthood. In most circumstances, device closure is reasonable and preferable for an uncomplicated isolated ostium secundum ASD and this would be appropriate in this patient. Management should be individualized; some patients prefer operative intervention because of the extended follow-up data available.

Observation is not recommended in an otherwise healthy patient with an ASD and significant left-to-right shunt. Prolonged observation will increase the risk of long-term complications, such as atrial fibrillation, progressive right heart enlargement, and associated progressive tricuspid valve regurgitation.

The 2007 American Heart Association guideline for the prevention of infective endocarditis has major revisions from previous guidelines. Prophylaxis is now limited to cardiac conditions with the highest risk of adverse outcome from infective endocarditis, including prosthetic heart valves; prior history of infective endocarditis; unrepaired cyanotic congenital heart disease; repaired congenital heart defects with prosthetic material or device, whether placed by surgery or by catheter intervention (for 6 months after the procedure); repaired congenital heart disease with residual defects; and cardiac "valvulopathy" in a transplanted heart.

Endocarditis prophylaxis is not recommended for patients with an uncomplicated ASD.

Warfarin anticoagulation is not indicated in this patient with an ASD. She has not had any atrial arrhythmias and has had no features to suggest a paradoxical embolism.

> **KEY POINT**
>
> - An atrial septal defect should be closed if there is evidence of a left-to-right shunt with a pulmonary flow to systemic flow ratio that is greater than or equal to 1.5:1.0, volume overload of right-sided cardiac chambers, or symptoms related to the defect.

Bibliography

Warnes CA, Williams RG, Bashore TM, et al. ACC/AHA 2008 Guidelines for the Management of Adults with Congenital Heart Disease: a report of the American College of Cardiology/American Heart Association Task Force on Practice Guidelines (writing committee to develop guidelines on the management of adults with congenital heart disease). Circulation. 2008;118(23):e714-833. [PMID: 18997169]

Item 73   Answer: B

Educational Objective: Use heart disease risk assessment to inform patient management.

This patient with metabolic syndrome has an intermediate risk of coronary artery disease (CAD) in the next 10 years. Interventions to reduce his risk of future CAD events are indicated. The patient is an active cigarette smoker, his blood pressure is in the prehypertension range, and his LDL cholesterol level is elevated. Appropriate risk factor modification includes weight loss, smoking cessation, and exercise with clinical re-evaluation in 3 to 6 months.

Although this patient has prehypertension, defined as a systolic blood pressure of 120 to 139 mm Hg or a diastolic blood pressure of 80 to 89 mm Hg, pharmacologic treatment of prehypertension is not recommended and has not been shown to reduce the risk of CAD events.

Statin therapy is not indicated for this patient at this time. Although the National Cholesterol Education Program (NCEP) recommends a goal LDL cholesterol level of 130 mg/dL (3.4 mmol/L) or less for patients with an intermediate risk of CAD, this goal for this patient may be achieved with lifestyle changes. His LDL cholesterol level should be remeasured approximately 3 months after institution of these changes.

Lipoprotein(a) and homocysteine levels are considered to be conditional risk factors for CAD. The use of conditional risk factors is not currently supported or recommended for cardiovascular risk estimation. The association between conditional risk factors and CAD is limited by the lack of standardized assays, the correlation of these risk factors with other major risk factors, and a lack of randomized trials demonstrating that the treatment of these conditional risk factors reduces the risk of CAD.

Exercise stress testing is not recommended for the estimation of cardiovascular risk in an asymptomatic patient. In patients with diabetes mellitus who are beginning an exercise program, exercise testing has been recommended.

> **KEY POINT**
>
> - For patients with low or moderate (<20%) 10-year risk of a coronary artery disease event, lifestyle modifications are recommended initially, with follow-up in 3 to 6 months.

Bibliography

Chobanian AV, Bakris GL, Black HR, et al; National Heart, Lung, and Blood Institute Joint National Committee on Prevention, Detection, Evaluation, and Treatment of High Blood Pressure; National High Blood Pressure Education Program Coordinating Committee. The Seventh Report of the Joint National Committee on Prevention, Detection, Evaluation, and Treatment of High Blood Pressure: The JNC 7 Report [erratum in JAMA. 2003;290(2):197.]. JAMA. 2003;289(19):2560-2572. [PMID: 12748199]

Item 74   Answer: B

Educational Objective: Manage acute myocarditis.

This patient has acute myocarditis, manifesting with flu-like systemic symptoms, chest pain, elevated troponin level, and reduced systolic function. The presentation of myocarditis is quite variable, ranging from asymptomatic to cardiogenic shock. Electrocardiographic findings may be variable as well, including findings mimicking acute coronary syndrome or myocardial infarction. Atrial or ventricular arrhythmias may be seen as well. Echocardiographic findings may show either global hypokinesis or regional wall motion abnormalities, the latter mimicking acute myocardial infarction. This patient's electrocardiogram demonstrates atrial tachycardia with 2:1 conduction. The initial laboratory screening for specific and treatable causes of myocarditis is negative. There is no specific treatment for idiopathic (also called lymphocytic) myocarditis other than supportive care and standard therapy for heart failure; thus, therapy with an angiotensin-converting enzyme (ACE) inhibitor such as captopril and a β-blocker such as carvedilol would be appropriate to start at this time.

Amiodarone is not indicated at this time because although an atrial tachyarrhythmia is present, it is not causing hemodynamic compromise and is well tolerated by the patient. The tachyarrhythmia is likely related to the acute illness and will likely resolve as the myocarditis resolves. If the tachyarrhythmia causes hemodynamic instability, cardioversion or rate- or rhythm-controlling medications should be considered.

There is no evidence for benefit of immunosuppression in acute myocarditis in recent randomized controlled trials, so methylprednisolone or other immunosuppressive agents would not be indicated.

It sometimes can be difficult distinguishing acute coronary syndrome from myocarditis. This patient's elevated cardiac enzymes indicate acute myocardial injury, which could be caused by myocardial infarction or myocarditis. Furthermore, in myocarditis, the electrocardiogram and echocardiogram can show focal abnormalities mimicking acute myocardial infarction. In this patient, however, the electrocardiogram shows only poor precordial R-wave progression without evidence for acute myocardial infarction, and the echocardiogram does not show focal wall motion abnormalities. Finally, the subacute appearance of flu-like symptoms and fever in a young person without risk factors for coronary artery disease is more compatible with myocarditis than coronary artery disease. Therefore, reperfusion therapy, including thrombolytic therapy with tissue plasminogen activator, is not correct.

Although various infections have been associated with myocarditis, there is little evidence to support bacterial infection in this patient. Sepsis can be associated with elevated cardiac biomarkers and systolic dysfunction that is reversible; however, this patient does not appear septic (she is not hypotensive, her leukocyte count is not significantly elevated, and her temperature is only slightly elevated). Therefore, treatment with antibiotics such as vancomycin and ceftriaxone is not indicated at this time. A potential cause of infectious cardiomyopathy is HIV infection. However, cardiomyopathy in this setting is typically asymptomatic or presents as chronic heart failure, rather than presenting acutely, as with this patient. If an infectious etiology were identified that would require specific treatment, standard treatment for heart failure would still be indicated.

KEY POINT

- The primary treatment for acute myocarditis is supportive care and standard treatment for systolic heart failure, including therapy with angiotensin-converting enzyme inhibitors and β-blockers.

Bibliography

Dec GW Jr, Waldman H, Southern J, Fallon JT, Hutter AM Jr, Palacios I. Viral myocarditis mimicking acute myocardial infarction. J Am Coll Cardiol. 1992;20(1):85-89. [PMID: 1607543]

Item 75   Answer: C

Educational Objective: Manage antiplatelet therapy following coronary stent placement.

Two types of coronary stents are used in the coronary vessels: bare metal and drug-eluting stents. Drug-eluting stents are coated with a medication that reduces the occurrence of in-stent restenosis. Dual antiplatelet therapy with clopidogrel and aspirin is mandatory following placement of a coronary stent to reduce sudden thrombotic occlusion of the stent. Clopidogrel is required for 1 month for bare metal stents and for 1 year for drug-eluting stents. In some highly compliant patients with bare-metal stents who are at low risk for bleeding, continuing clopidogrel for up to 1 year may be considered. Premature discontinuation of clopidogrel is associated with stent thrombosis. To reduce the occurrence of stent thrombosis, health care providers should only consider discontinuation of clopidogrel after direct discussion with the primary cardiologist. For patients with established atherosclerosis and in the absence of contraindications, aspirin should be continued indefinitely.

Because this patient received a bare metal stent, continuing clopidogrel for at least another 2 weeks and aspirin indefinitely is the correct answer. Discontinuing clopidogrel now is incorrect because 2 weeks of clopidogrel therapy is not sufficient to allow complete endothelialization or healing of the stent. Clopidogrel and aspirin should not be continued indefinitely. The risk of bleeding may exceed any benefit from the antithrombotic prophylaxis. Aspirin monotherapy is not sufficient to prevent stent thrombosis.

KEY POINT

- Clopidogrel should be continued for at least 1 year following placement of a drug-eluting stent and for at least 1 month following placement of a bare metal stent.

Bibliography

Grines CL, Bonow RO, Casey DE Jr, et al. Prevention of premature discontinuation of dual antiplatelet therapy in patients with coronary artery stents: a science advisory from the American Heart Association, American College of Cardiology, Society for Cardiovascular Angiography and Interventions, American College of Surgeons, and American Dental Association, with representation from the American College of Physicians. Circulation. 2007;115(6):813-818. [PMID: 17224480]

Item 76   Answer: A

Educational Objective: Manage coronary artery disease in a patient with contraindications to β-blockers.

Based upon the prolonged episode of chest pain and normal initial serum troponin level, this patient most likely has an acute coronary syndrome. Standard initial treatment includes aspirin, heparin, and a β-blocker. However this patient has severe chronic obstructive pulmonary disease (COPD), with her most recent FEV_1 documented at less than 30% predicted. Use of oral or intravenous β-blockers must therefore be considered carefully. The available evidence suggests that cardioselective β-blockers given to patients with COPD do not produce a significant short-term reduction in airway function or increase the incidence of COPD exacerbations. Given their benefit in conditions such as heart failure, coronary artery disease, and hypertension, cardioselective β-blockers should be considered for patients with COPD but administered with careful monitoring because data concerning long-term administration are not available No systematic reviews of cardioselective β-blockers in very severe COPD (<30% predicted FEV_1) have examined their safety and effectiveness. For this patient with severe COPD, a calcium channel blocker, such as verapamil or diltiazem, should probably be used instead of metoprolol.

Labetalol is a nonselective β-blocker and selective postsynaptic α₁-blocker. Labetalol is not approved for the treatment of acute coronary syndrome, and because it is a nonselective β-blocker, it would be a poor choice for a patient with COPD who needs β-blockade. Dyspnea and wheezing, probably due to spasm of bronchial smooth muscle, have been associated with labetalol therapy.

Ranolazine is indicated for the treatment of chronic stable angina with continued symptoms despite therapy with nitrates and a calcium channel blocker or β-blocker. In this patient, it would not be appropriate to initiate ranolazine during an acute episode of chest pain. It might be reasonable to consider ranolazine if the patient fails to respond adequately to combined therapy with nitrates and calcium channel blockers.

KEY POINT

- In patients with unstable angina who have contraindications to β-blockers, calcium channel blockers should be used.

Bibliography

Opie LH, Yusuf S, Kübler W. Current status of safety and efficacy of calcium channel blockers in cardiovascular diseases: a critical analysis based on 100 studies. Prog Cardiovasc Dis. 2000;43(2):171-196. [PMID: 11014332]

Item 77   Answer: B

Educational Objective: Evaluate new-onset heart failure.

An echocardiogram should be obtained in all patients with newly diagnosed or suspected heart failure to define whether the heart failure is systolic or diastolic and whether there are any structural or functional abnormalities that may be causing the heart failure (such as regional wall abnormalities, pericardial disease, or valvular abnormality). All of these issues may have a significant impact on management and prognosis. For example, several echocardiographic studies have shown that the extent of left ventricular cavity size, left and right ventricular ejection fractions, and the presence of diastolic dysfunction are predictors of survival.

B-type natriuretic peptide (BNP) is a hormone synthesized by the cardiac ventricles in response to increased wall stress due to pressure or volume overload. BNP assays have become a useful tool in the diagnosis of acute heart failure and differentiating it from noncardiac causes of dyspnea. A patient with a BNP concentration below 100 pg/mL is unlikely to have acute heart failure, whereas a patient with a concentration higher than 500 pg/mL has a high likelihood of having heart failure. BNP level will likely be elevated in this patient, confirming the presence of volume overload. Whereas BNP level can be helpful in differentiating heart failure from noncardiac causes of dyspnea in the acute setting, there is little ambiguity as to the patient's clinical status at this time. The physical examination,

history, and chest radiograph concordantly suggest volume overload and heart failure, and a BNP level confirming this would not be helpful. Furthermore, BNP cannot be used to differentiate between systolic and diastolic heart failure or identify functional abnormalities or potentially reversible causes of heart failure.

A radionuclide ventriculogram would accurately assess ventricular ejection fraction but would not provide other cardiac structural or functional information that may impact management.

Ischemia is a major cause of left ventricular dysfunction. Given the potential significant benefits of revascularization in appropriate candidates, including improved ventricular function and reduced morbidity and mortality, diligent evaluation for revascularizable CAD should be undertaken for most patients with heart failure. The American College of Cardiology/American Heart Association guidelines recommend coronary angiography for heart failure patients with angina or significant ischemia who are candidates for revascularization. This procedure is also reasonable to evaluate patients presenting with heart failure and no contraindications to revascularization who have chest pain less typical for angina and who have not had their coronary anatomy evaluated. Angiography is also a reasonable approach for heart failure patients without chest pain but with known or suspected coronary artery disease. A stress test would be appropriate in this patient if there were a higher clinical suspicion for coronary disease or ischemia causing new-onset heart failure. However, given the lack of anginal symptoms, the patient's relatively young age, and lack of risk factors, clinical suspicion at this point is low.

KEY POINT

- An echocardiogram should be obtained in all patients with newly diagnosed or suspected heart failure.

Bibliography

Hunt SA; American College of Cardiology; American Heart Association Task Force on Practice Guidelines (Writing Committee to Update the 2001 Guidelines for the Evaluation and Management of Heart Failure). ACC/AHA 2005 guideline update for the diagnosis and management of chronic heart failure in the adult [erratum in J Am Coll Cardiol. 2006;47(7):1503-1505.]. J Am Coll Cardiol. 2005;46(6):e1-82. [PMID 16168273]

Item 78   Answer: B

Educational Objective: Evaluate a patient with ongoing chest pain and normal wall motion on echocardiography.

An acute coronary syndrome is the first diagnostic concern in this patient, but the echocardiogram shows normal overall and regional ventricular function while she is experiencing chest pain, making ischemia or infarction very unlikely. Heart failure is an unlikely cause of acute dyspnea with normal overall left ventricular systolic function. The combination of symptoms with physical findings of asymmetric leg edema, elevated central venous pressure, tachypnea, and tachycardia suggests the possibility of pulmonary embolism, so the next test should be a CT pulmonary angiography to look for pulmonary emboli.

Cardiac MRI provides detailed images of cardiac anatomy and is an accurate method to assess myocardial viability and coronary anatomy and diagnose aortic dissection but is less accurate for the diagnosis of pulmonary embolism, the most likely diagnosis in this case. In addition, because a cardiac MRI study can be lengthy and limits the ability to monitor the patient, it is not ideal in an unstable patient with ongoing chest pain.

A normal echocardiogram between episodes of chest pain does not rule out unstable angina because wall motion returns to normal between ischemic episodes. However, this patient had no wall motion abnormalities during her ongoing chest pain. Because an acute coronary syndrome is highly unlikely, coronary angiography is not indicated as the next diagnostic test.

A resting radionuclide perfusion study can be helpful in the diagnosis of coronary ischemia when the electrocardiogram is nondiagnostic but does not provide additive information to that already obtained by echocardiography.

Transesophageal echocardiography is not sensitive for detection of pulmonary emboli but may be useful in acute chest pain when aortic dissection is suspected. Ascending aortic dissection is often associated with acute aortic regurgitation, myocardial ischemia, cardiac tamponade or hemopericardium, and hemothorax or exsanguination. Considerable (>20 mm Hg) variation in systolic blood pressure in the arms may be present. Descending thoracic aortic aneurysm is more commonly associated with splanchnic ischemia, renal insufficiency, lower extremity ischemia, or focal neurologic deficit due to spinal cord ischemia. This woman has no physical findings to suggest this diagnosis.

KEY POINT

- **Normal wall motion on echocardiography during chest pain excludes coronary ischemia or infarction.**

Bibliography

Galasko GI, Barnes SC, Collinson P, Lahiri A, Senior R. What is the most cost-effective strategy to screen for left ventricular systolic dysfunction: natriuretic peptides, the electrocardiogram, hand-held echocardiography, traditional echocardiography, or their combination? Eur Heart J. 2006;27(2):193-200. [PMID: 16267076]

Item 79   Answer: D

Educational Objective: Recognize the physical examination findings of patent ductus arteriosus.

This patient most likely has a patent ductus arteriosus. The ductus arteriosus connects the aorta and pulmonary artery during fetal life. Persistence of the ductus arteriosus after birth is associated with maternal rubella infection. Patients with a moderately sized patent ductus arteriosus may present with symptoms of heart failure, with enlarged heart chambers on the left side. The patient has features of a large left-to-right shunt with associated left heart enlargement characterized by a displaced left apical impulse. These findings suggest that the shunt is beyond the atrial level and rules out an atrial septal defect. The systolic and diastolic (continuous) murmur is most consistent with a patent ductus arteriosus.

It is uncommon to find someone with an unrepaired patent ductus arteriosus in the United States; however, this patient was born in North Africa, and she did not have access to health care. This patient would require hemodynamic cardiac catheterization assessment of pulmonary vascular resistance prior to considering intervention. Patent ductus arteriosus closure should be avoided in patients with irreversible pulmonary vascular disease. If the resistance is low, then percutaneous intervention could be considered and would result in reduction of the left ventricular size.

The patient is not cyanotic; therefore, an atrial septal defect with pulmonary valve stenosis is unlikely. In addition, a continuous murmur would not be expected in a patient with atrial septal defect and pulmonary valve stenosis. The systolic murmur would be consistent with a pulmonary outflow murmur and possibly with pulmonary valve stenosis, but there was no fixed splitting of the S_2, a characteristic finding in atrial septal defect.

The absence of cyanosis makes Eisenmenger syndrome unlikely. In addition, most patients with Eisenmenger syndrome have an unremarkable physical examination with the exception of an ejection click, accentuated pulmonic component of the S_2, and cyanosis. The presence of systolic and diastolic murmurs (a continuous murmur) and the palpable murmur suggest that Eisenmenger syndrome is not the correct diagnosis.

Rheumatic mitral valve disease with mitral stenosis and regurgitation may present with both a systolic and diastolic murmur and symptoms of dyspnea. It is also commonly noted in regions such as Africa, where rheumatic heart disease is more common than in the United States. The physical examination findings of a systolic and diastolic palpable murmur as well as a continuous murmur, however, are not characteristic of mitral stenosis and regurgitation.

Ventricular septal defect may cause left ventricular volume overload, as is suggested in this patient; however, patients with a ventricular septal defect characteristically have a systolic murmur associated with a thrill that obliterates the S_2, whereas a diastolic component is minimal or absent. A large ventricular septal defect causing volume overload may be associated with a displaced left ventricular impulse and mitral diastolic flow rumble.

KEY POINT

- **Unrepaired patent ductus arteriosus can cause left heart volume overload and symptoms of heart failure owing to a long-standing left-to-right shunt at the pulmonary level.**

Bibliography

Warnes CA, Williams RG, Bashore TM, et al. ACC/AHA 2008 Guidelines for the Management of Adults with Congenital Heart Disease: a report of the American College of Cardiology/American Heart Association Task Force on Practice Guidelines (writing committee to develop guidelines on the management of adults with congenital heart disease). Circulation. 2008;118(23):e714-833. [PMID: 18997169]

Item 80   Answer: B

Educational Objective: Diagnose prosthetic valve hemolytic anemia.

This patient has mild exertional dyspnea despite valve replacement for her aortic stenosis. Her dyspnea has improved from her preoperative status. Echocardiography demonstrates normal valve motion with mild paravalvular regurgitation. Significant paravalvular regurgitation identified by echocardiography may result from improper implantation of a valve, partial dehiscence of the valve, or prosthetic valve endocarditis. However, mild paravalvular regurgitation along the sewing ring is a common postoperative finding and would be an unlikely primary cause of cardiopulmonary symptoms or fatigue.

This patient has evidence of hemolysis with anemia, consisting of increased serum lactate dehydrogenase, decreased serum haptoglobin, and schistocytes seen on the blood smear. In addition, there is an increased reticulocyte count, indicating increased erythrocyte production. Mild hemolytic anemia is common in patients with prosthetic heart valves, but can be more severe in up to 10% to 20% of patients. Hemolytic anemia is more common in those with paravalvular regurgitation and those with mechanical valves. Clinical features include fatigue, anemia, new murmur, and, in more severe cases, jaundice and heart failure. Most cases of hemolytic anemia are subclinical, identified only by laboratory data. Symptomatic hemolytic anemia can usually be treated with oral iron and folate replacement, although more severe cases may warrant blood transfusion or recombinant human erythropoietin. Rarely, patients will require valve reoperation if hemolysis is due to significant valve dysfunction or progressive paravalvular regurgitation.

Complications of prosthetic valves include structural valve deterioration, valve thrombosis, embolism, bleeding, pannus formation, and endocarditis. This patient has maintained therapeutic levels of anticoagulation, and valve thrombosis is unlikely. Valve dehiscence or dysfunction should be suspected in patients who develop symptoms of heart failure with significant valve regurgitation. There are no clinical signs of heart failure and she has no history of fever, infectious exposures, or laboratory evidence of infection, making endocarditis less likely.

Pannus formation is a slowly growing fibrous overgrowth fixed on the prosthesis, causing valve dysfunction. In this patient, valve hemodynamics are consistent with a normally functioning prosthesis. Although the transaortic velocity of 3.4 m/s with an aortic valve area of 1.5 cm^2 would normally suggest obstruction of aortic outflow, valve hemodynamics of an aortic prosthesis are generally mildly increased over those of native valves because the sewing ring and prosthetic leaflets occupy space in the valve annulus.

In rare cases, prosthesis mismatch may occur when the inserted valve prosthesis is too small relative to patient size, recreating the outflow obstruction present preoperatively. The main hemodynamic consequence is persistence of significant transvalvular gradients through what is otherwise a normally functioning prosthesis. There is no echocardiographic evidence of valve obstruction, making prosthesis mismatch unlikely. Because prosthesis mismatch has been associated with decreased survival, sudden cardiac death, and decreased quality of life, and treatment in symptomatic patients is reoperation, careful intraoperative selection of correct prosthesis size at the time of initial surgery is warranted.

KEY POINT

- **Mild hemolysis is commonly seen in patients with a normally functioning mechanical valve, particularly in the presence of paravalvular regurgitation.**

Bibliography

Bonow RO, Carabello BA, Kanu C, et al. ACC/AHA 2006 guidelines for the management of patients with valvular heart disease: a report of the American College of Cardiology/American Heart Association Task Force on Practice Guidelines (writing committee to revise the 1998 Guidelines for the Management of Patients With Valvular Heart Disease): developed in collaboration with the Society of Cardiovascular Anesthesiologists: endorsed by the Society for Cardiovascular Angiography and Interventions and the Society of Thoracic Surgeons [erratum in Circulation. 2007;115(15):e409.]. Circulation. 2006;114(5):e84-231. [PMID: 16880336]

Item 81   Answer: D

Educational Objective: Understand the role of measuring biomarkers of inflammation in the prediction of cardiovascular risk.

This patient needs no further testing or treatment at this time. He is a healthy man with a low risk (<10%) of a cardiovascular event within the next 10 years based on the Framingham Risk Equation. Although he has a family history of premature coronary artery disease, the independent effect of a positive family history is difficult to assess because familial influences on risk status may be mediated in part by blood pressure and serum lipoprotein levels.

In recent years, the role of inflammation in the atherosclerotic disease process has become well established. All stages of the initiation and growth of the atherosclerotic plaque may be considered an inflammatory response to injury. C-reactive protein (CRP), a nonspecific, acute-phase reactant of systemic inflammation, satisfies a number of characteristics for a potentially useful risk marker, including standardized assay, independence from established risk factors, and association with cardiovascular disease end points in observational studies. Prospective population-based studies have shown consistent dose-response relationships between high-sensitivity CRP levels and the risk of incident coronary artery disease.

A randomized, placebo-controlled trial (JUPITER) evaluated whether cholesterol-lowering treatment with rosuvastatin in patients with elevated high-sensitivity CRP (≥2 mg/L), LDL cholesterol less than 130 mg/dL (3.4 mmol/L), and few other cardiovascular risk factors reduced the risk of a first cardiovascular event. The results demonstrated that after approximately 2 years of treatment, the statin group had a relative risk reduction of 47% in cardiovascular events. However, the absolute risk reduction was relatively small (1.2%), which resulted in treating 82 people for nearly 2 years to prevent one event. There was also an increased incidence of physician-reported diabetes mellitus in the statin-treated group. Finally, patients in this study were older (median age, 66 years), so the results may not be applicable to this patient. At present, high-sensitivity CRP levels may be used at the discretion of the physician for directing further therapy of patients with an intermediate (10%-20%) Framingham 10-year risk of a cardiovascular event.

Because this patient is at low, rather than intermediate, risk, initiating either daily aspirin or a statin based on his elevated CRP level is incorrect. Exercise electrocardiographic testing is not indicated for routine screening of asymptomatic patients, regardless of risk of cardiovascular disease.

KEY POINT

- **High-sensitivity C-reactive protein levels may be used to direct further therapy of patients with an intermediate (10%-20%) 10-year risk of a coronary artery disease event.**

Bibliography

Ridker PM, Danielson E, Fonseca FAH, et al; JUPITER Study Group. Rosuvastatin to prevent vascular events in men and women with elevated C-reactive protein. N Engl J Med. 2008;359(21):2195-2207. [PMID: 18997196]

Item 82   Answer: B

Educational Objective: Diagnose familial long QT syndrome.

This patient most likely has congenital long QT syndrome (LQTS), suggested by recurrent syncope triggered by activity, a prolonged QT interval on electrocardiogram (580 msec), and a family history of early sudden death. Her mother is probably affected; it is unfortunately not uncommon for LQTS patients to be misdiagnosed with a seizure disorder. Cardiac events in LQTS patients include syncope and cardiac arrest due to torsade de pointes ventricular tachycardia. Ninety percent of congenital LQTS cases are caused by mutations in three genes, and triggers of events vary by genotype. Corrected QT intervals are considered abnormal if greater than 440 msec in men and 450 to 460 msec in women, but there is substantial overlap among normal patients and abnormal LQT gene carriers.

LQTS type 1 is the most common type of congenital LQTS (45%-55% of cases) and is caused by mutations in KCNQ1, the α subunit of the delayed rectifier potassium channel (IKs). LQTS type 1 patients experience the majority of their events during exercise. Events during swimming may be specific for LQT1 mutations. LQTS type 2 (35%-45% of cases of LQTS) is caused by mutations in the KCNH2/HERG gene, which codes for IKr, the rapid component of the delayed rectifier potassium channel. This phenotype is similar to acquired LQTS, which is caused by drugs that prolong the QT interval by blockade of IKr. Cardiac events in LQTS type 2 are usually precipitated by emotional arousal, exercise, or loud or sudden noises. LQTS type 3 (8%-10% of cases) is caused by gain-of-function mutations in the sodium channel gene (SCN5A). The QT interval is usually quite prolonged, and events often occur during sleep. The risk of a cardiac event in LQTS is related to age, sex, QTc interval, genotype, and specific mutation. β-Blockers are most protective in LQTS type 1 patients, as compared to those with LQTS type 2 or type 3. All patients with congenital LQTS should be treated with a β-blocker, regardless of symptoms. Patients with recurrent syncope or cardiac arrest on β-blockers are candidates for defibrillator placement.

The Brugada syndrome is characterized by a pseudo right bundle branch block pattern with ST-segment elevation on the electrocardiogram and ventricular arrhythmias. Loss-of-function mutations in the SCN5A gene are present in approximately 30% of patients.

Another inherited arrhythmic disorder is the short QT syndrome, which carries a high risk of sudden cardiac death. The syndrome is characterized by an autosomal dominant pattern of inheritance, a short QT interval (<300 msec), atrial fibrillation occurring at a young age, and an increased risk of death due to ventricular fibrillation. The abnormally prolonged QT interval in this patient makes this diagnosis unlikely.

The Wolff-Parkinson-White syndrome is characterized by ventricular preexcitation (short PR interval and delta wave) and symptomatic tachycardia. Owing to the rapid conduction properties of some accessory pathways, atrial fibrillation can be a life-threatening arrhythmia in these patients due to rapidly conducting atrial fibrillation degenerating to ventricular fibrillation. Although patients with Wolff-Parkinson-White syndrome have an increased risk of sudden cardiac death, it is very unusual for this to be the first symptomatic manifestation of the syndrome.

KEY POINT

- **Clinical differences in triggers of arrhythmic events may suggest the underlying gene defect of congenital long QT syndrome; this has implications for outcome and drug management.**

Bibliography
Sauer AJ, Moss AJ, McNitt S, et al. Long QT syndrome in adults. J
Am Coll Cardiol. 2007;49(3):329-337. [PMID: 17239714]

Item 83 Answer: C

Educational Objective: Manage new-onset heart failure with hemodynamic compromise.

This patient presents with a new-onset, unexplained, hemodynamically significant heart failure. Although endomyocardial biopsy is generally not indicated in the evaluation of heart disease, it may prove critical in diagnosing unusual conditions, such as giant cell myocarditis, in which a histologic diagnosis dictates management. Endomyocardial biopsy is recommended in patients with new-onset heart failure (<2 weeks) with hemodynamic compromise and in those with new-onset heart failure of 2 weeks' to 3 months' duration associated with a dilated left ventricle and new ventricular arrhythmias, Mobitz type II second- or third-degree atrioventricular heart block, or failure to respond to usual care within 1 to 2 weeks. Giant cell myocarditis is a rare, idiopathic cause of fulminant or subacute-onset heart failure. Most patients with giant cell myocarditis present with heart failure (75%), but a substantial minority may present with ventricular arrhythmia (14%) or heart block (5%). Diagnosis is made by endomyocardial biopsy and is characterized by the presence of multinucleated giant cells with eosinophils and myocyte necrosis. Prognosis is very poor, and urgent evaluation for cardiac transplantation is recommended, although giant cell myocarditis can recur in the transplanted heart.

Patients with giant cell myocarditis may be so hemodynamically unstable and are generally felt to have such a poor prognosis that implantation of a ventricular assist device may be necessary as a bridge to cardiac transplantation. Given the rarity of the disease and significant survivor bias in published series and case reports, there are no large randomized prospective trials to provide definitive guidance regarding immunosuppressive therapy; currently, practice varies by center.

A biventricular pacemaker is indicated for treatment of patients with left ventricular ejection fraction less than or equal to 35%, QRS duration 120 msec or greater, sinus rhythm, and New York Heart Association (NYHA) class III or IV symptoms (that is, symptoms with mild activity or at rest) on optimal medical therapy for heart failure. Although this patient does have a reduced ejection fraction and NYHA class IV symptoms, he does not meet the other criteria of a prolonged QRS duration and being on optimal medical therapy. In any case, the patient's hemodynamic instability precludes this elective or semi-elective procedure.

Cardiac MRI can be useful in diagnosing infiltrative or inflammatory cardiomyopathies. In this case, however, the patient is too unstable to undergo MRI. In addition, given the clinical suspicion for giant cell myocarditis, endomyocardial biopsy is the gold standard for diagnosis.

Endomyocardial biopsy can be performed in the cardiac catheterization laboratory, where personnel and resources are available for management of cardiogenic shock. If necessary, endomyocardial biopsy can also be performed at bedside under transthoracic echocardiographic guidance.

An implantable defibrillator is indicated for hemodynamically significant ventricular arrhythmias in the setting of reduced ejection fraction. This patient's ventricular arrhythmias and hemodynamic instability are likely the result of an underlying acute cardiomyopathic process (giant cell myocarditis) that requires urgent treatment with cardiac transplantation, possibly preceded by ventricular assist device implantation. In addition, the patient's extreme instability precludes any sort of elective or semi-elective procedure such as an implantable defibrillator placement, and in a case such as this, an implantable defibrillator would only induce repeated shocks without treating the underlying disease process.

KEY POINT

- Endomyocardial biopsy is recommended in patients with new-onset heart failure (>2 weeks) and hemodynamic compromise.

Bibliography
Cooper LT, Baughman KL, Feldman AM, et al. The role of endomyocardial biopsy in the management of cardiovascular disease: a scientific statement from the American Heart Association, the American College of Cardiology, and the European Society of Cardiology. Endorsed by the Heart Failure Society of America and the Heart Failure Association of the European Society of Cardiology. J Am Coll Cardiol. 2007;50(19):1914-1931. [PMID 17980265]

Item 84 Answer: B

Educational Objective: Treat diastolic hypertension in a patient with diabetes mellitus and coronary artery disease.

Increasing the dosage of lisinopril is the most appropriate option for this patient. This patient has diabetes mellitus, coronary artery disease, and hypertension, with persistent elevation of the diastolic blood pressure despite pharmacologic therapy. Based on these risk factors, he has a high risk of a recurrent cardiovascular event within the next 10 years. His goal blood pressure for reducing this risk, based on JNC-7 recommendations, is less than 130/80 mm Hg. He therefore needs additional antihypertensive therapy.

The patient's current medications for treatment of hypertension are appropriate in the setting of diabetes mellitus and coronary artery disease. Angiotensin-converting enzyme (ACE) inhibitor therapy has been shown to reduce the risk of diabetic nephropathy independent of blood pressure lowering. In patients with coronary artery disease, both ACE inhibitors and β-blockers have been found to reduce the risk of recurrent cardiovascular events.

Lowering diastolic blood pressure should be gradual and cautious in patients with coronary artery disease or diabetes mellitus and in those who are older than 60 years, to avoid the possibility of inducing myocardial ischemia. Although lower systolic blood pressure measurements are associated with better outcomes in ischemic heart disease, there is inconsistent evidence that excessive diastolic blood pressure lowering may worsen cardiac outcomes.

The patient's metoprolol dosage should not be increased because he has bradycardia and first-degree atrioventricular block, both of which are relative contraindications to increased β-blocker therapy.

As yet there are no large comparative trials of ACE inhibitors and angiotensin receptor blockers (ARBs) in patients with type 2 diabetes. Both drugs appear to have cardioprotective effects that are independent from blood pressure control, and both are beneficial in patients with nephropathy. Most experts recommend beginning with an ACE inhibitor and switching to an ARB if the patient cannot tolerate the ACE inhibitor, usually because of cough. In patients with persistent proteinuria despite maximally tolerated dosages of an ACE inhibitor (or alternatively, an ARB), the drug from the opposite class can be added (while monitoring the serum creatinine and potassium concentrations). In most studies, the combination of an ACE inhibitor and an ARB produced greater reduction in protein excretion than did either drug alone. Since the patient is tolerating the lisinopril, there is no indication to change to an ARB. Because the patient does not have evidence of microalbuminuria, the addition of losartan to lisinopril is not indicated.

> **KEY POINT**
> - The blood pressure goal for patients with diabetes mellitus is less than 130/80 mm Hg.

Bibliography

Rosendorff C, Black HR, Cannon CP, et al. Treatment of hypertension in the prevention and management of ischemic heart disease: a scientific statement from the American Heart Association Council for High Blood Pressure Research and the Councils on Clinical Cardiology and Epidemiology and Prevention [erratum in Circulation. 2007;116(5):e121.]. Circulation. 2007;115(21):2761-2788. [PMID: 17502569]

Item 85   Answer: A

Educational Objective: Manage the timing of intervention for chronic aortic regurgitation.

This is a young, asymptomatic patient with a bicuspid aortic valve and significant aortic regurgitation. Transthoracic echocardiography demonstrates a dilated left ventricle, mildly decreased systolic function, and a moderately dilated ascending aorta. Asymptomatic patients with severe aortic regurgitation who develop left ventricular dilation or systolic dysfunction are at increased risk of sudden cardiac death, death, and heart failure. Therefore, if there is progression in left ventricular size or a decline in the ejection fraction, patients should be referred for aortic valve replacement. The prognosis of asymptomatic patients with severe

aortic regurgitation but with normal left ventricular size and function is excellent. Therefore, the American College of Cardiology/American Heart Association valvular heart disease guidelines recommend surgery in asymptomatic patients with severe aortic regurgitation when the left ventricular end-systolic dimension reaches 55 mm or the ejection fraction is less than 60%. This patient, therefore, is a candidate for valve replacement. In asymptomatic patients who do not meet surgical criteria, serial echocardiography is warranted to assess for disease progression.

Ascending aortic dilation leads to annular dilation and significant regurgitation in approximately 15% to 20% of patients with a bicuspid aortic valve, which increases the risk of aortic dissection and rupture. Most patients with severe aortic regurgitation and adverse hemodynamic effects on the ventricle are symptomatic. Surgical valve replacement is indicated in symptomatic patients because the mortality rate for severe, untreated, symptomatic aortic regurgitation exceeds 10% per year. Concurrent ascending aortic replacement should be performed if the ascending aorta diameter exceeds 4.5 cm.

Digoxin and diuretics may be used initially to relieve symptoms of heart failure, but are not indicated in asymptomatic patients.

Because pharmacologic afterload reduction (vasodilator therapy) with nifedipine or angiotensin-converting enzyme inhibitors may reduce regurgitant volume and improve forward stroke volume, these medications are a reasonable initial choice for antihypertensive therapy in patients who also have aortic regurgitation. However, outcome data on use of vasodilator therapy alone for aortic regurgitation are not conclusive. For asymptomatic patients with normal systolic function and mild regurgitation, vasodilator therapy is not recommended. For asymptomatic patients with normal systolic function and severe regurgitation, vasodilator therapy may be considered, but medical therapy does not supplant surgical intervention. Surgery should not be withheld if any surgical criteria are otherwise met.

In patients with significant aortic regurgitation and equivocal symptoms, exercise-induced increases in pulmonary systolic pressure of more than 60 mm Hg (or a 25 mm Hg increase over baseline) identified during treadmill stress echocardiography suggest hemodynamic significance and may lead to earlier referral for surgical intervention. In this patient, however, ventricular dilation and decreased ejection fraction are adequate criteria for recommending surgery.

> **KEY POINT**
> - Valve replacement surgery is recommended for asymptomatic patients with a bicuspid aortic valve and severe aortic regurgitation when the left ventricular end-systolic diameter reaches 55 mm or the left ventricular ejection fraction is less than 60%.

Bibliography

Ortiz JT, Shin DD, Rajamannan NM. Approach to the patient with bicuspid aortic valve and ascending aorta aneurysm. Curr Treat Options Cardiovasc Med. 2006;8(6):461-467. [PMID: 17078910]

Item 86   Answer: B

Educational Objective: Evaluate chronic stable angina.

Coronary angiography is the most appropriate option in this patient with continued anginal symptoms despite optimal medical therapy. The COURAGE trial found that a routine strategy of coronary angiography and revascularization compared with optimal medical therapy provided no benefit in patients with chronic stable angina. However, this patient remains highly symptomatic despite optimal medical therapy, and therefore would benefit from coronary angiography, which would allow direct evaluation of coronary anatomy and possibly percutaneous coronary intervention or surgical revascularization. Coronary revascularization is beneficial in patients with chronic stable angina and the following conditions: angina pectoris refractory to medical therapy; a large area of ischemic myocardium and high-risk criteria on stress testing; high-risk coronary anatomy, including left main coronary artery stenosis or three-vessel disease; and significant coronary artery disease with reduced left ventricular systolic function. In appropriately selected patients, revascularization, either with a percutaneous coronary intervention or coronary artery bypass grafting surgery, has been shown to reduce angina, increase longevity, and improve left ventricular performance.

For patients with unstable angina, admission to the coronary care unit and intravenous heparin and nitroglycerin would be beneficial. However, this patient has chronic stable angina, characterized by progressive exertional angina for 2 months without episodes of pain while at rest.

Exercise treadmill stress testing would not be useful for this patient's management as it would only confirm the known diagnosis of coronary artery disease. Results of an exercise stress test would not influence therapeutic decisions.

The effectiveness of ranolazine for the treatment of chronic stable angina has been demonstrated in several randomized trials, but its role is still undergoing definition. Most experts recommend its use for angina that is refractory to standard therapy. Ranolazine produces a dose-dependent increase in the QT interval, and is contraindicated in patients with preexisting QT-interval prolongation, liver disease, and in combination with drugs that prolong the QT interval or are inhibitors of CYP3A4, such as diltiazem and verapamil. Ranolazine also prolongs the half-life of digoxin and simvastatin, and these drugs may require dose reduction. Therefore, initiation of ranolazine in this patient is less desirable than coronary angiography and potential revascularization.

> **KEY POINT**
>
> - Coronary angiography is indicated in patients with chronic stable angina who experience lifestyle-limiting angina despite optimal medical therapy.

Bibliography

Boden WE, O'Rourke RA, Teo KK, et al; COURAGE Trial Research Group. Optimal medical therapy with or without PCI for stable coronary disease. N Engl J Med. 2007;356(15):1503-1516. [PMID: 17387127]

Item 87   Answer: A

Educational Objective: Diagnose coarctation of the aorta.

This patient has classic features of aortic coarctation. He has a pulse delay between the upper and lower extremities (radial artery to femoral artery delay). The blood pressure in the lower extremities, when measured, will be lower than the blood pressure noted in the upper extremities. The patient also has an ejection click and an early systolic murmur consistent with a bicuspid aortic valve, which is present in more than 50% of patients with aortic coarctation. The systolic and diastolic murmurs noted over the back are related to collateral vessels, which also cause the sign of rib notching, seen on this patient's chest radiograph on the inferior surface of the posterior upper thoracic ribs bilaterally.

Essential hypertension is a common cause of systemic hypertension, but the physical examination features of this patient are not explained by this diagnosis. In addition, a family history of hypertension is common in patients with essential hypertension.

Pheochromocytoma causes paroxysmal hypertension in about half of affected patients; other pheochromocytomas present similar to patients with essential hypertension. The signs and symptoms of pheochromocytoma are variable. The classic triad of sudden severe headaches, diaphoresis, and palpitations carries a high degree of specificity (94%) and sensitivity (91%) for pheochromocytoma in hypertensive patients. The absence of all three symptoms reliably excludes the condition. Finally, the physical examination features in this patient do not reflect this diagnosis.

Renovascular hypertension due to fibromuscular disease of the renal arteries usually presents in patients younger than 35 years of age. Atherosclerotic renovascular disease is more common in older patients and is frequently associated with vascular disease in other vessels (carotid or coronary arteries and peripheral vessels). Azotemia is often observed in patients with atherosclerotic renovascular hypertension. Renal artery stenosis cannot explain this patient's cardiac and peripheral vascular examination findings.

- **Coarctation of the aorta should be suspected in a young patient presenting with systemic hypertension.**

Bibliography

Warnes CA, Williams RG, Bashore TM, et al. ACC/AHA 2008 Guidelines for the Management of Adults with Congenital Heart Disease: a report of the American College of Cardiology/American Heart Association Task Force on Practice Guidelines (writing committee to develop guidelines on the management of adults with congenital heart disease). Circulation. 2008;118(23):e714-833. [PMID: 18997169]

Item 88   Answer: D

Educational Objective: Evaluate tricuspid regurgitation.

The most appropriate diagnostic test for this patient is ventilation-perfusion lung scanning. This patient has tricuspid regurgitation and significant pulmonary hypertension with evidence of pressure overload on the right ventricle. Pulmonary hypertension with right ventricular enlargement and tricuspid valve annular dilation can lead to significant regurgitation of an otherwise normal tricuspid valve. Pulmonary hypertension may occur when abnormalities in left heart valvular or myocardial function (systolic or diastolic) cause pulmonary venous hypertension. Additional causes of pulmonary hypertension include chronic hypoxic pulmonary disorders (such as chronic obstructive pulmonary disease, interstitial lung disease, or sleep apnea) and chronic thromboembolic disease. Pulmonary hypertension may occur in association with anorectic drug use, HIV infection, chronic liver disease, or collagen vascular disease. In the absence of identifiable risk factors, pulmonary hypertension may be idiopathic. A diagnosis of idiopathic primary pulmonary arterial hypertension requires exclusion of secondary and associated causes of pulmonary hypertension. Additionally, right heart catheterization is also needed in order to demonstrate elevated pulmonary vascular resistance.

Numerous diagnostic tests may be used to evaluate a patient with suspected pulmonary hypertension. Pulmonary function tests are needed to identify and characterize underlying lung disease. Ventilation-perfusion scanning is used to evaluate patients for chronic thromboembolic disease. A normal scan has greater than 90% sensitivity in excluding chronic thromboembolic disease and a similarly high specificity. Although helpful in the evaluation of acute pulmonary embolism, CT angiography is not known to be sufficiently sensitive for detection of chronic thromboembolism. Blood tests are performed to evaluate potential liver disease, HIV infection, or collagen vascular disease. A right heart catheterization confirms the presence of pulmonary hypertension and allows for calculation of pulmonary vascular resistance. Some patients require left heart catheterization as well.

Cardiac magnetic resonance (CMR) imaging is useful when evaluating primary myocardial abnormalities (such as an infiltrative disease), ventricular volumes, or assessing three-dimensional imaging of congenital heart disease. In this patient, transthoracic images do not suggest congenital heart disease. CMR imaging would not be the next imaging study of choice.

Exertional dyspnea may be an angina equivalent and stress echocardiography could be considered. However, the patient's age, relative paucity of cardiovascular risk factors, and abnormal transthoracic echocardiogram findings (right ventricular enlargement and pulmonary hypertension) argue against an ischemic cause for her symptoms. A ventilation-perfusion lung scan is the appropriate next diagnostic test.

Transesophageal echocardiography to evaluate for tricuspid valve vegetations would be indicated if there were a strong clinical suspicion for endocarditis. This patient's clinical presentation, with an absence of corroborating history, fever, or an elevated leukocyte count, does not suggest endocarditis.

- **Pulmonary hypertension may lead to right ventricular enlargement, tricuspid valve annular dilation, and regurgitation in an otherwise normal tricuspid valve.**

Bibliography

McLaughlin VV, McGoon MD. Pulmonary arterial hypertension. Circulation. 2006;114(13):1417-1431. [PMID: 17000921]

Item 89   Answer: B

Educational Objective: Evaluate peripheral arterial disease.

The patient is a heavy smoker with a clinical history suggestive for peripheral arterial disease. Additionally, he has some physical findings (hair loss, diminished pulses) that support this diagnosis. His ankle-brachial index (0.98), however, is not diagnostic of peripheral arterial disease. Given the strong clinical suspicion and the onset of the patient's symptoms with exercise, it would be reasonable to repeat the measurements for the ankle-brachial index immediately following a graded exercise test targeted to the onset of the patient's symptoms. A decrease of the ankle-brachial index by 20% after exercise suggests significant peripheral arterial disease.

Although the patient has a physically demanding job, it is unlikely that his current symptoms are simply due to muscular strain given the clinical findings of hair loss and diminished pulses and his risks for peripheral arterial disease. Treatment with an NSAID, therefore, is incorrect.

The normal neurologic examination suggests against significant cord or root compression, and the onset of the patient's symptoms with exertion and rapid relief with rest are not typical of spinal stenosis. The discomfort of spinal stenosis, or *pseudoclaudication*, is similar to that described for peripheral arterial disease. However, the symptoms are most often provoked by prolonged standing in an erect posture and are relieved with sitting or flexion at the waist. Therefore, MRI of the lumbosacral spine would not be appropriate.

The patient is not sedentary, nor does he have a known malignancy or hypercoagulable state, prior vascular injury, or asymmetric lower extremity edema. A deep venous thrombosis is unlikely to explain his current symptoms, and venous duplex ultrasonography of the lower extremities is not indicated.

KEY POINT

- When high clinical suspicion for peripheral arterial disease persists despite normal resting ankle-brachial index, exercise ankle-brachial index is a reasonable secondary test.

Bibliography

Stein R, Hriljac I, Halperin JL, Gustavson SM, Teodorescu V, Olin JW. Limitation of the resting ankle-brachial index in symptomatic patients with peripheral arterial disease. Vasc Med. 2006;11(1):29-33. [PMID: 16669410]

Item 90   Answer: D

Educational Objective: Recognize cardiac contraindications to pregnancy.

Pulmonary arterial hypertension (PAH) carries a very high risk of death during pregnancy, with an estimated maternal mortality rate of 30% to 50%. Thus, pregnancy is contraindicated in patients with severe PAH, even when asymptomatic. This patient should be counseled to avoid pregnancy because of PAH; if an unplanned pregnancy occurs, termination is recommended.

Bosentan, an endothelin receptor antagonist, is effective in improving symptoms in patients with PAH; however, it is teratogenic and is contraindicated for use during pregnancy.

If a patient with PAH gets pregnant and declines the recommendation for termination, cautious monitoring and admission to a high-risk pregnancy unit would be reasonable. Some groups have advocated cesarean delivery for patients with PAH who decide to continue with the pregnancy.

Anticoagulation has been advised by some groups for pregnant patients with PAH, but this is usually administered late in the pregnancy when the patient is hospitalized. There are no data to support the routine use of low-molecular-weight heparin or aspirin during pregnancy in patients with PAH.

KEY POINT

- Severe pulmonary arterial hypertension is a contraindication to pregnancy and carries an estimated maternal mortality rate of 30% to 50%.

Bibliography

Siu SC, Sermer M, Colman JM, et al; Cardiac Disease in Pregnancy (CARPREG) Investigators. Prospective multicenter study of pregnancy outcomes in women with heart disease. Circulation. 2001;104(5):515-521. [PMID: 11479246]

Item 91   Answer: A

Educational Objective: Evaluate a patient at intermediate risk of coronary disease using high-sensitivity C-reactive protein level.

Assessing high-sensitivity C-reactive protein (CRP) level would be an appropriate test to further stratify this patient's cardiovascular risk. This 61-year-old asymptomatic man has an intermediate (18%) 10-year risk of myocardial infarction or coronary death, according to the Framingham risk score, which is based on his age, sex, lipid levels, and blood pressure. In addition to improved blood pressure control, risk factor reduction in this patient would include lowering LDL cholesterol and raising HDL cholesterol levels. According to NCEP III guidelines, his goal LDL cholesterol level is 130 mg/dL (3.4 mmol/L). Lipid-lowering therapy is appropriate if his LDL cholesterol remains elevated after a 3-month trial of a low-fat diet, exercise, and weight reduction. However, given his adverse reaction to statins, the decision to try another lipid-lowering medication is not straightforward in this patient; therefore, additional risk factor evaluation would be helpful.

Elevated serum high-sensitivity CRP levels are an independent cardiovascular risk factor for myocardial infarction, stroke, and cardiovascular death, and are associated with development of metabolic syndrome and diabetes mellitus (low risk, <0.1 mg/dL [1.0 mg/L]; average risk, 0.1-0.3 mg/dL [1.0-3.0 mg/L]; high risk, >0.3 mg/dL [3.0 mg/L]). The JUPITER trial was designed to evaluate whether rosuvastatin therapy lowers cardiovascular risk in a primary prevention trial of subjects with elevated high-sensitivity CRP levels, but normal LDL levels. After approximately 2 years of treatment, patients in the statin group had a relative risk reduction of 47% in cardiovascular events. The absolute risk reduction, however, was relatively small (1.2%). At present, high-sensitivity CRP levels may be used at the discretion of the physician for directing further therapy of patients with an intermediate (10%-20%) Framingham 10-year risk of a cardiovascular event.

CT coronary angiography is useful for visualization of the proximal coronary arteries in selected patients with atypical or questionable symptoms who are at intermediate risk of coronary disease. However, the radiation dose is high and intravenous contrast is needed, which should be avoided in this patient with a creatinine level at the upper limit of normal.

Echocardiography is helpful in many types of cardiac disease, but this patient has no evidence of heart failure and no murmur on examination, and there are no other signs or symptoms to suggest structural heart disease. Left ventricular hypertrophy may be present due to hypertension, but the degree of left ventricular hypertrophy would not affect medical management.

An exercise stress test is not appropriate in an asymptomatic, nondiabetic patient without known coronary disease because the specificity in this setting is low.

Bibliography
Ridker PM, Danielson E, Fonseca FA, et al; JUPITER Study Group. Rosuvastatin to prevent vascular events in men and women with elevated C-reactive protein. N Engl J Med. 2008;359(21):2195-1207. [PMID: 18997196]

Item 92   Answer: D
Educational Objective: Treat aortic atheroma.

This patient has had a transient ischemic attack and has complex ascending aortic atheromas. The presence of an ascending aortic atheroma of 4 mm or greater in diameter increases the risk of recurrent stroke. There is debate as to whether warfarin or antiplatelet monotherapy is superior for risk reduction, and as no direct comparative study has been completed, either choice would be appropriate.

While intensive lipid-lowering therapy has not been studied specifically in patients with cerebrovascular events and aortic atheroma, treatment with 40 mg/d of pravastatin in the CARE trial was associated with a clinically significant reduction in the risk for stroke.

Aortic stenosis and mitral annular calcification are often associated findings in patients with identified ascending aortic atheromas. However, this patient's presenting symptoms are not principally due to aortic stenosis. Aortic arch endarterectomy or combined aortic valve and root replacement would carry a very high risk, especially given the necessity of heart-lung bypass and a recent cerebrovascular event. A decision to proceed with surgery should be predicated upon symptoms referable to aortic stenosis, such as angina, syncope or heart failure, in conjunction with demonstration of a severely stenotic valve.

Carotid endarterectomy is beneficial for symptomatic patients with recent nondisabling carotid artery ischemic events and ipsilateral 70% to 99% carotid artery stenosis. It may be considered in patients with stenosis of 50% to 69% if the patient is likely to live for 5 years or longer. Carotid endarterectomy has not demonstrated benefit for patients with stenosis of less than 50%.

Based upon autopsy studies, a patent foramen ovale (PFO) is present in up to 15% of the general population. The presence of a PFO does not establish causality, and in the presence of a clinically demonstrated established risk factor for stroke (aortic atheroma), closure of the PFO would carry some procedural risk and may not address the root cause of the transient ischemic attack. PFO closure is not indicated as initial therapy for a first cerebrovascular event.

Bibliography
Kronzon I, Tunick PA. Aortic atherosclerotic disease and stroke. Circulation. 2006;114(1):63-75. [PMID: 16818829]

Item 93   Answer: A
Educational Objective: Manage anticoagulation during pregnancy in a patient with a mechanical prosthetic valve.

Warfarin has a low molecular weight and crosses the placenta, causing fetal anticoagulation. Thus, the risk of spontaneous abortion, prematurity, embryopathy, stillbirth, and fetal intracranial hemorrhage are increased. Warfarin use throughout pregnancy until near term, however, does provide the lowest risk for maternal complications and death and is the primary treatment used in most countries outside of the United States. Warfarin embryopathy is a concern when warfarin is administered during the first trimester; however, when the dose of warfarin is less than 5 mg daily, the risk of embryopathy decreases to below 10%.

There is controversy regarding the best anticoagulation regimen for the pregnant patient with a mechanical valve prosthesis, balancing the safety to mother and fetus. No single agent has been demonstrated to be the agent of choice. Meticulous monitoring and dose adjustment of all anticoagulation regimens is required during pregnancy.

Low-dose aspirin can be safely used during pregnancy but does not provide adequate anticoagulation coverage alone or in conjunction with clopidogrel for a patient with a mechanical valve prosthesis. It is not known whether clopidogrel crosses the placenta, and its safety during pregnancy has not been determined.

Fondaparinux, which indirectly inactivates factor Xa selectively via an antithrombin-dependent mechanism, is approved for the prevention of venous thromboembolism after major orthopedic surgery and major abdominal surgery. Fondaparinux has also been approved for the treatment of pulmonary embolism and deep venous thrombosis. Fondaparinux is not approved for the prevention of mechanical valve–related thrombosis in either pregnant or nonpregnant patients.

Low-molecular-weight heparin (LMWH) does not cross the placenta and has demonstrated no teratogenic effects. However, controversy persists regarding the best management, and there is uncertainty about the safety of LMWH in pregnant patients with mechanical valve prostheses. Weight-based LMWH is not adequate for anticoagulation in the pregnant patient. The anti–factor Xa level of activity should be monitored weekly or biweekly and the dose adjusted according to the level.

> **KEY POINT**
>
> - Warfarin use throughout pregnancy until near term provides the lowest risk for maternal complications and death in women with mechanical heart valves.

Bibliography
Stout KK, Otto CM. Pregnancy in women with valvular heart disease. Heart. 2007;93(5):552-558. [PMID: 16905631]

Item 94   Answer: A

Educational Objective: Diagnose decompensated heart failure in a patient with a relatively low B-type natriuretic peptide level.

This patient has acute heart failure, despite his relatively low B-type natriuretic peptide (BNP) level. Evidence for decompensated heart failure includes jugular venous distention, pulmonary crackles, an S_3, and peripheral edema. Although the presence of jugular venous distention, abdominal jugular reflux, pulmonary crackles, S_3, and lower extremity edema all increase the likelihood of heart failure, these findings often do not predict the hemodynamic impairment in chronic heart failure. For example, pulmonary crackles may reflect the rapidity of onset of heart failure, rather than the degree of volume overload. Two signs have prognostic value: elevated jugular venous pressure and an S_3 are each independently associated with adverse outcomes, including progression of heart failure. BNP levels are affected by many factors and may be elevated with cardiovascular conditions other than heart failure, such as acute myocardial infarction and pulmonary embolism. Obesity is associated with lower BNP levels and, in this patient, the BNP level is relatively low due to his extreme obesity. The exact mechanisms that cause lower BNP levels in obese individuals have not been elucidated. BNP levels are higher in the settings of renal failure, older age, and female sex.

Although the patient has findings suggestive of acute pulmonary embolism, such as tachycardia and tachypnea, the presence of crackles and an S_3 suggests left-sided heart failure, which would not be expected as a result of pulmonary embolism. If a pulmonary embolism were so significant as to cause the patient's right-sided heart failure symptoms (that is, acute cor pulmonale), hypotension would very likely be present, but is not.

Cor pulmonale would typically present with a chronic rather than acute course and generally occurs in the setting of established pulmonary disease, such as emphysema or interstitial lung disease. This patient does not have any documented history of pulmonary disease. As cor pulmonale is right-sided heart failure due to pulmonary hypertension of various causes, right-sided failure symptoms predominate. While this patient does demonstrate right-sided

heart failure symptoms (jugular venous distention, peripheral edema), he also demonstrates left-sided failure symptoms (crackles) and absence of other supporting evidence for right-sided heart failure (tricuspid regurgitation murmur, right ventricular heave).

Although this patient does have risk factors for myocardial infarction, which can certainly present atypically in a patient with diabetes (such as with new-onset heart failure in the absence of typical chest pain), there is no evidence on the electrocardiogram to support recent myocardial infarction. The electrocardiogram shows only sinus tachycardia, without pathologic Q waves or suspicious ST changes.

> **KEY POINT**
>
> - B-type natriuretic peptide levels are generally lower in obese persons, even those with acute heart failure.

Bibliography
Daniels LB, Clopton P, Bhalla V, et al. How obesity affects the cutpoints for B-type natriuretic peptide in the diagnosis of acute heart failure. Results from the Breathing Not Properly Multinational Study. Am Heart J. 2006;151(5):999-1005. [PMID: 16644321]

Item 95   Answer: B

Educational Objective: Manage symptomatic aortic stenosis.

This patient's clinical examination and echocardiogram are consistent with severe aortic stenosis. The primary indication for aortic valve replacement in aortic stenosis patients is cardiopulmonary symptoms. End-stage manifestations for symptomatic aortic stenosis are angina, syncope, and heart failure, but initially, most patients present with exertional dyspnea. This patient's description of decreased exercise tolerance and dyspnea is consistent with symptomatic disease. Clinical vigilance in history-taking is essential as disease progression in aortic stenosis is slow (over decades), and many patients attribute symptoms to "old age." In patients who are asymptomatic, clinical follow-up to monitor for disease progression (every 6-12 months) is reasonable. In severe, symptomatic aortic stenosis, valve replacement improves long-term survival and quality of life.

Age is not a contraindication for valve replacement. Elderly patients with aortic stenosis who undergo aortic valve replacement have a postsurgical life expectancy equivalent to their age-matched peers without aortic stenosis. Given that after symptom onset, average survival without valve replacement is only 2 to 3 years, medical therapy alone is insufficient. Therefore, valve replacement is indicated in any symptomatic patient, regardless of age. As in any patient, the decision to proceed with valve replacement in an elderly patient should be tempered by comorbidities such as advanced malignancy. Postoperative outcome is less favorable in patients with systolic dysfunction. However, if the etiology of systolic dysfunction is increased afterload, function often improves with relief of the outflow obstruction.

Patients with cardiovascular risk factors under consideration for valve replacement should undergo preoperative coronary angiography so that bypass graft surgery can be performed concurrently with valve replacement if needed.

Percutaneous aortic balloon valvuloplasty is not routinely performed in patients with calcific aortic stenosis. Serious complications occur in more than 10% of procedures, and restenosis or recurrent symptoms occur within a year in most patients.

Patients with aortic stenosis are especially sensitive to changes in their central blood volume and preload. In the absence of physical examination signs supporting the diagnosis of fluid overload, switching from hydrochlorothiazide to furosemide is not indicated and may result in acute clinical deterioration of this patient.

KEY POINT

- **The primary indication for valve replacement in aortic stenosis is onset of cardiac signs and symptoms, such as angina, syncope, exertional dyspnea, or heart failure.**

Bibliography

Bonow RO, Carabello BA, Kanu C, et al. ACC/AHA 2006 guidelines for the management of patients with valvular heart disease: a report of the American College of Cardiology/American Heart Association Task Force on Practice Guidelines (Writing committee to Develop Guidelines on the Management of Patients with Valvular Heart Disease): developed in collaboration with the Society of Cardiovascular Anesthesiologists: endorsed by the Society for Cardiovascular Angiography and Interventions and the Society of Thoracic Surgeons [erratum in Circulation. 2007;115(15):e409.]. Circulation. 2006;114(5):e84-231. [PMID: 16880336]

Item 96   Answer: B

Educational Objective: Advise a patient on lifestyle modification to reduce the risk of cardiovascular disease.

This woman has several risk factors for cardiovascular disease, including obesity (BMI ≥30), her family history, her sedentary lifestyle, and her smoking status. When faced with the possibility of multiple interventions for cardiovascular disease risk factor management, it is often important to counsel the patient regarding the relative benefit of each intervention and to address the risk factors and interventions sequentially. However, there are also data to suggest that addressing multiple risk factors sequentially is not superior to and may be inferior to a simultaneous approach. Women who are current smokers have a 3-fold higher risk of cardiovascular disease compared with women who have stopped smoking or have never smoked. Surprisingly, the duration of smoking does not correlate with risk of future cardiovascular disease. (It does, however, correlate with risk of smoking-related cancers.) In addition, the risk of cardiovascular disease drops rapidly after smoking cessation, with the greatest relative reduction occurring in the first 5 years of stopping. Therefore, although this patient has

a 32 pack-year history of smoking, smoking cessation now will immediately and significantly reduce her risk of cardiovascular disease. With regard to her risk of having a cardiovascular event, the Framingham risk estimate is calculated to be 3% over the next 10 years (low risk) compared with less than 1% if she were a nonsmoker.

Other important lifestyle considerations include regular exercise, a healthy diet, and maintaining a healthy weight. Although the presence of these positive behavioral factors has been associated with a lower risk of cardiovascular events, lifestyle interventions have not conclusively been shown to reduce the risk of cardiovascular events.

The U.S. Preventive Services Task Force (USPSTF) recommends against the use of estrogen or estrogen plus progestin for the prevention of chronic diseases after menopause. The Women's Health Initiative showed at least a trend toward an increased risk with the use of estrogen or estrogen-progestin for breast cancer, coronary artery disease, stroke, venous thromboembolism, dementia and cognitive decline, and urinary incontinence; quality-of-life measures were not clinically improved with hormone use. However, this patient has been taking hormones for several years without a cardiovascular event, and stopping hormone therapy in this circumstance has not been shown to reduce the risk of a future cardiovascular event. However, there are other reasons for her to attempt discontinuation of hormone replacement therapy and this should be discussed with the patient.

KEY POINT

- **The risk of a cardiovascular event is reduced rapidly (within 5 years) of smoking cessation in women.**

Bibliography

Kenfield SA, Stampfer MJ, Rosner BA, Colditz GA. Smoking and smoking cessation in relation to mortality in women. JAMA. 2008;299(17):2037-2047. [PMID: 18460664]

Item 97   Answer: D

Educational Objective: Manage a patient at risk for sudden death from cardiac sarcoidosis.

This patient has a probable family history of sudden cardiac death, and her recurrent episodes of syncope are consistent with a cardiac etiology, as evidenced by the lack of associated prodromal symptoms and no evidence of seizure activity. Jugular venous distention and pedal edema are consistent with right-sided heart decompensation. Furthermore, electrocardiography shows conduction abnormalities, and 24-hour monitoring demonstrates ventricular ectopy and nonsustained ventricular tachycardia. A prior thallium stress test showed no ischemia but did reveal patchy myocardial uptake. This is a nonspecific finding but can be seen in cardiac sarcoidosis. Further findings support a clinical diagnosis of sarcoidosis in this patient, namely the maculopapular eruptions and chest radiograph findings of hilar lymphadenopathy and infiltrates. Endomyocardial biopsy findings of noncaseating granulomata confirm cardiac sarcoidosis.

Young black women have an apparent increased frequency for sarcoidosis as compared with other race and/or sex cohorts. Thus, this patient's race, sex, and age are characteristic for patients who more commonly present with sarcoidosis. Sudden death accounts for up to 65% of deaths due to cardiac sarcoidosis, presumably caused by ventricular tachyarrhythmias or conduction block. Symptomatic or electrocardiographically evident arrhythmias or conduction abnormalities typically become evident prior to sudden cardiac death. This patient's history of recurrent syncope, ventricular tachycardia, conduction abnormalities, and family history of sudden death place her at high risk for sudden death. The most appropriate management for this patient is placement of an implantable cardioverter-defibrillator (ICD), which has defibrillation and pacing capabilities for treatment of ventricular tachyarrhythmias and bradyarrhythmias, respectively.

Amiodarone has not been shown to effectively reduce the incidence of sudden cardiac death. Thus, as an isolated agent it does not have a role in prophylaxis of sudden death. However, in patients with an ICD, amiodarone can be used to reduce the frequency of episodes of ventricular tachycardia and subsequent firing of the ICD.

Cardiac magnetic resonance (CMR) imaging is useful for detection of localized myocardial high-intensity areas due to cardiac sarcoidosis and, when performed with late gadolinium enhancement, has a reported sensitivity of 100% and specificity of 78% for the disease. In this patient with confirmed cardiac sarcoidosis by endomyocardial biopsy, however, CMR imaging is not indicated. CMR imaging is a useful screening technique, but owing to the possibility of false-positive results, biopsy may still be necessary to determine the need for an ICD.

Electrophysiologic testing identifies patients with cardiac sarcoidosis who are likely to have sustained ventricular tachyarrhythmias or sudden death. However, such testing should be reserved for those patients who are stratified prior to testing in an intermediate-risk group. This patient is at high risk for sudden cardiac death based on documented cardiac involvement from sarcoidosis, syncope, nonsustained ventricular tachycardia on 24-hour ambulatory monitoring, and family history of sudden death. Thus, a negative electrophysiologic study would likely be a false negative and, therefore, would not obviate the need for an ICD.

A permanent pacemaker would not protect against sudden death from ventricular tachyarrhythmias and thus would not be sufficient treatment for this patient.

KEY POINT

- **The most appropriate management for patients with cardiac sarcoidosis who are at high risk for sudden death is placement of an implantable cardioverter-defibrillator.**

Bibliography

Mehta D, Lubitz SA, Frankel Z, et al. Cardiac Involvement in Patients with Sarcoidosis: Diagnostic and Prognostic Value of Outpatient Testing. Chest. 2008;133(6):1426-1435. [PMID: 18339784]

Item 98   Answer: B
Educational Objective: Treat reversible heart block.

This patient most likely has Lyme carditis. The presence of the characteristic skin rash, erythema migrans, with or without a history of tick bite in an endemic region, has a probability greater than 80% of being caused by *Borrelia burgdorferi* infection, and is sufficient to support a decision to treat Lyme disease empirically without laboratory confirmation. Although antibiotics have not been shown to improve resolution of cardiac symptoms, it is recommended that patients with cardiac symptoms or advanced heart block be admitted for monitoring and antibiotic therapy. The preferred antibiotic regimen is intravenous ceftriaxone until the heart block resolves, followed by a 21-day course of oral therapy. The discovery of Lyme disease in any stage should prompt antibiotic treatment since early phases may regress spontaneously but leave patients at risk for later (neurologic or rheumatic) stages. The recommended 3-week course of treatment seems to reduce the chance of disease progression dramatically.

Lyme carditis is manifested by acute-onset, high-grade atrioventricular conduction defects that may occasionally be associated with myocarditis. Carditis occurs in 5% to 10% of patients with Lyme disease, usually within a few weeks to months after infection. Cardiac involvement can occur in isolation or with other symptoms of the disease. Atrioventricular block can present in any degree, and progression to complete heart block is often rapid. Prognosis is good, with usual resolution of atrioventricular block within days to weeks. This patient has complete heart block, as evidenced by a faster sinus rate than the escape rhythm, and no relationship between the atrial and ventricular electrical activity. In some patients, heart block is the first and only manifestation of Lyme disease, but the diagnosis can be confirmed by a positive IgM and IgG antibody response to *B. burgdorferi*. Lyme serologic testing should be considered in any patient with unexplained high-grade atrioventricular block, particularly in patients with potential tick exposure living in endemic areas.

Electrophysiology study is not indicated, since it does not provide additional prognostic information. Atrioventricular block is usually within the node, but sinoatrial and His-Purkinje involvement have also been described.

Erythromycin is considered a third-line agent for the treatment of Lyme disease, as it is less effective than penicillin or cephalosporin drugs. However, oral erythromycin can be used for patients with erythema migrans who are intolerant of amoxicillin, doxycycline, and cefuroxime.

Most cases of Lyme carditis resolve spontaneously, and neither temporary nor permanent pacemaker therapy is needed. Temporary pacing would be required if the patient were hemodynamically unstable with bradycardia. However, this rarely occurs in the setting of Lyme carditis. Indications for permanent pacemaker placement would include persistent high-grade atrioventricular block.

KEY POINT

- Lyme carditis is manifested by acute-onset, high-grade atrioventricular conduction defects that may occasionally be associated with myocarditis.

Bibliography

Bratton RL, Whiteside JW, Hovan MJ, Engle RL, Edwards FD. Diagnosis and treatment of Lyme disease. Mayo Clin Proc. 2008;83(5):566-571. [PMID: 18452688]

Item 99   Answer: E

Educational Objective: Evaluate suspected coronary artery disease using the appropriate stress test.

This 68-year-old woman has cardiac risk factors of smoking and hypertension (with an elevated systolic blood pressure on therapy), resulting in an intermediate Framingham risk score (18% likelihood of a coronary event in 10 years). In addition, she has atypical chest pain, so further evaluation is appropriate. An exercise stress test is recommended in patients with a normal baseline electrocardiogram (ECG) who are able to exercise because it provides information about exercise tolerance and hemodynamic response to exercise.

There are concerns that ECG stress testing in women, compared with men, has a lower sensitivity and specificity for the diagnosis of coronary disease. Stress testing with imaging by echocardiography and radionuclide perfusion imaging have been found to be more accurate in women. However, this approach is controversial, and current guidelines continue to recommend a standard ECG treadmill test as the first approach. If this patient were taking a β-blocker for hypertension control, it would need to be withheld prior to the stress test because a stress test requires that the patient achieve 85% of maximum predicted heart rate to be diagnostic. Additional blood pressure control before the test also is needed, as high blood pressure may result in the need to prematurely terminate the test.

An adenosine nuclear perfusion stress test is contraindicated in patients with significant bronchospastic disease and hence is not the correct choice for a patient with asthma. Whenever possible, exercise stress testing is preferred over pharmacologic stress testing because of the additional physiologic information on exercise tolerance and the blood pressure and heart rate response to exercise.

Coronary angiography would only be appropriate if the patient were presenting with an acute coronary syndrome or after an abnormal stress test.

A coronary artery calcium score is measured from noncontrast CT images. Although it correlates with cardiovascular risk, it is not a direct measure of the severity of luminal coronary disease. It can be helpful in furthering the risk stratification of selected asymptomatic patients but would not provide information on the cause of this patient's chest pain.

Dobutamine stress echocardiography is an appropriate choice in patients who are unable to exercise and are not hypertensive at rest. This patient is able to exercise, so treadmill testing is the more appropriate choice. If dobutamine stress testing were performed, her hypertension would need to be better controlled first.

KEY POINT

- Exercise electrocardiographic stress testing is the primary approach to the diagnosis of coronary artery disease in patients who can exercise and have a normal resting electrocardiogram.

Bibliography

Mieres JH, Shaw LJ, Arai A, et al. Role of noninvasive testing in the clinical evaluation of women with suspected coronary artery disease: consensus statement from the Cardiac Imaging Committee, Council on Clinical Cardiology, and the Cardiovascular Imaging and Intervention Committee, Council on Cardiovascular Radiology and Intervention, American Heart Association. Circulation. 2005;111(5):682-696. [PMID: 15687114]

Item 100   Answer: B

Educational Objective: Recognize mitral regurgitation associated with a repaired ostium primum atrial septal defect.

The patient has clinical features of mitral regurgitation, including a displaced cardiac apex, and a grade 3/6 holosystolic murmur is noted at the apex and radiates to the axilla. In addition, the electrocardiogram demonstrates findings of first-degree atrioventricular block (prolonged PR interval) and left axis deviation where the QRS complex is positive in lead I but negative in lead aVF; these are typically seen in a patient with an ostium primum atrial septal defect due to abnormal development and location of the conduction tissue. The past history of an atrial septal defect closed surgically, the physical examination findings demonstrating mitral regurgitation, together with the electrocardiographic features, would suggest that the patient had an ostium primum atrial septal defect and now has mitral regurgitation related to a residual cleft. Ostium primum atrial septal defects are generally associated with a cleft in the mitral valve. Patients often have associated mitral regurgitation that progresses after closure of the atrial septal defect if the mitral valve is not repaired at the time of operative intervention. Additional findings may include left ventricular outflow tract obstruction and tricuspid regurgitation related to a tricuspid valve cleft.

Aortic stenosis is characterized by small and late carotid pulsations, a sustained apical impulse, and a late-peaking systolic murmur best heard at the second right intercostal space. The murmur characteristically radiates to one or both carotid arteries. The electrocardiogram in aortic stenosis demonstrates left ventricular hypertrophy.

Patients with pulmonary valve stenosis demonstrate a parasternal impulse due to right ventricular pressure overload. The apical impulse is not displaced. An ejection click and a systolic murmur are noted over the second left intercostal space. The murmur increases in intensity during inspiration due to the increased systemic venous return. No diastolic murmur is noted. The electrocardiogram in pulmonary valve stenosis demonstrates right axis deviation and findings of right ventricular hypertrophy.

There are no definite features associated with a residual atrial septal defect in this patient, such as a parasternal impulse due to right heart enlargement. Fixed splitting of the S_2 and tricuspid rather than mitral regurgitation would be expected in a patient with residual atrial septal defect; this would cause a holosystolic murmur at the left sternal border that increases in intensity with inspiration.

KEY POINT

- **Patients with ostium primum atrial septal defect with a mitral valve cleft that is not closed at the time of initial repair often present with symptoms of severe mitral regurgitation and require late mitral valve repair or replacement.**

Bibliography
Webb G, Gatzoulis MA. Atrial septal defects in the adult: recent progress and overview. Circulation. 2006;114(15):1645-1653. [PMID: 17030704]

Item 101   Answer: B

Educational Objective: Treat hypovolemia in a patient with chronic heart failure.

A high B-type natriuretic peptide (BNP) level typically reflects volume overload; however, factors other than volume status may also influence BNP levels, including renal failure, older age, and female sex, all of which are associated with relative increases in BNP independent of heart failure or volume status. In this patient, the elevated BNP level is related to a decreased glomerular filtration rate associated with prerenal azotemia, although any cause of renal failure—whether volume related or not—is associated with a relative increase in BNP level. There is no evidence other than the elevated BNP level to suggest volume overload; rather, the evidence points to volume depletion, including her recently increased blood urea nitrogen and serum creatinine levels, rapid weight loss, tachycardia, and possibly, her blood pressure, which is relatively low for her. Volume depletion in this patient is presumably due to overdiuresis related to the increase in furosemide dose, which would improve with intravenous fluids and an adjustment to furosemide dose.

The utility of using BNP levels to guide outpatient management of heart failure is still being studied. The multi-center TIME-CHF trial showed no benefit to BNP-guided therapy over symptom-guided therapy for patients 75 years or older in either overall survival, survival free of all-cause hospitalizations, or survival free of hospitalizations for heart failure.

This patient's chronic atrial fibrillation is currently not optimally rate controlled, although this is likely a function of volume depletion. The tachycardia is not causing hemodynamic instability, so there is no urgency for establishing rate control with diltiazem. Rate control will likely be restored with volume repletion.

Because this patient's renal insufficiency is likely related to volume depletion and she is not hemodynamically unstable, inotropic support with milrinone is not needed at this time. If the patient were unstable, with signs of low cardiac output and hypoperfusion (such as shock liver, altered mental status, or significant hypotension), inotropic support in addition to intravenous fluids would be appropriate.

This patient does not have evidence for significant heart failure decompensation such as elevated jugular venous pressure, an S_3, and pulmonary crackles, and therefore does not need acute afterload reduction with nesiritide. Furthermore, because the primary problem is intravascular volume depletion, additional vasodilation would only worsen hypotension.

KEY POINT

- **B-type natriuretic peptide levels are elevated in the setting of renal insufficiency.**

Bibliography
Pfisterer M, Buser P, Rickli H, et al; TIME-CHF Investigators. BNP-guided vs symptom-guided heart failure therapy: the Trial of Intensified vs Standard Medical Therapy in Elderly Patients With Congestive Heart Failure (TIME-CHF) randomized trial. JAMA. 2009;301(4):383-392. [PMID: 19176440]

Item 102   Answer: D

Educational Objective: Treat symptomatic peripheral arterial disease.

The patient has symptomatic left infrapopliteal arterial disease, confirmed by ankle-brachial index and segmental plethysmography. A supervised program of regular, repeated exercise to the point of near-maximal pain significantly increases pain-free walking time and walking distance in patients with symptomatic peripheral arterial disease. Additionally, for infrapopliteal disease, a supervised exercise program is more effective over the long-term than percutaneous revascularization and is less expensive. Patients with severe ischemic heart disease, severe valvular heart disease, or known large aortic aneurysms must be considered carefully and individually before prescription of exercise, but there are no other vascular contraindications in patients without threatened limb loss.

When significant inflow disease is present, revascularization may help provide better distal flow and relief of symptoms referable to infrapopliteal disease. This patient demonstrates no femoral or lower abdominal bruits to suggest inflow disease involving the distal aorta or iliac or common femoral arteries, nor does the patient have thigh or buttock claudication, which might also suggest inflow disease. This patient does not have ischemic pain at rest and does not have evidence on physical examination of ischemic ulceration or gangrene. In addition to an ankle-brachial index of greater than 0.4, these features suggest that this patient does not have critical limb ischemia. Urgent revascularization for limb salvage is, therefore, unnecessary as a first therapeutic endeavor.

Medical treatment with cilostazol, a phosphodiesterase inhibitor, is effective in increasing pain-free and overall walking distance and is recommended for patients with lifestyle-limiting claudication. However, cilostazol is contraindicated in patients with heart failure or left ventricular systolic dysfunction. Chronic use of oral phosphodiesterase inhibitors (not specifically cilostazol) for inotropic therapy in patients with heart failure has been associated with increased mortality.

Percutaneous treatment or surgical bypass should be reserved for patients with threatened limb loss or for patients with short-distance or lifestyle-limiting claudication who have failed to benefit from conservative therapy. Infrapopliteal disease is more often occlusive and involves smaller caliber vessels, both of which make surgical revascularization potentially a more durable solution when intervention is needed. Although drug-eluting stents are being used with increasing frequency for the treatment of infrapopliteal disease, long-term outcomes are not yet known.

KEY POINT

- A supervised exercise program can provide substantial symptomatic benefit to selected patients with claudication.

Bibliography

Treesak C, Kasemsup V, Treat-Jacobson D, Nyman JA, Hirsch AT. Cost-effectiveness of exercise training to improve claudication symptoms in patients with peripheral arterial disease. Vasc Med. 2004;9(4):279-285. [PMID: 15678620]

Item 103   Answer: A

Educational Objective: Treat prosthetic valve endocarditis.

This patient has a mechanical aortic valve with severe aortic regurgitation. She has symptoms of heart failure with hypoxia and pulmonary hypertension. Acute severe aortic regurgitation is a surgical emergency, necessitating valve replacement, particularly with symptoms of heart failure.

Despite the absence of obvious vegetations on her echocardiogram, there is evidence of endocarditis (abnormal murmur, severe valve regurgitation, fever, and an elevated leukocyte count). In more severe infections, a paravalvular

abscess can develop around adjacent structures, predisposing to bradyarrhythmias. Patients with fever and a prosthetic valve should be treated presumptively for endocarditis unless a clear alternative source of infection is present. Surgery should not be delayed to complete an antibiotic course if surgical criteria are met, however, given the grim prognosis if the infected valve is left untreated. Empiric broad-spectrum antibiotics should be instituted after obtaining blood cultures from multiple sites. Subsequently, antibiotics can be tailored for the etiologic organism once isolated.

An intra-aortic balloon pump is absolutely contraindicated in this patient with severe aortic regurgitation because diastolic inflation of the balloon would exacerbate aortic regurgitation.

This patient has severe aortic regurgitation with hyperdynamic left ventricular function and an increased pulse pressure. Inotropic therapy (dobutamine or milrinone) is not indicated, and may promote worsening hypotension due to vasodilation. The probable source of her hypotension is sepsis. Although her acute management may necessitate vasopressor support, surgery is the most urgent intervention needed.

Thrombolytic therapy is a potential treatment for prosthetic valve thrombosis. Prosthetic valve dysfunction should be considered as a possible etiology for this patient's acute presentation; however, her clinical course is not consistent with acute prosthetic valve thrombosis. She has been compliant with warfarin therapy and the INR is currently therapeutic, decreasing the likelihood of an acute thrombosis. Serum lactate dehydrogenase and haptoglobin concentrations are normal in this patient, arguing against hemolysis due to prosthetic valve dysfunction. Finally, there was no evidence of valvular thrombosis on the transthoracic echocardiogram.

KEY POINT

- Patients with fever and a prosthetic valve should be treated presumptively for endocarditis unless a clear alternative source of infection is present.

Bibliography

Habib G, Thuny F, Avierinos JF. Prosthetic valve endocarditis: current approach and therapeutic options. Prog Cardiovasc Dis. 2008;50(4):274-281. [PMID: 18156006]

Item 104   Answer: D

Educational Objective: Recognize absolute and relative contraindications to thrombolytic therapy for ST-elevation myocardial infarction patients.

The patient is experiencing an acute inferior wall ST-elevation myocardial infarction (STEMI). The treatment for an acute STEMI is either revascularization or thrombolytic therapy. Relative contraindications to thrombolytic therapy include pregnancy, poorly controlled hypertension, prior ischemic stroke more than 3 months ago, prolonged cardiopulmonary resuscitation within 3 weeks, recent (within 2 to 4 weeks) internal bleeding, active peptic ulcer disease, and current use of anticoagulants (warfarin). Absolute contraindications include any prior intracerebral hemorrhage, known cerebrovascular lesion (arteriovenous malformation), ischemic stroke within 3 months, suspected aortic dissection, active bleeding (excluding menses), and significant closed head or facial trauma within 3 months. The patient presented has two relative contraindications for thrombolytic therapy—uncontrolled hypertension and a prior stroke. She is currently hemodynamically stable without cardiogenic shock. Despite the inherent time delays, the best treatment approach would be to transfer her to a nearby facility where percutaneous coronary intervention could be performed. Current data suggest that a time delay of less than 60 minutes is acceptable in transferring patients for percutaneous coronary intervention.

Aggressive medical therapy would not be the correct option for this patient given the electrocardiographic findings, her relatively young age, and the ability to transfer her to a nearby hospital to receive appropriate care.

Transfer for coronary artery bypass graft surgery would not be the correct option given that the patient's coronary anatomy has not yet been defined. Most patients presenting with a STEMI can be treated effectively with percutaneous coronary intervention. Bypass surgery in the setting of an acute infarction is therefore rarely performed.

> **KEY POINT**
> - **Absolute and relative contraindications to thrombolytic therapy should be reviewed in all patients being considered for thrombolytic therapy.**

Bibliography

Boden WE, Eagle K, Granger CB. Reperfusion strategies in acute ST-segment elevation myocardial infarction: a comprehensive review of contemporary management options. J Am Coll Cardiol. 2007;50(10):917-929. [PMID: 17765117]

Item 105   Answer: D

Educational Objective: Manage a patient with New York Heart Association functional class III or IV heart failure.

This patient has symptoms consistent with New York Heart Association (NYHA) class III functional status (symptoms develop with mild activity), and she does not appear volume-overloaded on examination. Spironolactone is indicated for treatment of severe (NYHA functional class III or IV) systolic heart failure in addition to standard therapy with angiotensin-converting enzyme (ACE) inhibitors, β-blockers, and diuretics as needed. The addition of spironolactone is associated with a 30% relative reduction in mortality. Given the risk of side effects, care should be taken in observing appropriate guidelines for use of spironolactone.

Serum creatinine and potassium levels should be serially monitored. In the RALES trial, patients were excluded if their creatinine level was greater than 2.5 mg/dL (190.8 µmol/L) in men or 2.0 mg/dL (152.6 µmol/L) in women or their potassium level was greater than 5 meq/L (5 mmol/L).

It is generally not recommended to add angiotensin receptor blocker therapy to ACE inhibitor therapy. The risk of adverse side effects, such as hyperkalemia and hypotension, is increased, and there is no definitive benefit in mortality or morbidity.

In black patients with NYHA class III or IV heart failure, the addition of hydralazine with isosorbide dinitrate to standard heart failure therapy (ACE-inhibitors, β-blockers, and diuretics as needed) is indicated for additional survival benefit. This patient is not black; therefore, hydralazine is not indicated. In addition, hydralazine possibly would not be well tolerated because of her relatively low blood pressure.

The addition of metolazone to loop diuretic therapy can be useful to increase diuretic effectiveness. However, this patient appears euvolemic (no jugular venous distention, clear lungs, no edema, no S_3) while on her current diuretic regimen, so enhanced diuresis is not needed. Also, in this patient, excessive diuresis may result in worsening of her chronic kidney disease and the development of hyperkalemia.

> **KEY POINT**
> - **Spironolactone, angiotensin-converting enzyme inhibitors, and β-blockers are indicated for treatment of New York Heart Association class III and IV heart failure.**

Bibliography

Pitt B, Zannad F, Remme WJ, et al. The effect of spironolactone on morbidity and mortality in patients with severe heart failure. Randomized Aldactone Evaluation Study Investigators. N Engl J Med. 1999;341(10):709-717. [PMID: 10471456]

Item 106   Answer: B

Educational Objective: Manage a patient with cardiogenic shock.

Placement of a pulmonary artery catheter can assist in assessing volume status, intracardiac filling pressures, and cardiac output in selected patients with decompensated heart failure. If hypovolemia is present, volume resuscitation with intravenous fluids is indicated, whereas if volume overload is present, intravenous diuretics are warranted. Elevated intracardiac filling pressures will likely be improved with a combination of diuresis and afterload reduction. A low cardiac output indicates primary cardiogenic shock, and inotropic agents may be needed to augment myocardial contractility and thus cardiac output. The patient's central venous and pulmonary capillary wedge pressures demonstrate that she is reasonably euvolemic.

Her cardiac output is very low, and the increased creatinine and aminotransferase levels are evidence for end-organ hypoperfusion. To improve cardiac output and thus end-organ perfusion, an intravenous inotrope such as milrinone is indicated. Milrinone is a phosphodiesterase inhibitor and does not produce inotropic effects via interaction with β-receptors. Intravenous inotropic agents are indicated only for short-term treatment of cardiogenic shock, or in selected patients who are receiving palliative care or bridging to cardiac transplantation. Long-term treatment with intravenous inotropic agents does not improve clinical outcomes and, in fact, likely increases mortality. In general, although β-blockers can frequently be continued at unchanged or reduced doses during hospitalization for heart failure decompensation, when the decompensation is severe enough to cause cardiogenic shock, it is recommended to stop the β-blocker to avoid its negative inotropic effects.

The patient is not volume overloaded at this time; therefore, diuresis with furosemide is not indicated. Furthermore, the patient is hypotensive, with clinical consequences of hypotension (renal and hepatic insufficiency), and diuresis would likely worsen the hypotension. The patient is not hypovolemic; therefore, infusion of normal saline is not needed and may contribute to clinical worsening if the heart cannot manage the increased preload.

Nesiritide is recombinant B-type natriuretic peptide and has natriuretic, diuretic, and vasodilatory properties. Although nesiritide has been demonstrated to produce favorable hemodynamic effects in patients with decompensated heart failure, its effects on long-term morbidity (particularly in regard to renal function) and mortality are still being evaluated. Because nesiritide lowers blood pressure, its use is contraindicated in the setting of hypotension or cardiogenic shock, as is present in this patient.

Anemia is often present in heart failure patients and may have many causes, including chronic disease and renal failure. Although the patient's hemoglobin level has decreased in the past month, the decrease is within the range of normal variation. The patient's shock cannot be attributed to blood loss, as there is no history to support acute blood loss and the hemodynamic values do not indicate a volume-depleted state. Thus, packed erythrocyte transfusion would not be indicated.

KEY POINT

- **Positive inotropic agents such as dobutamine or milrinone can be used to correct low cardiac output and improve perfusion in patients with cardiogenic shock.**

Bibliography

Reynolds HR, Hochman JS. Cardiogenic shock: current concepts and improving outcomes. Circulation. 2008;117(5):686-697. [PMID: 18250279]

Item 107   Answer: A

Educational Objective: Differentiate an ischemic and viable limb from one requiring amputation.

Acute arterial occlusion is manifested by the "five P's"—pain, paresthesia, absent pulses, paralysis, and pallor; the viability of an acutely threatened limb is determined by the severity of these clinical characteristics. Improvement in pain, as occurred in this patient, should not be taken as a reassuring sign, but rather as a sign of progressive neurologic deficit due to ischemia. This patient has an immediately threatened limb as demonstrated by marked motor and sensory deficits and the absence of arterial Doppler signals, but with the presence of intact venous signals and some residual motor function (class IIb acute ischemia). Emergency surgical revascularization is necessary if the limb is to be saved.

The venous system, like the arterial system, can be evaluated by ultrasound to demonstrate flow. When venous flow can be demonstrated by this technique without demonstrable arterial flow (class II acute ischemia), then either arterial flow is occurring in major vessels at undetectably low velocities, or there is flow in smaller collateral vessels only. In either circumstance, the presence of a venous flow signal demonstrates that there is some small degree of blood flow into the threatened limb. Decisions regarding treatment must be predicated upon vascular flow signals and sensorimotor dysfunction.

In patients with class I acute limb ischemia (moderate to severe claudication but no rest pain, audible venous and arterial Doppler signals), antiplatelet therapy along with systemic anticoagulation with heparin is indicated. Patients with transient sensory deficits and no motor weakness are typically considered for intra-arterial thrombolytic therapy. This patient has marked motor and sensory deficits and his limb is immediately threatened; he needs emergency surgical revascularization.

Patients with anesthesia, paralysis, and loss of vascular flow signals (class III ischemia) have irreversible ischemia and prompt amputation is required. Patients with less dense sensorimotor defects and intact venous flow signals (class IIb ischemia) may obtain limb salvage, but only with immediate revascularization. Patients without sensorimotor loss and with evidence of intact vascular flow (class IIa ischemia) are more likely to obtain limb salvage, but only with prompt vascular intervention.

KEY POINT

- **In patients with acute limb ischemia with mild to moderate weakness and sensory loss that extends beyond the toes (class IIb ischemia), limb salvage is only possible with immediate revascularization.**

Bibliography

Norgren L, Hiatt WR, Dormandy JA, et al. Inter-Society Consensus for the Management of Peripheral Arterial Disease (TASC II). Eur J Vasc Endovasc Surg. 2007;33 Suppl 1:S1-75. [PMID: 17140820]

Item 108 Answer: D

Educational Objective: Manage sick sinus syndrome.

This patient has symptomatic sick sinus syndrome (SSS) with correlation of symptoms and bradycardia. Like many patients with SSS, she also has atrial fibrillation. Her history of rapidly conducted atrial fibrillation suggests she will continue to require atrioventricular nodal blockade for rate control while in atrial fibrillation. In addition, she has coronary artery disease, which is an indication for β-blocker therapy. Treatment of SSS is directed at symptoms; correlation of symptoms with arrhythmia is essential. Symptomatic sinus node dysfunction is an indication for pacemaker placement, even if the bradycardia occurs as a consequence of drug therapy, if there is no acceptable alternative.

SSS comprises a collection of pathologic findings that result in bradycardia. These include sinus arrest, sinus exit block, and sinus bradycardia. Approximately 50% of patients with SSS also have associated supraventricular tachycardia, most often atrial fibrillation or atrial flutter. The tachycardia-bradycardia syndrome is characterized by rapid ventricular conduction during episodes of atrial fibrillation, but resting bradycardia between episodes. This combination makes management of intermittent tachycardia difficult without pacemaker backup. SSS is common in the elderly, and because symptoms can be intermittent or nonspecific, misdiagnosis can occur.

Amiodarone is not an appropriate choice for this patient. Although it may reduce the risk of symptomatic episodes of atrial fibrillation, it is likely to worsen sinus node dysfunction.

A β-blocker is indicated in this patient with a previous myocardial infarction to reduce her risk of recurrent myocardial infarction and cardiovascular mortality, and it should not be discontinued. In addition, the β-blocker provides atrioventricular nodal blockade necessary for rate control during atrial fibrillation. Metoprolol, therefore, should not be discontinued.

The patient has no signs or symptoms of heart failure or other indications for echocardiogram.

KEY POINT

- Symptomatic sinus node dysfunction is an indication for pacemaker placement, even if the bradycardia occurs as a consequence of drug therapy, if there is no acceptable alternative.

Bibliography

Gregoratos G, Abrams J, Epstein AE, et al. ACC/AHA/NASPE 2002 guideline update for implantation of cardiac pacemakers and antiarrhythmia devices: summary article: a report of the American College of Cardiology/American Heart Association Task Force on Practice Guidelines (ACC/AHA/NASPE Committee to Update the 1998 Pacemaker Guidelines). Circulation. 2002;106(16):2145-2161. [PMID: 12379588]

Item 109 Answer: A

Educational Objective: Manage a patient with diastolic heart failure.

The patient's history and echocardiogram are consistent with heart failure with preserved systolic function; that is, she has symptoms of heart failure in the setting of normal systolic function and no valvular abnormalities. She has hypertension, which predisposes to the development of left ventricular hypertrophy and impaired ventricular relaxation. The primary treatment goals in diastolic heart failure are to treat the underlying cause and to manage any potentially exacerbating factors, which commonly include tachycardia, hypertension, and ischemia. This patient's blood pressure is still not optimally controlled, and adding candesartan would be appropriate at this time.

Blockade of neurohormonal activation, including the renin-angiotensin-aldosterone system, in heart failure with preserved systolic function is beneficial in reducing salt and water retention, as well as ameliorating adverse cardiac remodeling, cellular fibrosis, and hypertrophy. One of the few large, randomized prospective trials examining treatments for heart failure with preserved systolic function demonstrated that the angiotensin receptor blocker candesartan reduced heart failure–related hospitalizations but not mortality in patients with heart failure with preserved systolic function.

Digoxin is a positive inotropic agent that is used in the treatment of symptomatic systolic heart failure. There are currently no data to support the use of digoxin for the treatment of diastolic heart failure.

The patient currently appears euvolemic, and does not need the additional diuresis that would be caused by switching from hydrochlorothiazide to furosemide.

Although additional hypertension control is indicated at this time, and increasing metoprolol would be helpful in that regard, it would be a less optimal choice than adding an angiotensin receptor blocker. The data regarding the impact of metoprolol on morbidity and mortality in diastolic dysfunction are less robust, and in this particular patient, the heart rate is already bradycardic, which limits further increases in metoprolol dosage.

KEY POINT

- The angiotensin receptor blocker candesartan has been shown to reduce heart failure–related hospitalizations but not mortality in patients with diastolic heart failure.

Bibliography

Yusuf S, Pfeffer MA, Swedberg K, et al; CHARM Investigators and Committees. Effects of candesartan in patients with chronic heart failure and preserved left-ventricular ejection fraction: the CHARM-Preserved Trial. Lancet. 2003;362(9386):777-781. [PMID: 13678871]

Item 110   Answer: B

Educational Objective: Exclude noncardiac conditions in the evaluation of a patient with a possible ST-elevation myocardial infarction.

This patient's chest pain, which began suddenly at rest and radiates to the back, is suggestive of aortic dissection. An acute aortic syndrome should be suspected in any patient who presents with sudden severe thoracic pain. Ascending aortic dissection is often associated with acute aortic regurgitation, myocardial ischemia, cardiac tamponade or hemopericardium, and hemothorax or exsanguination. Considerable (>20 mm Hg) variation in systolic blood pressure in the arms may be present. An aortic dissection should be excluded in a patient with a suggestive history prior to initiating antithrombotic therapy or thrombolytic therapy.

Imaging tests that can confirm or exclude the diagnosis of aortic dissection include contrast-enhanced CT, transesophageal echocardiography, and thoracic magnetic resonance angiography. All three approaches have similar accuracy, and the choice of imaging method largely depends on availability, operator experience, and coexisting conditions.

Medical therapy for an acute coronary syndrome would not be indicated in the setting of an aortic dissection but would be appropriate once the diagnosis of aortic dissection has been ruled out.

Thrombolytic therapy would be contraindicated and potentially fatal in a patient with an aortic dissection. In addition, the electrocardiogram of this patient demonstrates left ventricular hypertrophy and only 0.5-mm ST-segment elevation (most likely secondary to the left ventricular hypertrophy), which does not meet criteria for thrombolytic therapy (1 mm of ST-segment elevation in two contiguous leads).

Transthoracic echocardiography has limited utility for the evaluation of the thoracic aorta for dissection; however, it may suggest the diagnosis in patients referred for other indications, such as new aortic regurgitation, proximal ascending dissection flap, or hemopericardium.

KEY POINT

- **Multiple imaging tests can confirm or exclude the diagnosis of aortic dissection, including contrast-enhanced CT, transesophageal echocardiography, and thoracic magnetic resonance angiography.**

Bibliography

Nienaber CA, von Kodolitsch Y, Nicolas V, et al. The diagnosis of thoracic aortic dissection by noninvasive imaging procedures. N Engl J Med. 1993;328(1):1-9. [PMID: 8416265]

Item 111   Answer: C

Educational Objective: Diagnose hypertrophic cardiomyopathy.

This patient has a systolic murmur. The most common diagnoses to consider in the differential diagnosis include a primary valve source, such as a bicuspid aortic valve, aortic stenosis, mitral valve prolapse, and a benign murmur. Other cardiac abnormalities associated with a systolic murmur include hypertrophic cardiomyopathy, ventricular septal defect, and aortic coarctation.

In this patient, the physical examination is most consistent with hypertrophic cardiomyopathy. The systolic murmur of hypertrophic cardiomyopathy is caused by turbulent flow and obstruction in the left ventricular outflow tract from the thickened interventricular septum. In severe cases, systolic anterior motion of the mitral valve apparatus into the left ventricular outflow tract contributes to the systolic murmur. If mitral valve leaflet coaptation is affected, there may be concurrent mitral regurgitation. The stand-to-squat maneuver and passive leg lift transiently increase venous return (preload), which increases left ventricular chamber size and volume. As a consequence, there is less relative obstruction and turbulence in the left ventricular outflow tract, decreasing murmur intensity. The Valsalva maneuver and the squat-to-stand maneuver transiently decrease venous return, with the septum and anterior mitral leaflet brought closer together. Turbulent flow—and the murmur—are increased. Handgrip exercise increases afterload and decreases the relative pressure gradient across the left ventricular outflow tract, so murmur intensity for hypertrophic cardiomyopathy is decreased. Transthoracic echocardiography can confirm a diagnosis of hypertrophic cardiomyopathy.

Aortic coarctation in an adult is characterized by hypertension and a continuous or late systolic murmur that may be heard over the back. Because pulses distal to the aortic obstruction are decreased, aortic coarctation is also associated with abnormal differences in upper and lower extremity blood pressures. The carotid upstroke is normal in coarctation.

The murmur of aortic stenosis is an early systolic murmur that often radiates superiorly, toward the carotid arteries. Hypertrophic cardiomyopathy is associated with rapid upstrokes of the carotid arteries, helping to distinguish it from aortic stenosis (of either a bicuspid or tricuspid aortic valve), which is associated with a carotid artery pulsation that has a slow up-rise and is diminished in volume.

The murmur associated with mitral valve prolapse and regurgitation is a holosystolic to late systolic murmur that is apically located and associated with a midsystolic click. In a patient with mitral valve prolapse, the Valsalva maneuver moves the click murmur complex earlier in systole and may increase the intensity of the murmur. Similarly, decreased preload (smaller left ventricular chamber size) increases systolic buckling of the valve leaflets, and the murmur lengthens or intensifies. The carotid upstroke is normal in mitral valve prolapse.

The murmur associated with a ventricular septal defect is a harsh systolic murmur located parasternally that radiates to the right sternal edge and may be associated with a palpable thrill but no change in the carotid artery pulsation. Maneuvers that increase afterload, such as isometric handgrip exercise, increase the left-sided murmurs of mitral regurgitation and ventricular septal defect.

KEY POINT

- **Maneuvers that increase preload (stand-to-squat and passive leg lift) decrease the murmurs of hypertrophic cardiomyopathy and mitral valve prolapse.**

Bibliography

Etchells E, Bell C, Robb K. Does this patient have an abnormal systolic murmur? JAMA. 1997;277(7):564-571. [PMID: 9032164]

Item 112 Answer: A

Educational Objective: Determine the risks associated with pregnancy in a woman with tetralogy of Fallot.

Women with tetralogy of Fallot have an increased risk of having offspring with congenital anomalies. Approximately 15% of women with tetralogy of Fallot have chromosome 22q11.2 microdeletion, which raises the risk of having a child with congenital heart disease substantially, from 4% to 6% in affected women without the microdeletion to approximately 50% in those with the microdeletion. There is a reasonable chance that this patient with tetralogy of Fallot and dysmorphic features is 22q11.2 microdeletion–positive. Screening for the chromosome 22q11.2 microdeletion should be considered in women with tetralogy of Fallot to determine the risk of having an offspring with congenital heart disease, and this would be an appropriate test for this patient. Patients with conotruncal abnormalities (tetralogy of Fallot, pulmonary artery atresia, truncus arteriosus) are recognized to be at increased risk for having the 22q11.2 microdeletion. Although dysmorphic features may suggest an increased chance of having the microdeletion, this genetic defect cannot be reliably assessed by physical examination, and so additional testing would be necessary to determine the risk. It would be appropriate to do this testing prior to pregnancy in order to provide comprehensive pregnancy counseling.

The patient is asymptomatic, has preserved ventricular function, and no history of cardiovascular symptoms or arrhythmia; therefore, cardiovascular decompensation or arrhythmia during pregnancy would be relatively unlikely (<10%).

Cyanosis is a recognized handicap to fetal growth, with resultant low-birth-weight infants and increased fetal morbidity. This patient has repaired tetralogy of Fallot, is not cyanotic, and is on no concerning medications. The fetal birthweight should not be reduced based on maternal congenital heart disease.

KEY POINT

- **In patients with tetralogy of Fallot and 22q11.2 microdeletion, the chance of an offspring being born with congenital heart disease is approximately 50%.**

Bibliography

Beauchesne LM, Warnes CA, Connolly HM, et al. Prevalence and clinical manifestations of 22q11.2 microdeletion in adults with selected conotruncal anomalies. J Am Coll Cardiol. 2005;45(4):595-598. [PMID: 15708709]

Item 113 Answer: D

Educational Objective: Manage acute abdominal aortic aneurysm.

The patient's clinical presentation—severe abdominal or back pain with syncope followed by vague discomfort—is typical for a ruptured abdominal aortic aneurysm (AAA) that has been locally contained, preventing his immediate death. The sentinel event of severe sudden back pain associated with loss of consciousness marks the occurrence of rupture. Symptoms after that time are likely due to either local irritation and inflammation related to the rupture and hemorrhage or to expansion of the aneurysm against adjacent structures. Leukocytosis and anemia are common. A CT scan should be performed for diagnosis, and the aneurysm should be repaired emergently.

This patient has several risk factors for AAA, including the major risk of cigarette smoking. The incidence of AAA is higher in men than in women and in whites versus blacks, and it increases with age. Hypertension and hyperlipidemia probably contribute to the risk of AAA development to a lesser degree.

Contained rupture of AAA, when misdiagnosed, is most often mistaken for renal colic, acute myocardial infarction, or diverticulitis. Renal colic may produce severe pain in the lower back, flank, or groin. Typically, the pain waxes and wanes. It is unlikely that renal colic would present with syncope, and the normal urinalysis also makes this diagnosis unlikely.

Acute myocardial infarction can be associated with syncope, and the electrocardiogram is not always diagnostic, particularly if there are findings such as left ventricular hypertrophy, which may obscure subtle abnormalities. However, the presence of abdominal and lower back pain rather than chest pain makes this diagnosis less likely.

Diverticulitis would present with crampy abdominal pain, most commonly in the left lower quadrant, often associated with a change in bowel habits. Leukocytosis may be present. Syncope associated with the onset of pain would be a very unusual presentation for this entity.

- **Abdominal pain, back pain, and syncope often herald an abdominal aortic aneurysm rupture.**

Bibliography

Schermerhorn ML, O'Malley AJ, Jhaveri A, Cotterill P, Pomposelli F, Landon BE. Endovascular vs. open repair of abdominal aortic aneurysms in the Medicare population. N Engl J Med. 2008;358(5):464-474. [PMID: 18234751]

Item 114   Answer: D

Educational Objective: Manage ventricular septal defect following ST-elevation myocardial infarction.

Mechanical complications occur in roughly 0.1% of patients with ST-elevation myocardial infarction (STEMI) and usually occur 2 to 7 days after infarction. Late complications following STEMI include cardiogenic shock, ventricular septal defect, mitral regurgitation, free wall rupture, and left ventricular thrombus. This patient's progressive hypotension, respiratory distress, and new systolic murmur and thrill suggest either ischemic mitral regurgitation or a ventricular septal defect. Either mitral regurgitation or a ventricular septal defect can result in a prominent v wave in the pulmonary capillary wedge pressure tracing. However, only a ventricular septal defect results in the "step-up" in oxygen saturation from the right atrium to the right ventricle seen in this patient. Following echocardiography to confirm the diagnosis, this patient should undergo emergent surgery to repair the defect. Although treatment for a ventricular septal defect is emergent surgery, in-hospital mortality remains high at approximately 60%.

Emergent pericardiocentesis would be indicated in the setting of pericardial tamponade that may occur following a STEMI from hemorrhagic pericarditis or free wall rupture. Pericardial tamponade from rupture of the left ventricular free wall usually leads to sudden hypotension and death. Ventricular free wall rupture typically occurs 1 to 4 days after acute myocardial infarction; rarely, it occurs up to 3 weeks after myocardial infarction. Patients usually present with cardiovascular collapse, tamponade, or pulseless electrical activity. Right heart catheterization demonstrates diastolic pressure elevation and equalization of pressures from the right atrium, right ventricle, and pulmonary capillary wedge with reduced cardiac output. Echocardiography shows a pseudoaneurysm or localized pericardial effusion; in some patients, the rupture site can be visualized.

Mitral valve repair would be the correct answer for a patient with severe ischemic mitral regurgitation. The patient presented has a post-infarction ventricular septal defect and not ischemic mitral regurgitation. Ischemic mitral regurgitation presents with a new systolic murmur following a large myocardial infarction. Whereas pulmonary artery catheter tracings may also show an elevated pulmonary capillary wedge pressure with prominent v waves, there would not be a step-up in oxygen saturation

from the right atrium to the right ventricle. This finding is diagnostic for a ventricular septal defect.

A massive pulmonary embolism may produce cardiovascular collapse and hypoxemia but cannot explain the new systolic murmur, left heart failure, prominent v wave, and step-up of oxygen saturation. Therefore, a pulmonary artery thrombectomy is not indicated.

- **A ventricular septal defect following an ST-elevation myocardial infarction results in a new systolic murmur and a "step-up" in oxygen saturation from the right atrium to the right ventricle.**

Bibliography

Poulsen SH, Praestholm M, Munk K, Wierup P, Egeblad H, Nielsen-Kudsk JE. Ventricular septal rupture complicating acute myocardial infarction: clinical characteristics and contemporary outcome. Ann Thorac Surg. 2008;85(5):1591-1596. [PMID: 18442545]

Item 115   Answer: B

Educational Objective: Manage a patient with atrial fibrillation with a rapid ventricular response.

This patient should undergo atrioventricular node ablation and pacemaker placement. In patients with atrial fibrillation, the ventricular rate is dependent on the electrical conduction properties of the atrioventricular node. Appropriate ventricular rate control is essential in order to avoid symptoms and to prevent a tachycardia-related cardiomyopathy. This patient is asymptomatic despite high ventricular rates that are persisting despite multiple atrioventricular nodal blocking agents. In addition, he has discontinued β-blockers due to side effects. When heart rate control is inadequate despite maximum tolerated atrioventricular nodal blockade, a rhythm control strategy must be reconsidered. Rhythm control usually requires antiarrhythmic drugs, which may also be poorly tolerated due to side effects and toxicities. Procedural options for rate control include ablation of the atrioventricular node and His bundle, with permanent pacemaker placement. This is the most common nonpharmacologic approach for rate control, and has been shown to be safe and effective in many studies. Demonstrated outcomes in patients after atrioventricular nodal ablation include improved quality of life, ventricular function, and exercise capacity, as well as decreased heart failure episodes, hospital admissions, and use of antiarrhythmic drugs.

Preliminary data suggest that, in a highly selected group of patients, radiofrequency ablation of atrial fibrillation may be appropriate as first-line treatment of atrial fibrillation prior to pharmacologic treatment. However, the technique of radiofrequency ablation for atrial fibrillation is still evolving, and there is a risk for significant complications. Radiofrequency ablation for atrial fibrillation, therefore, is not the best option for this patient.

Amiodarone is the most efficacious antiarrhythmic medication, but has a low likelihood of inducing primary conversion to sinus rhythm, so it is not the best option for this patient. Although it can provide effective rate control, the risks of adverse effects outweigh its benefits for this indication. In this patient, there is no indication for an antiarrhythmic drug for maintenance of sinus rhythm, since he is asymptomatic from the atrial fibrillation. He has also requested to not take more medications.

In refractory symptomatic patients, the maze surgical approach may be considered. This procedure consists of making multiple atrial incisions to reduce the effective size of the atria, thereby preventing formation and maintenance of atrial fibrillation wavelets. A recent review of the maze procedure cited efficacy of 99% in preventing recurrence of atrial fibrillation; however, several centers have shown a significant mortality rate with this operation, ranging from 1% to 3%. This procedure is particularly well suited for patients undergoing cardiac surgery for other reasons and would not be the first consideration in this patient.

KEY POINT

- **Atrioventricular nodal (junctional) ablation with pacemaker placement is a safe and effective non-pharmacologic rate control option in patients with rapidly conducted atrial fibrillation.**

Bibliography

Lim KT, Davis MJ, Powell A, et al. Ablate and pace strategy for atrial fibrillation: long-term outcome of AIRCRAFT trial. Europace. 2007;9(7):498-505. [PMID: 17491103]

Item 116   Answer: B

Educational Objective: Recognize complications that occur after repair of tetralogy of Fallot.

This patient has a history of tetralogy of Fallot with previous repair, which usually involves placement of a transannular pulmonary outflow tract patch. This causes severe pulmonary valve regurgitation, which is confirmed by the presence of a diastolic murmur that increases with inspiration, a parasternal impulse (right ventricular enlargement), and elevated central venous pressure. The holosystolic murmur at the left lower sternal border is characteristic of tricuspid regurgitation. Long-standing pulmonary valve regurgitation causes right ventricular enlargement and tricuspid annular dilatation with resultant regurgitation. The tricuspid regurgitation causes right atrial enlargement and increases the risk of atrial arrhythmias. The chest radiograph demonstrates features of right heart enlargement with a prominent right heart border (right atrium) and absence of the retrosternal air space (right ventricular enlargement). A right-sided aortic arch is also noted, which is present in 25% of patients with tetralogy of Fallot.

Tetralogy of Fallot is the most common form of cyanotic congenital heart disease, accounting for approximately 10% of all congenital defects. Although these defects have

been successfully repaired for more than 50 years, most patients with repaired tetralogy of Fallot have cardiac residua that may manifest with symptoms of dyspnea, heart failure, or arrhythmias years after repair. Life-long informed surveillance is recommended for patients with repaired tetralogy of Fallot. Patients with repaired tetralogy of Fallot are at increased risk of developing atrial arrhythmias due to atrial enlargement and prior atrial surgical incisions. These patients are also at risk of developing ventricular arrhythmias, which result primarily from dilatation and dysfunction of the right ventricle. Arrhythmias are a major cause of morbidity and mortality in patients with repaired tetralogy of Fallot.

Aortic valve regurgitation may occur in patients with repaired conotruncal abnormalities, such as tetralogy of Fallot. These patients may demonstrate progressive enlargement of the aorta and, eventually, aortic valve regurgitation may occur. The physical examination findings in this patient suggest pulmonary valve regurgitation rather than aortic valve regurgitation. The murmur of aortic regurgitation does not vary with respiration and is best heard in the second left intercostal space and down the left sternal border and would not cause right ventricular enlargement with a parasternal impulse. The pulse pressure is normal in this patient, and in a patient with aortic regurgitation, a wide pulse pressure would be expected.

A holosystolic murmur at the left sternal border that increases with inspiration is characteristic of tricuspid regurgitation rather than mitral valve regurgitation.

Residual or recurrent ventricular septal defect also occurs in patients with prior tetralogy of Fallot repair. A ventricular septal defect causes a loud systolic murmur that obliterates the S_2 and is often associated with a palpable thrill. A displaced apical left ventricular impulse and mitral diastolic flow rumble would suggest a hemodynamically important ventricular septal defect causing volume overload.

Right ventricular outflow tract obstruction occurs commonly after repair of tetralogy of Fallot. However, the primary features include right ventricular hypertrophy rather than right heart enlargement. In addition, this patient's murmurs of tricuspid and pulmonary valve regurgitation would suggest that right ventricular outflow tract obstruction is not the cause of the patient's current clinical deterioration. The murmur of pulmonary stenosis is an early systolic murmur that increases with inspiration and is heard best at the second left intercostal space. It is associated with a loud P_2 heart sound that is sometimes palpable.

KEY POINT

- **Pulmonary valve regurgitation is the most common residua after repair of tetralogy of Fallot.**

Bibliography

Warnes CA, Williams RG, Bashore TM, et al. ACC/AHA 2008 Guidelines for the Management of Adults with Congenital Heart Disease: a report of the American College of Cardiology/American

Heart Association Task Force on Practice Guidelines (writing committee to develop guidelines on the management of adults with congenital heart disease). Circulation. 2008;118(23):e714-833. [PMID: 18997169]

Item 117 Answer: B
Educational Objective: Treat severe heart failure.

Barring contraindications, treatment with an angiotensin-converting enzyme (ACE) inhibitor and a β-blocker is indicated for all patients with systolic heart failure, for morbidity and mortality benefit. For patients with New York Heart Association (NYHA) functional class III or IV symptoms, spironolactone is also indicated for additional survival benefit. Even patients with severe heart failure (NYHA functional class III-IV) generally tolerate β-blocker therapy. Because patients with severe heart failure are at highest risk for morbidity and mortality, the absolute reduction in events is greatest in this subgroup. In general, β-blockers should not be initiated when a patient is acutely decompensated or volume overloaded because initiation of therapy is associated with a transient decline in cardiac output. However, β-blockers can be initiated and tolerated once euvolemia or near-euvolemia has been established. β-Blockers can usually be continued during decompensated states of heart failure if the patient was previously stable while on β-blocker therapy, unless the decompensation is severe to the degree of cardiogenic shock. β-Blocker therapy with carvedilol should be carefully reintroduced into this patient's medical regimen.

Routine combined treatment with an ACE inhibitor and an angiotensin-receptor blocker (ARB), such as candesartan, for heart failure is not recommended. There are no definitive data to support improvement in clinical outcomes, and the risk of complications, such as hyperkalemia, is increased. Although it has not been established definitively whether ARBs should be substituted for or added to ACE inhibitor therapy for heart failure, ARBs are a reasonable substitute for patients who are intolerant of ACE inhibitors because of cough.

Clopidogrel is an antiplatelet agent indicated for treatment after intracoronary stenting or non–ST-elevation myocardial infarction, neither of which applies to this patient. Beyond those indications, there is no indication for treatment of heart failure with clopidogrel.

There are no definitive data to support routine use of anticoagulation with warfarin for treatment of systolic heart failure outside of standard indications for anticoagulation such as atrial fibrillation, intracardiac thrombus, or thromboembolic disease.

KEY POINT

- β-Blockers should not be initiated when a patient with heart failure is acutely decompensated or volume overloaded.

Bibliography

Packer M, Fowler MB, Roecker EB, et al; Carvedilol Prospective Randomized Cumulative Survival (COPERNICUS) Study Group. Effect of carvedilol on the morbidity of patients with severe chronic heart failure: results of the carvedilol prospective randomized cumulative survival (COPERNICUS) study. Circulation. 2002;106(17):2194-2199. [PMID: 12390947]

Item 118 Answer: B
Educational Objective: Manage severe mitral regurgitation.

The best management option in this patient is an exercise treadmill echocardiogram. Management of patients with chronic mitral regurgitation requires periodic evaluation of regurgitation severity and left ventricular size and function. In determining the need for mitral valve surgery, quantitative echo Doppler measurements are now integrated with qualitative assessment of regurgitation severity. Diagnostic criteria for severe mitral regurgitation include a vena contracta width ≥7 mm, a regurgitant orifice area ≥0.4 cm^2, a regurgitant volume ≥60 mL, and a regurgitant fraction ≥50%. This patient's echocardiographic criteria are consistent with severe mitral regurgitation. This patient remains asymptomatic despite the new finding of chordal rupture and worsening of mitral regurgitation since the last echocardiographic study.

The interval change and borderline pulmonary hypertension in this patient indicate a probable need for surgery; however, timing of surgery is not clear. In asymptomatic patients with severe mitral regurgitation, surgery is indicated if adverse hemodynamic effects from the regurgitant valve develop. Clinical markers that should prompt surgical intervention include left ventricular enlargement or dysfunction (end-systolic dimension >40 mm and ejection fraction <60%), new-onset atrial fibrillation, pulmonary arterial systolic pressure >50 mm Hg, or an exercise-associated increase in pulmonary pressures (increase of approximately 25 mm Hg over baseline). Otherwise, asymptomatic patients with severe, chronic mitral regurgitation but normal left ventricular size and function can be reevaluated with periodic 6- to 12-month monitoring. This patient's left ventricular size and function do not meet criteria for surgery. This patient admits to a sedentary lifestyle and does not exercise regularly. Therefore, reliably gauging cardiopulmonary symptoms from history alone would be difficult. Exercise treadmill echocardiography would provide objective data on exercise tolerance. Severely limited exercise duration would imply she has symptomatic mitral regurgitation. Additionally, pulmonary pressure response to exercise can be assessed. Exercise-induced increases in pulmonary arterial systolic pressure of 25 mm Hg over baseline pressures suggest hemodynamic significance and should lead to earlier surgical referral.

Coronary angiography is not indicated in this asymptomatic 42-year-old patient with no anginal symptoms, a paucity of cardiovascular risk factors, and a low pretest probability of coronary artery disease.

Surgical intervention for chronic mitral regurgitation includes valve repair (annuloplasty) or valve replacement. Which procedure to perform depends on multiple factors, including mitral regurgitation etiology, mitral valve anatomy, and the severity of left ventricular dysfunction. When feasible, mitral valve annuloplasty is preferred over replacement. Annuloplasty attempts to preserve the functional components of the mitral valve, including the subvalvular apparatus and leaflets with their attachment to the papillary muscles, resulting in improved postoperative left ventricular function with avoidance of the risks associated with prosthetic valves. In patients whose valve is not amenable to annuloplasty repair, valve replacement with either mechanical or bioprosthetic valves should be performed.

KEY POINT

- **Clinical markers that should prompt surgical intervention in asymptomatic patients with severe mitral regurgitation include left ventricular enlargement or dysfunction, atrial fibrillation, pulmonary pressures over 50 mm Hg, or an exercise-associated increase in pulmonary pressures.**

Bibliography

Supino PG, Borer JS, Schuleri K, et al. Prognostic value of exercise tolerance testing in asymptomatic chronic nonischemic mitral regurgitation. Am J Cardiol. 2007;100(8):1274-1281. [PMID: 17920370]

Item 119   Answer: A

Educational Objective: Treat acute decompensated heart failure.

This patient demonstrates evidence of volume overload (edema, crackles, jugular venous distention, orthopnea), low cardiac output (rising creatinine level, hypotension, cool extremities), and other markers of decompensated heart failure (S_3, hyponatremia). The immediate goal of therapy is to improve cardiac output (and therefore systemic perfusion) by administering an inotropic agent such as dobutamine. Appropriate uses of inotropic agents include temporary treatment of diuretic-refractory acute heart failure decompensations or as a bridge to definitive treatment, such as revascularization or cardiac transplantation. Inotropic agents also may be appropriate as a palliative measure in patients with end-stage heart failure. Inotropic agents increase the risk of sudden cardiac death and therefore can only be used in a monitored setting or for palliation in patients with end-stage disease.

Although the patient has volume overload, intravenous furosemide would not be the next appropriate step because immediate diuresis would likely exacerbate hypotension and renal insufficiency. Diuresis would be appropriate once

his blood pressure has increased as a result of administering an inotropic agent such as dobutamine.

Although nesiritide has shown favorable short-term hemodynamic changes in patients with acute decompensated heart failure, definitive longer-term benefits have not been demonstrated, and, in fact, there is evidence for increased risk of renal failure and mortality. In addition, because nesiritide is a pure vasodilator, administration would not be appropriate in the setting of significant hypotension.

β-Blockers, such as carvedilol, reduce morbidity and mortality in patients with heart failure, and initiation is generally well tolerated even in severe heart failure. Initiation prior to discharge from hospitalization for heart failure is well tolerated and results in superior adherence to practice guidelines. However, initiation of a β-blocker is not appropriate during acute decompensated heart failure because the immediate effect of negative inotropy would exacerbate the patient's low-output state. β-Blockers should be initiated once the patient is in a euvolemic, stable clinical state, which can include the predischarge time period.

KEY POINT

- **In patients with acute decompensated heart failure, administration of an inotropic agent such as dobutamine can improve cardiac output and therefore systemic perfusion.**

Bibliography

Ko DT, Hebert PR, Coffey CS, et al. Adverse effects of beta-blocker therapy for patients with heart failure: a quantitative overview of randomized trials. Arch Intern Med. 2004;164(13):1389-1394. [PMID: 15249347]

Item 120   Answer: D

Educational Objective: Manage perioperative anticoagulation in a prosthetic valve patient undergoing noncardiac surgery.

Prosthetic mechanical valves require continuous, lifelong anticoagulation with warfarin to reduce valve thrombosis. Periprocedural anticoagulation management for mechanical valves is dependent on the patient's clinical history and cardiac position of the valve. In this patient with an aortic prosthetic valve and without a history of prior thromboembolism, warfarin can be discontinued without a heparin bridge 3 to 5 days before surgery.

Generally, transvalvular flow across mitral prostheses is lower than aortic prostheses; therefore, valves in the mitral position have a higher incidence of thrombosis in the setting of subtherapeutic anticoagulation. For aortic valve prostheses, transvalvular velocities are higher and thrombotic risk is lower. In higher-risk patients—those with mitral prostheses, multiple prosthetic valves, atrial fibrillation, or previous thromboembolic events—therapeutic-dose heparin as a bridge before and after the procedure to maintain therapeutic anticoagulation is recommended.

No bridging anticoagulation regimen is needed in low-risk patients such as this patient. Postoperative management of patients who are chronically maintained on anticoagulation typically includes starting intravenous unfractionated heparin and oral warfarin therapy as soon as surgical control of bleeding allows.

Although oral vitamin K reverses the anticoagulation effect of warfarin, achieving therapeutic anticoagulation after administration is often prolonged. Therefore, oral vitamin K is only recommended in patients with supratherapeutic INRs (over 5.0) if the patient is at increased risk of bleeding or if rapid reversal is needed, such as for urgent surgery. This patient's surgery is elective and rapid reversal of anticoagulation is not warranted. Clopidogrel is an antiplatelet agent and is not indicated for primary antithrombotic management of mechanical prosthetic valves.

KEY POINT

- Low-risk patients with mechanical valves (aortic prosthesis and no history of prior thromboembolism) undergoing noncardiac surgery can have warfarin discontinued without a heparin bridge 5 days prior to surgery.

Bibliography

Hirsh J, Guyatt G, Albers GW, Harrington R, Schünemann HJ; American College of Chest Physicians. Executive summary: American College of Chest Physicians Evidence-Based Clinical Practice Guidelines (8th Edition) [erratum in Chest. 2008;134(4):892.]. Chest. 2008;133(6 Suppl):71S-109S. [PMID: 18574259]

Index

Note: Page numbers followed by f and t denote figures and tables, respectively.
Test questions are indicated by a Q.

Abciximab, for acute coronary syndromes, 20
Abdominal aortic aneurysm, 90, Q15, Q113
ACE inhibitors
    for abdominal aortic aneurysm, 90
    angioedema due to, 31–33
    for aortic regurgitation, 74
    for coronary artery disease, 16
    for heart failure, 31–33, 32t
    for Marfan syndrome, 92
    for myocardial infarction, 24, 25
    in pregnancy, 100, 102t
    for restrictive cardiomyopathy, 43
Acute aortic syndromes, 92–93, 93t
Acute coronary syndromes, 18–25
    classification of, 18–19, 18f
    clinical presentation of, 18–19
    in diabetes mellitus, 2, 27–28
    treatment of, 19–25
    in women, 26–27
Acute limb ischemia, 97, 97f, 97t, 98t
Acute myocarditis, 41
Acute respiratory failure, mitral regurgitation after, 76
Adenosine
    for arrhythmias, 52, 56–57
    in pregnancy, 102t
    in stress testing, 6, 8t, 13, 13f
    for supraventricular tachycardia, 56–57
African Americans
    cardiovascular disease in, 2
    heart failure in, 34
Alcohol ablation, for hypertrophic cardiomyopathy, 47
Alcohol use/abuse, cardiovascular disease and, 4
Alteplase, for myocardial infarction, 22–23, 22f, 23t, 24
Ambulatory electrocardiography, for arrhythmias, 7, 10t
Amiodarone
    for arrhythmias, 52t, 53, 57. *See also specific arrhythmias*
    in pregnancy, 102t
    for supraventricular tachycardia, 57
Amlodipine
    for angina, 14
    for heart failure, 34–35
Amyloidosis
    cardiomyopathy in, 42, 42t, 44t
    treatment of, 44t
Analgesia, for pericarditis, 64–66, 65t
Anemia
    hemolytic, prosthetic valve, Q80
    iron deficiency, in congenital heart disease, 88, Q38
Aneurysm, aortic
    abdominal, 90, Q15, Q113
    thoracic, 90–91, 91t
Angina pectoris. *See also* Coronary artery disease
    chronic stable, 12–18, Q37, Q86
    in diabetes mellitus, 27
    drug therapy for, 14–15, 23
    evaluation of, Q62
    management of, 14, Q28, Q37, Q86
    refractory, 17
    revascularization procedures for, 16–17, 21–23, 27
    unstable, 18–21, 18f, 19f, 20t, Q9
    in women, 26
Angioedema, ACE inhibitor–related, 31–33
Angiography
    coronary, 6, 7, 8t, 9t
        in heart failure, 30
    indications for, 13–14
    in peripheral arterial disease, 94
    radionuclide, in cardiac examination, 5t, 6, 7, 8t
Angioplasty
    coronary artery, 16, 21–23, 22f, 23t, 25
        in diabetes mellitus, 28
        in women, 27
    in peripheral arterial disease, 96, 96t
Angiotensin-converting enzyme inhibitors. *See* ACE inhibitors
Angiotensin receptor blockers
    for heart failure, 31–32, 32t
    in pregnancy, 102t
    for restrictive cardiomyopathy, 43
Ankle-brachial index, 94, 95f
Ankylosing spondylitis, cardiovascular disease and, 3–4, 3t
Anthracyclines, cardiotoxicity of, 42t
Antianginal agents, 14–15
Antiarrhythmics, 52–53, 52t. *See also specific agents and arrhythmias*
Antibiotics
    for endocarditis, 79
    prophylactic, for valvular disease, 79, 80t
Anticoagulants
    for acute coronary syndromes, 21, 24
    for acute limb ischemia, 97
    for aortic atheroma, 89
    for atrial fibrillation, 53–54, 54t
    for heart failure, 40
    for mitral stenosis, 74
    for pericarditis, 66
    perioperative management of, 17–18, Q120
    in pregnancy, 100–101, 101f, 102t, Q93
    for prosthetic valves, 80
Anticonvulsants, in pregnancy, 103t
Antihypertensives, for peripheral arterial disease, 95
Antioxidants, coronary artery disease and, 11–12
Antiplatelet agents
    for acute coronary syndromes, 19, 20, 23, 24, 25
    for acute limb ischemia, 97
    for aortic atheroma, 89
    for atrial fibrillation, 54
    for coronary artery disease, 12, 15, 17, 19, 20
        in diabetes mellitus, 28
        in women, 26, 102t
    perioperative management of, 17–18, Q120
    for peripheral arterial disease, 95, 97
    in pregnancy, 102t
Antithrombotic therapy. *See* Thrombolysis
Aortic aneurysms
    abdominal, 90, Q15, Q113
    thoracic, 90–91, 91t
Aortic atheromas, 89, Q92
Aortic coarctation, 85–86, 85f, Q36, Q87
    murmur in, 71t, 85
    postoperative, 87
Aortic diameter, normal values for, 72t
Aortic disease, 89–93
    acute, 92–93, 93t
    in Marfan syndrome, 91
    in Takayasu arteritis, 92
Aortic dissection, 90–91, Q71
    in Marfan syndrome, 91
Aortic intramural hematoma, 92–93, Q30
Aortic override, in tetralogy of Fallot, 87–88, 87f
Aortic regurgitation, 71t, 72, 73t, 74, 75t, Q85
    acute, 76
    chronic, 76–77
Aortic root dilation, in Marfan syndrome, 91–92
Aortic root replacement

for aortic regurgitation, 74
for aortic stenosis, 74
Aortic sclerosis, 72–73
Aortic stenosis, 71t, 72–73, 72t, 73t, Q41, Q66, Q95
Aortic ulcer, atherosclerotic, 92–93
Aortic valve, bicuspid, 71t, 73–74, 85, Q56
Aortoiliac endovascular therapy, for peripheral arterial disease, 96, 96t
Arrhythmias, 49–61
    atrial fibrillation. *See* Atrial fibrillation
    atrial flutter, 52, 52t, 55–56, 55f, Q29
    atrial septal defect and, 82
    atrioventricular block, 49, 50f
    bradycardia, 49
    bundle branch block, 52
    cardioversion for. *See* Cardioversion
    clinical presentation of, 49
    diagnosis of, 7, 10t
    drug therapy for, 52–53, 52t
    evaluation of, 49
    in long QT syndrome, 60
    post–myocardial infarction, 24
    premature ventricular complexes, 58, Q68
    right ventricular dysplasia and, 41
    in short QT syndrome, 61
    in sick sinus syndrome, 49
    sudden cardiac death and, 59–61
    tachycardias, 50–53, 51f, 52t, 56–61, Q40. *See also* Tachycardia(s)
    in Wolff-Parkinson-White syndrome, 57–58
Arrhythmogenic right ventricular dysplasia, 41
Arterial bypass surgery
    coronary. *See* Coronary artery bypass grafting
    for peripheral arterial disease, 96, 96t
Arteriosclerosis. *See* Atherosclerosis
Arteritis
    giant cell, 3–4, 3t
    Takayasu, 3–4, 3t, 92
Arthritis, rheumatoid, cardiovascular disease and, 3–4, 3t
Ascending aorta, diameter of, 72t
Aspirin
    for acute coronary syndromes, 19, 20, 23, 25
    for aortic atheroma, 89
    for atrial fibrillation, 54
    for coronary artery disease, 12, 15, 17, 19, 20
        in diabetes mellitus, 27, 28
    for pericarditis, 64, 65t, 67t
    for peripheral arterial disease, 95
    in pregnancy, 102t
    for prosthetic valves, 80
Asystole, 60, 61
Atenolol
    for arrhythmias, 52t
    in pregnancy, 100, 102t
Atheromas, aortic, 89, Q92
Atherosclerosis. *See also* Cardiovascular disease; Coronary artery disease
    aortic, 89, Q92
        ulceration in, 92–93
    diagnosis of, 6–7, 8t–9t
    peripheral arterial disease and, 93–98
Athlete's heart, vs. hypertrophic cardiomyopathy, 46, 46t
Atorvastatin. *See also* Statins
    for peripheral arterial disease, 96
Atrial arrhythmias, atrial septal defect and, 82
Atrial fibrillation, 52, 53–55, 54t, Q70, Q115
    mitral stenosis and, 74–76
    in pregnancy, anticoagulants for, 100–101, 101f, 102t
    in Wolff-Parkinson-White syndrome, 57–58, 58f
Atrial flutter, 52, 52t, 55–56, Q29
Atrial myxomas, 47–48, 48f, Q18
Atrial septal defect, 81–83, 82f, Q54, Q72
    murmur in, 71t
    postoperative/postintervention, 87
Atrial septum, lipomatous hypertrophy of, 47–48
Atrial tachycardia, 56–57, 57f
Atrioventricular block, 49, 50f
Atrioventricular dissociation, 49
Atrioventricular junction ablation, for atrial fibrillation, 54
Atrioventricular nodal reentrant tachycardia, 56–57
Atrioventricular reentrant tachycardia, 56–57

in Wolff-Parkinson-White syndrome, 57–58
Azathioprine, for pericarditis, 67t

Bacterial endocarditis, 79, Q20
Balloon angioplasty, coronary artery, 16, 21–23, 22f, 23t, 25
    in diabetes mellitus, 28
    in women, 27
Balloon valvuloplasty, for pulmonary stenosis, 87
Behçet disease, cardiovascular disease and, 3–4, 3t
ß-blockers
    for abdominal aortic aneurysm, 90
    for acute aortic syndromes, 92
    for acute coronary syndromes, 19, 23, 25
        in diabetes mellitus, 27–28
    for angina, 14
    for arrhythmias, 52–53, 52t. *See also specific arrhythmias*
    for heart failure, 32t, 33
    for hypertrophic cardiomyopathy, 47
    for Marfan syndrome, 92
    for peripheral arterial disease, 95
    in pregnancy, 100, 102t
    for restrictive cardiomyopathy, 43
    for supraventricular tachycardia, 56, 57
Bicuspid aortic valve, 71t, 73–74, 85, Q56
Bioprosthetic valves, 80–81
Biopsy, endomyocardial, in heart failure, 30
Bisoprolol, for heart failure, 32t, 33
Bivalirudin, for acute coronary syndromes, 21
Biventricular pacemakers, 35–36, 35t
Blacks
    cardiovascular disease in, 2
    heart failure in, 34
Bradycardia, 49
Brugada syndrome, 60–61, 61f
B-type natriuretic peptide
    in heart failure, 29–30, 36
    in restrictive cardiomyopathy, 43
Bumetadine, for heart failure, 32t, 33–34
Bundle branch block, 52

Calcium, coronary artery, 6–7, 14
Calcium channel blockers
    for acute coronary syndromes, 19
    for angina, 14
    for arrhythmias, 52–53, 52t. *See also specific arrhythmias*
    for heart failure, 34–35
    in pregnancy, 102t
    for restrictive cardiomyopathy, 43
    for supraventricular tachycardia, 56, 57
Cancer
    cardiac, 47–48, 48f
    cardiotoxic chemotherapy in, 2–3
    cardiovascular disease and, 2–3
Candesartan, for heart failure, 31–33, 32t
Captopril
    for heart failure, 31–33, 32t
    in pregnancy, 102t
Cardiac arrest, 59–61. *See also* Sudden cardiac death
Cardiac arrhythmias. *See* Arrhythmias
Cardiac catheterization, 5t, 6
    in valvular disease, 70
    in ventricular septal defect, 84–85
Cardiac imaging, 5t, 6–7, 8t, 9t
Cardiac murmurs. *See* Heart murmurs
Cardiac resynchronization therapy, 35–36, 35t
Cardiac shunts, in congenital heart disease, 82–88. *See also specific defects*
Cardiac tamponade, 66–68
Cardiac tumors, 47–48, 48f, Q18
Cardiogenic shock
    in heart failure, 37–39, 38f
    management of, Q106
    post–myocardial infarction, 24

Cardiomyopathy, 40–47
  eosinophilic, 42t
  hypertrophic, 44–47, 45f, 45t–47t, 46f, Q8, Q111
    murmurs in, 71t
  ischemic, Q11
  peripartum, 99, Q4
  restrictive, 41–44, 42t, 44t, Q23
    vs. constrictive pericarditis, 68t
  tachycardia-mediated, 41
  Takotsubo, 40–41
Cardiopulmonary resuscitation, in cardiac arrest, 60
Cardiotoxic drugs, 2–3, 42t, Q49
Cardiovascular disease
  atherosclerotic. See Atherosclerosis; Coronary artery disease
  cancer and, 2–3
  diabetes mellitus and, 2, 27–28
  diagnosis of, 4–10
  epidemiology of, 1–4
  ethnicity and, 2
  hormone replacement therapy and, 26–27
  lifestyle factors and, 4, Q96
  mortality from, 1, 1f
  pregnancy in, 98–103
    drug therapy and, 100–101, 101f, 102t–103t
    management of, 98–99, 99t
    peripartum cardiomyopathy in, 99
    risk assessment for, 98–99, 99t, 100t
  prevention of, 11–12
  radiation-induced, 2–3, 42t, Q50, Q51
  risk factors for, 10–12
  risk management in, 4, Q96
  systemic inflammatory conditions and, 3–4, 3t
  in women, 1, 1f, 26–27
Cardioversion, 52, Q42
  for atrial fibrillation, 53–54
  for atrial flutter, 56
  for cardiac arrest, 60
  for supraventricular tachycardia, 57
  for tachycardia, 52
Carvedilol, for heart failure, 32t, 33
Catheter ablation, for supraventricular tachycardia, 57
Catheterization, cardiac, 5t, 6
  in valvular disease, 70
  in ventricular septal defect, 84–85
Cerebrovascular accident. See Stroke
CHADS$_2$ score, for atrial fibrillation, 54, 54t
Chemotherapy, cardiotoxic, 2–3
Chest pain
  in acute aortic syndromes, 92
  anginal. See Angina pectoris
  atypical, 18, Q27
  evaluation of, 18, Q22, Q78
  in myocardial infarction, 18, 23
    vs. in pericarditis, 62, 64t
  in pericarditis, 62–66, 63t, 64t
Cholesterol emboli, acute limb ischemia and, 97, 97f
Cigarette smoking. See Smoking
Cilostazol, for peripheral arterial disease, 96
Claudication, 93, 94t, 97
Clopidogrel
  for acute coronary syndromes, 21, 24, 25
  for coronary artery disease, 15–16, 17, 21
    in diabetes mellitus, 27
  for peripheral arterial disease, 95
  in pregnancy, 102t
Coarctation of aorta, 85–86, 85f, Q36, Q87
  murmur in, 71t, 85
  postoperative, 87
Cocaine, cardiovascular disease and, 4, Q35
Colchicine, for pericarditis, 64, 65t, 66, 67t
Complete heart block, 49, 51f
Computed tomography
  cardiac, 5t, 6, 7, 9t
  coronary, 6, 9t, 14
Computed tomography angiography, in peripheral arterial disease, 94
Congenital heart disease, 81–88
  atrial septal defect, 71t, 81–83, 82f, 87, Q54, Q72

coarctation of aorta, 71t, 85–86, 85f, 87, Q36, Q87
  cyanotic, 88
  Eisenmenger syndrome, 84, 88
  murmurs in, 70, 71t
  patent ductus arteriosus, 71t, 86, Q79
  patent foramen ovale, 83, 83f, Q45
  pregnancy in, 88, 99–103. See also Pregnancy, in cardiovascular disease
  previously operated, 87–88
  pulmonic stenosis, 71t, 86–88, 87f, Q6, Q61
  tetralogy of Fallot, 87–88, 87f, Q67, Q112, Q116
  ventricular septal defect. See Ventricular septal defect
Congestive heart failure. See Heart failure
Conivaptan, for heart failure, 40
Constrictive pericarditis, 43, 68–69, 68t, 69f, Q50
Coronary angiography, 6, 7, 8t, 9t
  in heart failure, 30
  indications for, 13–14
Coronary artery angioplasty, 16, 21–23, 22f, 23t
  in diabetes mellitus, 28
  in women, 27
Coronary artery bypass grafting, 16–17, 17t
  in diabetes mellitus, 28
  in women, 27
Coronary artery calcium score, 6–7, 14
Coronary artery disease. See also Heart disease
  acute coronary syndromes and, 18–25. See also Acute coronary syndromes
  angina in
    chronic stable, 12–18, Q37, Q86
    unstable, 18–21, 18f, 19f, 20t
  depression and, 12
  in diabetes mellitus, 2, 27–28
  diagnosis of, 6–7, 8t–9t, 12–14, 12t, 13f, Q10, Q57, Q91, Q99
  differential diagnosis of, 6
  lifestyle factors in, 12
  management of, 14–18, 15f, Q2, Q76
    antianginal agents in, 14–15
    coronary revascularization in, 16–17, 21–23, 27
    follow-up care in, 17–18
    vascular-protective agents in, 15–16
  noncardiac surgery in, 17–18
  prevention of, 11–12
  risk factors for, 10–12
  risk stratification in, 25, Q73, Q81
  in women, 1, 26–27
Coronary artery stents, 16, 17–18, Q75
  antiplatelet therapy for, 20
  drug-eluting, 17–18
  thrombosis of, 17
Coronary computed tomography, 6, 9t, 14
Coronary revascularization, 16–17, 21–23, 27
Cor pulmonale, 78
Corticosteroids, for pericarditis, 65t, 66, 67t
Counterpulsation, external enhanced
  for angina, 17
  for heart failure, 40
C-reactive protein, coronary artery disease and, 11
Cryptogenic stroke, patent foramen ovale and, 83
Cyanotic congenital heart disease, 88

Defibrillation, for cardiac arrest, 60
Defibrillators, implantable cardioverter, 35, 35t, Q42
  for hypertrophic cardiomyopathy, 47
  for ventricular arrhythmias, 61
Dental procedures, antibiotic prophylaxis for, 79, 80t
Depression, coronary artery disease and, 12
Diabetes mellitus
  cardiovascular disease and, 2, 27–28
  peripheral arterial disease and, 94, 94t, 95–96
Diet, coronary artery disease and, 11–12
Digitalis, for heart failure, 32t
Digoxin
  for arrhythmias, 52, 52t
  for atrial fibrillation, 53
  for heart failure, 32t, 34
  in pregnancy, 102t
Diltiazem
  for angina, 14
  for arrhythmias, 52t

in pregnancy, 102t
Dipyridamole
  in pregnancy, 102t
  in stress testing, 6, 8t, 13, 13f
Disopyramide
  for hypertrophic cardiomyopathy, 47
  in pregnancy, 102t
Diuretics
  for heart failure, 32t, 33–34, 40
  in pregnancy, 102t
  resistance to, 34
Dobutamine echocardiography, 6–7, 8t
  in valvular disease, 70
Dobutamine stress testing, 6, 8t, 13, 13f
Dofetilide, for arrhythmias, 52t, 53
Down syndrome, congenital heart disease in, 82, 84
Doxorubicin, cardiotoxicity of, 3
Dressler syndrome, 62
Drug abuse, cardiovascular disease and, 4, Q35
Drug therapy
  cardiotoxic, 2–3, 42t, Q49
  pulmonary hypertension due to, 78
  teratogenic, 100–101, 102t–103t
Ductus arteriosus, patent, 71t, 86, Q79
Dysrhythmias. See Arrhythmias

Echocardiography, 5–6, 5t, 8t
  in acute aortic syndromes, 92
  in aortic regurgitation, 76–77
  in cardiac tamponade, 67
  in congenital heart disease, 82–88. See also specific defects
  in constrictive pericarditis, 68, 69f
  dobutamine, 6–7, 8t, 70
  in endocarditis, 79
  in heart failure, 29, 36–37
  in mitral regurgitation, 76–77
  in pericardial effusion, 66, 67f
  in valvular disease, 70, 73t
Eisenmenger syndrome, 84, 88
Ejection fraction, normal values for, 72t
Electrocardiography
  in acute coronary syndromes, 18–25
  in arrhythmias, 7, 10t, 49. See also specific arrhythmias
  in heart failure, 29, 30
  in pericarditis, 63, 65t
  in stress testing, 6, 7t–10t, 12–13
    in diabetes mellitus, 27
    in heart failure, 30
    indications for, 12–13, 12t, 13t, 17
    in women, 26
Electronic pacemakers, 35–36, 35t, Q48
  for atrial fibrillation, 54–55
  for bradycardia, 49
Electrophysiologic studies, for arrhythmias, 10t
Embolism. See also Thrombosis/thromboembolism
  acute limb ischemia and, 97, 97t
  cholesterol, 97, 97f
  paradoxical, in atrial septal defect, 82, 83
Enalapril
  for aortic regurgitation, 74
  for heart failure, 31–33, 32t
  in pregnancy, 102t
Endarterectomy, for peripheral arterial disease, 96, 96t
Endocarditis, 79–80, 79t, Q20
  antibiotic prophylaxis for, 79, 80t
  in drug abusers, 4
  Löffler, 42t
  prosthetic valve, 79, 80–81, Q103
Endomyocardial biopsy, in heart failure, 30
Endomyocardial fibrosis, 42t, 44t
Eosinophilic cardiomyopathy, 42t
Eplerenone, for heart failure, 32t
Eptifibatide, for acute coronary syndromes, 20
Erythrocytosis, in cyanotic congenital heart disease, 88
Esmolol, in pregnancy, 100, 102t
Estrogen, cardiovascular disease and, 26–27
Ethnicity. See Race/ethnicity
Event monitoring, for arrhythmias, 7, 10t

Exercise
  coronary artery disease and, 12
  in hypertrophic cardiomyopathy, 47
  in peripheral arterial disease, 96
Exercise stress testing, 6, 7t, 8t, 9t, 10t, 12–13
  in diabetes mellitus, 27
  in heart failure, 30
  indications for, 12–13, 12t, 13t, 17
  in women, 26
External enhanced counterpulsation
  for angina, 17
  for heart failure, 40

Fabry disease, 42t
  treatment of, 44t
Familial long QT syndrome, 60, Q82
Felodipine
  for angina, 14
  for heart failure, 34–35
Ferrous gluconate, for iron deficiency, in congenital heart disease, 88
Ferrous sulfate, for iron deficiency, in congenital heart disease, 88
Fibrinolytics
  for coronary artery disease, in women, 26
  for prosthetic valve thrombosis, 81
Figure 3 sign, 85, 85f
Flecainide
  for arrhythmias, 52, 52t
  in pregnancy, 102t
Fluid management, in heart failure, 32t, 33–34, 40
Foramen ovale, patent, 83, 83f, Q45
Fosinopril, for heart failure, 31–33, 32t
Framingham risk score, 10–11
Free wall rupture, post–myocardial infarction, 24
Friction rub, 62
Furosemide, for heart failure, 32t, 33–34

Giant cell arteritis, 3–4, 3t
Giant cell myocarditis, 41
Glycoprotein IIb/IIIa inhibitors, for acute coronary syndromes, 20, 24

Headaches, migraine, patent foramen ovale and, 83
Heart. See also under Cardiac; Cardiovascular
  athlete's, vs. hypertrophic cardiomyopathy, 46, 46t
  tumors of, 47–48, 48f
Heart block
  complete, 49, 51f
  first-degree, 49
  reversible, 49, Q98
  second-degree, 49, 50f
Heart disease. See also Cardiovascular disease
  atherosclerotic. See Coronary artery disease
  congenital, 81–88. See also Congenital heart disease
  diagnosis of, 4–10
  epidemiology of, 1–4
  murmurs in, 70, 71t. See also Heart murmurs
  in pregnancy, 98–103. See also Pregnancy, in cardiovascular disease
  rheumatic, mitral stenosis and, 74–76
  structural, 4–6, 5t
  sudden cardiac death in, 59–61
  valvular, 69–81. See also Valvular heart disease
Heart failure, 29–40
  acute exacerbations of, 37–39
  in African Americans, 34
  B-type natriuretic peptide in, 36
  cardiogenic shock in, 37–39, 38f
  in cardiomyopathy, 40–47
  classification of, 31t
  decompensation in, 37–39, 38f
  diagnosis of, 4–6, 5t, 29–31, Q44, Q77, Q94
  follow-up in, 36
  management of, 31–40, 109, Q5, Q12, Q58, Q60, Q65, Q69, Q83, Q101, Q105, Q117, Q119
    in advanced refractory failure, 39–40
    in chronic failure, 36–40
    device therapy in, 35–36, 35t, 39, 39f, Q53
    drug therapy in, 31–35, 32t
    fluid management in, 32t, 33–34, 40
    investigational therapies in, 39–40

in newly diagnosed patients, 31–36
with preserved systolic function, 35, Q109
transplantation in, 39–40, 39t
post–myocardial infarction, 24
in pregnancy, 100, Q13. *See also* Pregnancy, in cardiovascular disease
prognosis in, 37
risk factors for, 29
serial assessment in, 36
stages of, 31t
in valvular heart disease, 69–70
Heart murmurs, 70, 71t, Q24
in congenital heart disease, 71t, 81–87. *See also specific defects*
diagnosis of, 4–6, 5t
in endocarditis, 79
in pregnancy, 6
in valvular disease, 70, 71t
Heart transplantation, 39–40, 39t
Hematoma, aortic intramural, 92–93, Q30
Hemochromatosis
cardiomyopathy in, 42t, 43
treatment of, 44t
Hemolytic anemia, prosthetic valve, Q80
Hemorrhage, intracerebral, thrombolytic-related, 24
Heparin
for acute coronary syndromes, 21, 23
for atrial fibrillation, 53–54
for pericarditis, 66
in pregnancy, 100–101, 101f, 102t
Hepatic disease, statins and, 16
Hereditary hemochromatosis
cardiomyopathy in, 42t, 43
treatment of, 44t
Homocysteine, coronary artery disease and, 11
Hormone replacement therapy, cardiovascular disease and, 26–27
Hydralazine
for heart failure, 33, 34
in pregnancy, 102t
Hypereosinophilic syndrome, treatment of, 44t
Hyperglycemia, in metabolic syndrome, 2
Hyperkalemia, spironolactone-related, 34
Hyperlipidemia
coronary artery disease and, 11
management of, Q21. *See also* Statins
in metabolic syndrome, 2, 11
peripheral arterial disease and, 94, 96
Hypertension. *See also* Cardiovascular disease
coronary artery disease and, 11
diastolic, management of, Q84
ethnicity and, 2
in metabolic syndrome, 2
in peripheral arterial disease, 95
pulmonary arterial
in pregnancy, 98–99, Q90
tricuspid regurgitation and, 78
Hypertrophic cardiomyopathy, 44–47, 45f, 45t–47t, 46f, Q8, Q111
murmurs in, 71t

Ibuprofen, for pericarditis, 64, 65t, 66
Imaging studies, 6–7, 8t, 9t
Implantable cardioverter defibrillators, 35, 35t, Q42
for hypertrophic cardiomyopathy, 47
for ventricular arrhythmias, 61
Infective endocarditis, 79, Q20
Inferior vena caval atrial septal defect, 82, 82f
Inflammation, in coronary artery disease, 11
Innocent flow murmur, 71t
Insulin resistance. *See also* Metabolic syndrome
cardiovascular disease and, 2, 11
Interatrial septum, lipomatous hypertrophy of, 47–48
Intermittent claudication, 93, 94t, 97
Intracardiac shunts, in congenital heart disease, 82–88
Intracerebral hemorrhage, thrombolytic-related, 24, 26
Intramural hematoma, aortic, 92–93
Intravenous drug use, endocarditis and, 4
Iron deficiency, in congenital heart disease, 88, Q38
Ischemia
acute limb, 97, 97f, 97t, 98t
myocardial

diagnosis of, 30
silent, 18, 27
Isosorbide dinitrate, for heart failure, 34
Isradipine, for angina, 14

Junctional escape rhythms, 49

Kawasaki disease, cardiovascular disease and, 3–4, 3t

Labetalol, in pregnancy, 100, 102t
Left atrial dimension, 72t
Left ventricular dysfunction, post–myocardial infarction, 24
Left ventricular end-diastolic dimension, 72t
Left ventricular end-systolic dimension, 72t
Left ventricular free wall rupture, post–myocardial infarction, 24
Left ventricular thrombus, post–myocardial infarction, 24
Lidocaine
for arrhythmias, 52t
in pregnancy, 102t
Limb claudication, 93, 94t, 97
Limb ischemia, acute, 97, 97f, 97t, 98t
Limb pressure recordings, in peripheral arterial disease, 94
Lipid-lowering agents
for abdominal aortic aneurysm, 90
for acute coronary syndromes, 21, 25, 28
for coronary artery disease, 16
for diabetes mellitus, 28
for peripheral arterial disease, 94, 96
Lipomatous hypertrophy of interatrial septum, 47–48
Lipoprotein(a), coronary artery disease and, 11
Lipoproteins, elevated serum. *See* Hyperlipidemia
Lisinopril
for heart failure, 31–33, 32t
in pregnancy, 102t
Livedo reticularis, 97, 97f
Liver disease, statins and, 16
Löffler endocarditis, 42t
Long QT syndrome, 60, Q82
Loop recording, for arrhythmias, 7, 10t
Losartan, for heart failure, 31–33, 32t
Low-density lipoproteins. *See also* Hyperlipidemia
in coronary artery disease, 11

Magnetic resonance angiography, in peripheral arterial disease, 94
Magnetic resonance imaging, cardiac, 5t, 6, 7, 8t, 9t
Mammary souffle, 71t
Marfan syndrome, 91–92, 91t
Metabolic syndrome
cardiovascular disease in, 2, 11
peripheral arterial disease in, 94t
Metoprolol
for arrhythmias, 52t
for heart failure, 32t, 33
for myocardial infarction, 23
in pregnancy, 100, 102t
Microcytosis, in cyanotic congenital heart disease, 88
Migraine, patent foramen ovale and, 83
Mitral regurgitation, 24, 71t, 73t, 75t, 76, 77–78, Q7, Q47, Q100, Q118
acute, 76
chronic, 77–78
post–myocardial infarction, 24, 76
Mitral stenosis, 71t, 73t, 74–76, 75t, Q3, Q33
Mitral valve prolapse, 71t, 77, 78
Mobitz type I heart block, 49, 50f
Mobitz type II heart block, 49, 50f
Murmurs. *See* Heart murmurs
Myectomy, for hypertrophic cardiomyopathy, 47
Myocardial disease
hypertrophic cardiomyopathy, 44–47
restrictive cardiomyopathy, 41–44
in systemic disease, 3t, 42–44, 42t, 44t
Myocardial infarction
in diabetes mellitus, 27–28
management of, Q26
mitral regurgitation after, 24, 76
non–ST-elevation, 18–21, 18f, 19f, 20t, Q16, Q17, Q32
pericarditis after, 62
right ventricular, 24–25, Q1

ST-elevation, 18, 18f, 21–25, 22f, 23t, Q19, Q46, Q63, Q104, Q110
  in women, 26–27
Myocardial ischemia
  diagnosis of, 30
  silent, 18, 27
Myocarditis
  acute, 41, Q74
  giant cell, 41
Myxomas, 47–48, 48f, Q18

Nesiritide, for heart failure, 40
Nifedipine
  for angina, 14
  for aortic regurgitation, 74
Nitrates
  for acute coronary syndromes, 19
  for angina, 14, Q28
  in pregnancy, 102t
Nitroprusside, in pregnancy, 102t
Non–ST-elevation myocardial infarction, 18–21, 18f, 19f, 20t, Q16, Q17, Q32
Nonsteroidal anti-inflammatory drugs, for pericarditis, 64–66, 65t, 67t
Noonan syndrome, 86
Nuclear myocardial perfusion, 8t, 9t
Nutritional supplements, coronary artery disease and, 11–12

Obesity
  coronary artery disease and, 11
  metabolic syndrome and, 2, 11
Omega-3 fatty acids, coronary artery disease and, 11–12
Ostium primum atrial septal defect, 81–82, 82f
Ostium secundum atrial septal defect, 81–83, 82f

Pacemakers, electronic, 35–36, 35t, Q48, Q53
  for atrial fibrillation, 54–55
  for bradycardia, 49
Pain
  chest. *See* Chest pain
  in peripheral arterial disease, 93, 94t
Palpitations, evaluation of, Q64
Papillary fibroelastomas, 47–48
Papillary muscle dysfunction/rupture, murmur in, 71t
Paradoxical embolism, in atrial septal defect, 82, 83
Paroxysmal atrial fibrillation, Q70
Paroxysmal supraventricular tachycardias, 52, 52t, 56–58
Patent ductus arteriosus, 71t, 86, Q79
Patent foramen ovale, 83, 83f, Q45
Percutaneous coronary intervention, 16, 17
  in diabetes mellitus, 28
  for myocardial infarction, 21–23, 22f, 23t, 25
  in women, 27
Percutaneous transluminal angioplasty, for peripheral arterial disease, 96
Percutaneous valvotomy, for mitral stenosis, 75
Pericardial disease, 62–69
Pericardial effusion, 66, 67f, Q52
  cardiac tamponade and, 66–68
  in pericarditis, 64
Pericardial friction rub, 62
Pericardiectomy, for restrictive pericarditis, 69
Pericardiocentesis
  for cardiac tamponade, 67
  for pericardial effusion, 66
Pericarditis
  acute, 62–66, 63t, 64t, Q25, Q43, Q55
  constrictive, 43, 68–69, 68t, 69f, Q50
  post–myocardial infarction, 62
  recurrent, 62, 66, 67t, Q34
Peripartum cardiomyopathy, 99, Q4
Peripheral arterial disease, 93–98
  acute limb ischemia in, 97, 97f, 97t, 98t
  claudication in, 84t, 93
  clinical presentation of, 93
  differential diagnosis of, 93
  management of, 94–97, Q102
    endovascular/surgical, 96–97, 96t
    medical, 96
    risk factor modification in, 94–96
  physical examination in, 94, Q89, Q107

risk factors for, 94, 94t
Pharmacologic stress testing, 6, 8t, 12–13, 13f
Phenytoin, in pregnancy, 103t
Phlebotomy, for cyanotic congenital heart disease, 88
Plethysmography, in peripheral arterial disease, 94
Polyarteritis nodosa, cardiovascular disease and, 3–4, 3t
Positron emission tomography (PET), cardiac, 7t, 8, 9t
Potassium channel blockers, for arrhythmias, 52–53, 52t
Prednisone, for pericarditis, 65t, 66, 67t
Pregnancy
  anticoagulation in, 100–101, 101f, 102t, Q93
  in cardiovascular disease, 98–103
    drug therapy and, 100–101, 101f, 102t–103t
    management of, 98–99, 99t, Q13, Q14
    peripartum cardiomyopathy in, 99
    risk assessment for, 98–99, 99t, 100t
  in congenital heart disease, 88, 99–103
  heart murmurs in, 6
  in Marfan syndrome, 91
  pulmonary arterial hypertension in, 98–99, Q90
Premature ventricular complexes, 58, Q68
Procainamide
  for arrhythmias, 52t
  in pregnancy, 103t
Propafenone
  for arrhythmias, 52, 52t
  in pregnancy, 103t
Propranolol
  for arrhythmias, 52t
  in pregnancy, 100, 102t
Prosthetic valves, 80–81, Q80. *See also* Valvular heart disease
  antibiotic prophylaxis for, 79, 80t
  endocarditis and, 79, 80–81, Q103
Pseudoclaudication, 93
Pulmonary arterial hypertension
  in pregnancy, 98–99, Q90
  tricuspid regurgitation and, 78
Pulmonary artery systolic pressure, normal values for, 72t
Pulmonic regurgitation, 71t, 87
Pulmonic stenosis, 71t, 86–87, Q6, Q61
  in tetralogy of Fallot, 87–88, 87f
Pulseless electrical activity, 61, 68

Quinapril, for heart failure, 31–33, 32t
Quinidine, in pregnancy, 103t

Race/ethnicity
  cardiovascular disease and, 2
  heart failure and, 34
Radiation exposure
  cardiomyopathy due to, 42t
  cardiovascular disease due to, 2–3, 42t, Q50, Q51
  from imaging studies, 7, 8t
Radiofrequency ablation
  for atrial fibrillation, 54–55
  for atrial flutter, 56
Radionuclide angiography, in cardiac examination, 5t, 6, 7, 8t
Ramipril, for heart failure, 31–33, 32t
Ranolazine, for angina, 14–15
Reperfusion therapy, for coronary artery disease, 16–17, 21–23, 25
  in diabetes mellitus, 28
  in women, 27
Respiratory failure, acute, mitral regurgitation after, 76
Restrictive cardiomyopathy, 41–44, 42t, 44t, Q23
  vs. constrictive pericarditis, 68t
Resuscitation, in cardiac arrest, 60
Reteplase, for myocardial infarction, 22–23, 22f, 23t, 24
Revascularization. *See* Reperfusion therapy
Rheumatic heart disease. *See also* Valvular heart disease
  mitral stenosis and, 74–76
Rheumatoid arthritis, cardiovascular disease and, 3–4, 3t
Right bundle branch block, in tetralogy of Fallot, 88
Right ventricular dysplasia, arrhythmogenic, 41
Right ventricular hypertrophy, in tetralogy of Fallot, 87–88, 87f
Right ventricular infarction, 24–25, Q1, Q63
Right ventricular outflow tract tachycardia, 59

Sarcoidosis
    cardiomyopathy in, 42–43, 42t, 44, 44t
    cardiovascular disease in, 3–4, 3t
    treatment of, 44t, Q97
Sarcomas, cardiac, 47–48
Scleroderma, cardiomyopathy in, 42t
Screening, for abdominal aortic aneurysm, 90
Seattle Heart Failure Model, 37
Segmental limb pressure recordings, in peripheral arterial disease, 94
Septal lipomatous hypertrophy, 47–48
Shock, cardiogenic
    in heart failure, 37–39, 38f
    management of, Q106
    post–myocardial infarction, 24
Short QT syndrome, 61
Shunts, in congenital heart disease, 82–88. See also specific defects
Sick sinus syndrome, 49, Q108
Sildenafil, and nitrates, 14
Silent ischemia, 18
    in diabetes mellitus, 27
Simvastatin. See also Statins
    for peripheral arterial disease, 96
Single photon emission computed tomography, cardiac, 7t, 8
Sinus node dysfunction, 49
Sinus venosus atrial septal defect, 82, 82f
Smoking
    cardiovascular disease and, 4
    peripheral arterial disease and, 94t
Sodium channel blockers, for arrhythmias, 52–53, 52t
Sotalol
    for arrhythmias, 52t, 53
    in pregnancy, 100, 102t
SPECT, cardiac, 7t, 8
Spinal cord stimulation, for angina, 17
Spinal stenosis, pseudoclaudication in, 93, Q39
Spironolactone, for heart failure, 32t, 34
Square root sign, 69
Statins
    for abdominal aortic aneurysm, 90
    for acute coronary syndromes, 21, 25
    for coronary artery disease, 16, 28
    for diabetes mellitus, 28
    for peripheral arterial disease, 94, 96
ST-elevation myocardial infarction, 18, 18f, 21–25, 22f, 23t, Q19, Q46, Q63, Q104, Q110
Stents
    coronary artery, 16, 17–18, Q75
        antiplatelet therapy for, 20
        drug-eluting, 17–18
        thrombosis of, 17
    for peripheral arterial disease, 96, 96t
Steroids, for pericarditis, 65t, 66, 67t
Stress testing
    in diabetes mellitus, 27
    electrocardiographic, 6, 7t–10t, 12–13, 12t, 13f
    in heart failure, 30
    indications for, 12–13, 12t, 13t, 17
    pharmacologic, 6, 8t, 12–13, 13f
    in women, 26, 27
Stroke
    aortic atheroma and, 89
    atrial fibrillation and, 54
    ethnicity and, 2
    patent foramen ovale and, 83
Structural heart disease, diagnosis of, 4–6, 5t
Substance abuse, cardiovascular disease and, 4, Q35
Sudden cardiac death, 59–61
Supraventricular tachycardia, 52, 52t, 56–58, Q14
Surgery
    antiplatelet therapy and, 17–18
    chronic anticoagulation and, 17–18, Q120
    noncardiac, in coronary artery disease, 17–18
Surgical maze procedures, for atrial fibrillation, 55
Syncope, evaluation of, 7, Q31
Systemic lupus erythematosus, cardiovascular disease and, 3–4, 3t
Systemic sclerosis
    cardiomyopathy in, 42t
    cardiovascular disease and, 3–4, 3t

Tachycardia(s), 50–53, 51f, 52t, 56–61
    atrial, 56–57, 57f
    atrioventricular nodal reentrant, 56–57
    atrioventricular reentrant, 56–57
        in Wolff-Parkinson-White syndrome, 57–58
    right ventricular outflow tract, 59
    supraventricular, 52, 52t, 56–58, Q14
    ventricular, 50–53, 51f, 52t, 59–61, Q40. See also Ventricular tachycardia
Tachycardia-bradycardia syndrome, 49
Tachycardia-mediated cardiomyopathy, 41
Tadalafil, and nitrates, 14
Takayasu arteritis, 3–4, 3t, 92
Takotsubo cardiomyopathy, 40–41
Tamponade, cardiac, 66–68
Tenecteplase, for myocardial infarction, 22–23, 22f, 23t, 24
Tetralogy of Fallot, 87–88, 87f, Q67, Q112, Q116
Thoracic aortic aneurysm, 90–91, 91t
Thrombolysis
    for acute limb ischemia, 97
    complications of, 24, 26
    for myocardial infarction, 21, 22f, 23t, 24
        in women, 26
Thrombolysis in Myocardial Infarction (TIMI) risk score, 20, 20t
Thrombosis/thromboembolism. See also Embolism
    acute limb ischemia and, 97, 97f, 97t
    in atrial fibrillation, 54
    in atrial septal defect, 82, 83
    left ventricular, post–myocardial infarction, 24
    prosthetic valve, 80, 81
    stent, 17
TIMI risk score, 20, 20t
Tirofiban, for acute coronary syndromes, 20
Toe-brachial index, 94
Torsemide, for heart failure, 32t, 33–34
Trandolapril, for heart failure, 31–33, 32t
Transesophageal echocardiography, 5t, 6. See also Echocardiography
Transplantation, heart, 39–40, 39t
Transthoracic echocardiography, 5–6, 5t. See also Echocardiography
Trastuzumab, cardiotoxicity of, 3
Tricuspid regurgitation, 71t, 78, Q88
Tricuspid stenosis, 71t
Tricuspid valve infection, in drug abusers, 4
Tumors, cardiac, 47–48, 48f, Q18
Turner syndrome, aortic coarctation in, 85

Ulcers, atherosclerotic aortic, 92–93
Ultrafiltration, for heart failure, 40

Vagal maneuvers, for supraventricular tachycardia, 56, 57
Valsalva maneuver, for supraventricular tachycardia, 56, 57
Valsartan, for heart failure, 31–33, 32t
Valvular heart disease, 69–81
    antibiotic prophylaxis for, 79, 80t
    aortic regurgitation in, 71t, 72, 73t, 74, 75t, 76–77, Q85
    aortic stenosis in, 71t, 72–73, 72t, 73t, Q41, Q66, Q95
    bicuspid aortic valve in, 71t, 73–74, 85, Q56
    diagnosis of, 69–70, 72f
    endocarditis and, 79, 80–81
    management of, 70, 73t
    mitral regurgitation in, 24, 71t, 73t, 75t, 76, 77–78, Q7, Q47, Q100, Q118
    mitral stenosis in, 71t, 73t, 74–76, 75t, Q3, Q33
    mitral valve prolapse in, 71t, 77, 78
    murmurs in, 70, 71t
    post–myocardial infarction, 24
    in pregnancy, anticoagulation for, 100–101, 101f, 102t. See also Pregnancy, in cardiovascular disease
    prosthetic valves for, 79, 80–81, 80t, Q80
    pseudostenosis in, 70
    pulmonic regurgitation in, 71t, 87
    pulmonic stenosis in, 71t, 86–87, 87f, Q6, Q61
    serial evaluation in, 70, 73t
    tricuspid regurgitation in, 71t, 78, Q88
    tricuspid stenosis in, 71t
Valvuloplasty, balloon, for pulmonary stenosis, 87
Vardenafil, and nitrates, 14
Vasodilators, for heart failure, 32t, 34
Vasopressin-receptor antagonists, for heart failure, 40

Ventricular assist devices, 39, 39t
Ventricular fibrillation, 57, 60–61, Q59
Ventricular hypertrophy, in tetralogy of Fallot, 87–88, 87f
Ventricular septal defect, 84–85, 84f, Q114
    murmur in, 71t, 84
    post–myocardial infarction, 24
    postoperative, 87
    in tetralogy of Fallot, 87–88, 87f
Ventricular tachycardia, 50–53, 51f, 52t, 59–61, Q40
    idiopathic, 59
    nonsustained, 59
    in structural heart disease, 59
    sudden cardiac death and, 59–61
    sustained, 59
Verapamil
    for angina, 14
    for arrhythmias, 52t
    for hypertrophic cardiomyopathy, 47
    in pregnancy, 102t

Walk test, in heart failure, 36
Warfarin
    for aortic atheroma, 89
    for atrial fibrillation, 54, 54t
    for pericarditis, 66
    in pregnancy, 100–101, 101f, 102t
    for prosthetic valves, 80
Wolff-Parkinson-White syndrome, 56, 57–58, 58f
Women, cardiovascular disease in, 1, 1f